being

female

Also by RITA BARON-FAUST

Breast Cancer: What Every Woman Should Know
Preventing Heart Disease: What Every Woman Should Know
Mental Wellness for Women

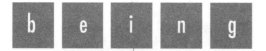

female

What Every Woman Should
Know About Gynecological Health

Rita Baron-Faust *with the Physicians of the New York University Medical Center Women's Health Service and the Department of Obstetrics and Gynecology*

WILLIAM MORROW AND COMPANY, INC.
New York

Illustrations on pages 8, 19, 25, 45, 58, 75, 80, 86, 88, 172, 217, 226, 227, 228 are copyrighted © 1995 by the American Society for Reproductive Medicine and reproduced by special permission.
   Illustrations on pages 5, 13, 18, 56, 287 are copyrighted © 1994 by Milex Products, Inc., and reproduced by special permission.

This book is not intended to substitute for the help and services of a trained professional. All matters regarding your health require medical consultation and supervision and following any of the advice in this book should be done in conjunction with the services of a qualified health professional.

The names and biographical characteristics of individuals profiled in this book have been changed to protect the privacy of the individuals concerned.

It is the policy of William Morrow and Company, Inc., and its imprints and affiliates, recognizing the importance of preserving what has been written, to print the books we publish on acid-free paper, and we exert our best efforts to that end.

               Library of Congress Cataloging-in-Publication Data
Baron-Faust, Rita.
     Being female : what every woman should know about
gynecological health / Rita Baron-Faust.
          p.   cm.
     Includes index.
     ISBN 0-688-12071-7
     1. Gynecology—Popular works.   2. Women—Health and hygiene.
I. Title.
RG121.B27   1998
618.1—dc21   97-37162
                                                             CIP

Printed in the United States of America

First Edition

1   2   3   4   5   6   7   8   9   10

BOOK DESIGN BY LISA STOKES

www.williammorrow.com

FOR MY GRANDMOTHERS,
Who managed in a different world
and
FOR MY MOTHER,
My dearest friend

i n t r o d u c t i o n

A revolution is taking place in women's health care. A decade ago, women's health was a sorely neglected area of both medical research and medical practice, and women's health care was often fragmented and inadequate. Now, there are myriad studies and clinical trials involving thousands of women across the country, led by the massive Women's Health Initiative. When we started the NYU Medical Center Women's Health Service in 1992, there were only a few dozen such programs across the country. Today, there are hundreds of facilities where women's diverse health needs can be met under one roof.

We started our own program in the Department of Obstetrics and Gynecology with the goal of providing an interdisciplinary facility for women's health care in an academic environment, utilizing the best of our gynecological, medical, radiological and surgical staffs. The program has since expanded to include Primary Care; a Maternal-Fetal Medicine Service to assist women with complicated pregnancies or who have experienced recurrent miscarriage and preterm deliveries; a comprehensive Oncology Service; Reproductive Services offering infertility evaluation and state-of-the-art in vitro fertilization technology; advanced diagnostic and screening services for breast, ovarian and uterine cancers, osteoporosis, gynecological abnormalities and a Menopause Unit to serve the needs of midlife women. With the construction of our freestanding women's health center at the Washington Square campus of New York University, we now offer a range of services to younger women.

The nonprofit Women's Health Service continues to support biomedical and clinical research by the NYU School of Medicine and NYU Medical Center, participate in clinical trials in a number of fields, and offer community outreach and education. The formation of Women's O.W.N. (Optimal Wellness Now) has enabled us to provide a wider range of community outreach programs. We have also added a Comprehensive Breast Center as part of our Kaplan Cancer Center. We hope to eventually clone our program and assist other medical centers in developing comprehensive health programs for women. Our ultimate mission is to provide "one-stop shopping" where women from all economic and social classes will be seen promptly and treated with sensitivity, and with consideration of their hectic family and work schedules.

Underlying all of our efforts, however, is the goal of preventive medicine. For while women outlive men, they still suffer more days of disability due to health problems than men, and the gender gap widens as women age. As physicians, we must begin to involve women at the earliest stages of their lives and to interest and educate them in good health and well-being. This education must start with a thorough understanding of their own reproductive anatomy and functioning, which is so well outlined in this book, the fourth volume in our series of women's health handbooks.

Most women regard their gynecologist as their primary care physician, and bring to their routine exams a wide range of concerns from sexually-transmitted diseases to osteoporosis. All too often, they leave with questions unanswered. This clear and comprehensive book will provide answers to questions women have about health issues that affect them across the lifespan. We hope it will educate women about their gynecological health in a way that will enable them to participate more fully in this most important area of health care.

—ROBERT H. MORRIS, M.D.
Director, New York University Medical Center
Women's Health Service

f o r e w o r d

Being male, I was frankly surprised to be asked to write the foreword to *Being Female*. I am uncertain where and when my interests in obstetrics and gynecology first appeared. I am the result of the last of my mother's seven pregnancies. The first of these resulted in my sister, but the next five ended in a variety of adverse pregnancy outcomes, including a stillbirth, a premature infant who succumbed to respiratory distress syndrome and three miscarriages. Perhaps the psychic scars left by these events in my mother's consciousness helped propel me into my chosen field. Having been trained in OB/GYN, I was better prepared than most husbands at dealing with my wife's first pregnancy—but as emotionally unprepared for the birth of my daughter as any other new dad. Similarly, despite an NIH grant to study menstruation, I was unable to discuss the topic with my own daughter. ("Get real, Dad!")

Fortunately, this book does not suffer from the same limitations in reaching women with crucial information about their gynecological health. Using actual patient histories as well as concise and clear presentations of current scientific knowledge, the author takes the reader through the entire spectrum of gynecological health. From fibroids to infertility, from sexually transmitted disease to ovarian cancer, women can obtain answers to a myriad of questions, learn to take better care of themselves, and more easily understand what their doctors are telling them. I can enthusiastically recommend this book to all my patients as well as to my mother, sister, wife and daughter. ("Get real, Dad!")

—CHARLES J. LOCKWOOD, M.D.
Chair of the Department of Obstetrics and Gynecology
New York University School of Medicine

f o r e w o r d

Being a woman and an obstetrician/gynecologist in practice for many years, as well as the mother of three daughters, furthering women's reproductive health and welfare, especially in the areas of health education and promotion, has become my special passion.

Having initially been trained by male physicians and esteemed colleagues, I have been puzzled to find patients expressing a strong preference for female doctors. There is no difference in the quality of my training and that of my male colleagues; we have both had the benefit of years of teaching and clinical experience. But women may be seeking another level of care and communication when choosing a physician. Perhaps some women are not comfortable broaching certain subjects, especially with a male physician. Or it may be that only another woman can provide commonsense and practical advice in intimate areas based on experiences that a man does not have, however skilled a physician he may be.

Unfortunately, until recently, the information and advice that male and female physicians had to offer their women patients were not based on either scientific or lay literature. While women comprise slightly more than 50 percent of the population, no serious studies on women patients actually existed until the late 1970s and 1980s. Before that time, information in many areas of health care was comprised of extrapolations of studies done on men, because women were excluded from clinical trials. But that situation is changing. As the number of female physicians has increased, a field of gender-based medicine has been created.

The first effective medication for menstrual cramps is credited to a female physician. The first definitive body of information on menopause and the years beyond was developed by a female physician. The area of perimenopause, still in its infancy, has been pioneered by women physicians. Perhaps this has come about through the same impetus driving female patients to seek out female doctors: to find out more about those things that are unique to ourselves as women.

The medical profession and the health care industry have now realized that women's health has been an area of neglect, as well as a potential market. As a result, many health initiatives and programs for women have sprung up across the country. As the average life expectancy for women continues to lengthen, it is of paramount importance to provide women with information to maintain and safeguard their health at all stages of life.

This is precisely why this book is so important. It is not only clear, factual, extensively researched, and beautifully written but also comes from the author's perspective as a woman. This perspective has prompted medical writer Rita Baron-Faust to include many issues not often discussed; the questions she has had as a woman patient have led her to seek out the expertise of a wide range of physicians and researchers for answers to give to other women. This book should serve as a valuable resource not only to women of all ages but to their obstetricians/gynecologists of both sexes.

—ILONA V. BRANDEIS, M.D., M.P.H.
Assistant Professor of Clinical OB/GYN
Director, N.Y. Reproductive Institute for Women with Disabilities, WC

acknowledgments

I am deeply grateful to New York University Medical Center, which has supported and nurtured this project over the past six years. The Department of Public Affairs, especially Peter Ferrara, Dan Perkes and Lynn Odell, have helped immensely. Drs. Robert Morris and Anthony Grieco have continued to give their enthusiastic support to these books and to me.

I am particularly indebted to Dr. Charles Lockwood, the chairman of the Department of Obstetrics and Gynecology, whose boundless energy, enthusiasm, accessibility and insightful comments have helped immeasurably with this complicated volume.

My gratitude also goes to the physicians in the Department of Obstetrics and Gynecology, especially Drs. Steven Goldstein, Bruce Young, Ilona Brandeis, Iffath Hoskins, and to Sandra Kammerman in the Department of Medicine, as well as many other physicians in the divisions of Maternal and Fetal Health and Reproductive Endocrinology, the In Vitro Fertilization Service and the Kaplan Cancer Center (especially Drs. Rita Demopoulos and Randy Stevens), who acted as medical advisers and helped me understand the wide-ranging field of gynecology, ensuring the scientific accuracy of often new and evolving material.

Special thanks to Michelle Marble and Alan Henderson of *Women's Health Weekly*, whose publication I have come to depend on; to my good friend Saralie Faivelson, the editor of *Medical Tribune for OB/GYNs*; to Penny Murphy and Greg Phillips at the American College of Obstetricians and Gynecologists for their assistance over the years; to Tina Hoff of the Kaiser Family Foundation and Susan Tew at the Alan Guttmacher Institute for providing tapes of joint media seminars I could not attend and for fielding questions; to the task force and the faculty of the American Medical Women's Association (AMWA) Advanced Curriculum in Women's Health, who allowed me to attend their three-day workshops in 1993 and 1994; to Joyce Zeitz and Jennifer Kelly at the American Society for Reproductive Medicine for their invaluable assistance and for providing many of the illustrations that enhance and clarify this material; and to the North American Menopause Society for providing abstracts and other materials. I especially appreciated the personal and technical insights provided by Mary Lou Ballweg of the Endometriosis Association, Cheryle B. Gartley, founder of the Simon Foundation for Continence, and Joanne Yount, Executive Director of the Vulvar Pain Foundation. And finally, to my longtime friends at the American Medical Association, including *JAMA* editor George Lundberg, M.D., Tom Toftey, Jeff Molter and others, for their help over the years.

I have learned so much about writing and publishing from my editor at William Morrow, Toni Sciarra, whose edits are practically invisible; my agent, Vicky Bijur, has been unfailingly enthusiastic and supportive.

Love and gratitude also go to my husband, Allen, for not minding (too much) all the out-of-town conference trips and the long, long hours that go into the research and writing of my books and for checking all the Web sites, phone numbers and other facts to be had on the Internet; to my son, Alexander, for being such a good "helper" in the office, and to my mother, who has made it possible for me to travel as much as I did in writing these books and who has read every single word of every book, with a sharp eye and an even sharper pencil.

Herbert A. Goldfarb, M.D.
Assistant Clinical Professor of
Medicine

Steven R. Goldstein, M.D.
Professor of Obstetrics and
Gynecology
Director, Gynecological Ultrasound
Unit

James A. Griffo, M.D.
Professor of Obstetrics and
Gynecology
Director, Division of Reproductive
Endocrinology

Frederick Licciardi, M.D.
Assistant Professor of OB/GYN,
Division of Reproductive
Endocrinology

Andrew McCullough, M.D.
Assistant Professor of Urology
Director, Male Sexual Health
Program

Louis A. Mucelli, M.D.
Clinical Instructor, Obstetrics and
Gynecology

Franco M. Muggia, M.D.
Anne Murnick and David H.
Cogan Professor of Oncology
Director, Kaplan Cancer Center

Lila E. Nachtigall, M.D.
Professor of Medicine
Director, Women's Wellness

Victor W. Nitti, M.D.
Assistant Professor of Medicine
Director of Female Urology

Valerie Peck, M.D.
Clinical Associate Professor of
Medicine
Metabolic Consultant, Bone
Densitometry,
NYU Women's Health Service

Robert F. Porges, M.D.
Professor and Vice Chairman,
Department of Obstetrics and
Gynecology
Director, Division of Pelvic
Reconstructive Surgery

John R. Quagliarello, M.D.
Associate Professor of Clinical
OB/GYN
Associate Director, Division of
Reproductive Endocrinology

Virginia Sadock, M.D.
Director, Graduate Program in
Human Sexuality
Clinical Professor of Psychiatry

Lisa B. Schwartz, M.D.
Assistant Professor of Obstetrics
and Gynecology

Randy E. Stevens, M.D.
Assistant Professor,
Codirector, Gynecologic Radiation
Oncology

Bruce K. Young, M.D.
Herbert R. Silverman/Henry R.
Silverman Professor of Obstetrics
and Gynecology

Director, Division of Maternal-
Fetal Medicine
Director, Obstetrical Services,
NYU School of Medicine
and NYU Medical Center

Robert C. Wallach, M.D.
Director, Gynecologic Oncology
Professor of Clinical Medicine

Livia S. Wan, M.D.
Director, Family Planning Division
Director, Division of Endoscopic
and Pelvic Surgery
Professor of OB/GYN

Leonard Wolf, M.D., F.A.C.O.G.,
F.R.C.O.G. (UK)
Associate Clinical Professor of
OB/GYN

The author also wishes to express gratitude to the following people who provided information, insight and peer review on the myriad aspects of women's gynecological and reproductive health during the research and writing of this book.

Nancy Alexander, M.D.
Special Assistant to the Director,
Office of Technology Transfer,
National Institutes of Health

Gloria A. Bachmann, M.D.
Professor and Chief,
Division of General Obstetrics and
Gynecology,
University of Medicine and
Dentistry of New Jersey–
Robert Wood Johnson Medical
School
Chief, OB/GYN Service,
Robert Wood Johnson University
Hospital

Mary Lou Ballweg
Founder and Executive Director,
Endometriosis Association

Robert L. Barbieri, M.D.
Kate Macy Ladd Professor of
Obstetrics and Gynecology

and Reproductive Biology
Chairman, Department of
OB/GYN, Harvard Medical School

Tamara G. Bavendam, M.D.
Associate Professor of Surgery/
Urology
Director, Center for Pelvic
Disorders,
Allegheny University of the Health
Sciences, Philadelphia

Barbara J. Berger, M.D.
Assistant Professor of Clinical
Medicine,
Albert Einstein College of Medicine

Beverly Saunders Biddle, M.H.A.
Executive Director,
National Lesbian and Gay Health
Association,
Washington, DC

Robert N. Butler, M.D.
Director, International Longevity Center,
Mount Sinai Medical Center,
New York

Joanna M. Cain, M.D.
Chairman, Department of Obstetrics and Gynecology,
Pennsylvania State University School of Medicine, Hershey, PA

Eugenia E. Calle, Ph.D.
Director, Analytic Epidemiology,
Epidemiology and Surveillance Research,
The American Cancer Society

Donald L. Chatman, M.D.
Clinical Associate Professor of OB/GYN,
Northwestern University School of Medicine,
Chicago, IL

Jaqueline E. Darroch, Ph.D.
Senior Vice-President,
The Alan Guttmacher Institute,
New York, NY

Jean Endicott, Ph.D.
Chief, Department of Research Assessment and Training,
New York State Psychiatric Institute, New York, NY

Ellen W. Freeman, Ph.D.
Director, PMS Program,
Research Professor in Obstetrics, Gynecology and Psychiatry,
University of Pennsylvania Hospital

Cheryle B. Gartley
Founder and President,
The Simon Foundation for Continence

Marla Jean Gold, M.D.
Assistant Professor of Medicine,
Medical College of Pennsylvania

David Grimes, M.D.
Professor and Vice Chairman,
Department of OB/GYN and Reproductive Sciences,
University of California,
San Francisco

Phillip Hanno, M.D.
Professor and Chairman,
Department of Urology,
Temple University School of Medicine

Richard U. Hausknecht, M.D.
Associate Clinical Professor of OB/GYN,
Mount Sinai School of Medicine

Sharon L. Hillier, Ph.D.
Associate Professor, University of Pittsburgh Department of OB/GYN and Reproductive Sciences
Director, Reproductive Infectious Disease Research,
Magee-Women's Hospital,
Pittsburgh, PA

Penelope J. Hitchcock, D.Vm.
Chief, Sexually Transmitted Diseases Branch,
National Institute of Allergy and Infectious Diseases (NIAID)

Ruth J. Katz, J.D., M.P.H.
Director, Public Health Programs,
Kaiser Family Foundation, Menlo
Park, CA

David L. Keefe, M.D.
Associate Professor of OB/GYN,
Division of Biology and Medicine,
Brown University
Director, Laboratory of
Reproductive Medicine,
Marine Biological Laboratory,
Woods Hole, MA

Luella Klein, M.D.
Charles Howard Candler Professor,
Department of Gynecology and
Obstetrics,
Emory University School of
Medicine, Atlanta

Susan Klugman, M.D.
Assistant Clinical Professor of
OB/GYN,
Albert Einstein College of
Medicine,
Montefiore Medical Center

June La Valleur, M.D.
Assistant Professor of OB/GYN
Director, Mature Woman's Center,
University of Minnesota Medical
School

Stanley C. Marinoff, M.D.
Director, Center for Vulvovaginal
Disorders
Clinical Professor of OB/GYN,
George Washington University
School of Medicine

William M. McCormack, M.D.
Professor of Medicine and
OB/GYN
Chief, Infectious Diseases Division,
State University of New York
Health Sciences Center at Brooklyn

Howard L. Minkoff, M.D.
Professor and Director, Maternal-
Fetal Medicine,
State University of New York
Health Sciences Center at Brooklyn

Daniel R. Mishell, M.D.
Professor and Chairman,
Department of of OB/GYN,
University of Southern California
School of Medicine, Los Angeles

Cynthia C. Morton, Ph.D.
William Lambert Richardson
Professor of Obstetrics, Gynecology
and Reproductive Biology,
and Professor of Pathology,
Harvard Medical School
Director of Cytogenetics, Brigham
and Women's Hospital, Boston

Anita L. Nelson, M.D.
Associate Professor of Obstetrics
and Gynecology,
University of California, Los
Angeles (UCLA) School of
Medicine
Medical Director, Women's Health
Care Clinic, Harbor-UCLA
Medical Center

Roberta Ness, M.D.
Director of Epidemiology of
Women's Health Program,
Graduate School of Public Health,
University of Pittsburgh

David L. Olive, M.D.
Chief of Reproductive
Endocrinology and Infertility,
Department of Obstetrics and
Gynecology,
Yale University School of Medicine

Herbert B. Peterson, M.D.
Branch Chief of Women's Health
and Fertility,
Centers for Disease Control and
Prevention
Clinical Professor of OB/GYN,
Emory University, Atlanta

David Phillips, Ph.D.
Senior Scientist,
The Population Council, New York

Vicki Ratner, M.D.
President,
Interstitial Cystitis Association

Sherry E. Rier, Ph.D.
Tracy H. Dickinson Research Chair
of the Endometriosis Association,
Department of Physiology,
Dartmouth Medical School,
Lebanon, NH

Gail Erlick Robinson, M.D.
Professor of Psychiatry, Obstetrics
and Gynecology,
University of Toronto

Allan Rosenfield, M.D.
Dean, Columbia University School
of Public Health
Professor of Public Health,
OB/GYN

Carolyn D. Runowicz, M.D.
Associate Professor of OB/GYN
Director, Division of Gynecologic
Oncology,
Montefiore Medical Center, New
York City

Nanette F. Santoro, M.D.
Associate Professor and
Director, Division of Reproductive
Endocrinology,
University of Medicine and
Dentistry of New Jersey–
Robert Wood Johnson Medical
School, Newark, NJ

Mark V. Sauer, M.D.
Director, Reproductive
Endocrinology and Assisted
Reproduction,
Columbia-Presbyterian Medical
Center, NY

Vicki L. Seltzer, M.D.
Chair, Department of OB/GYN,
Long Island Jewish Medical Center
Professor of OB/GYN
Albert Einstein College of Medicine

Sally K. Severino, M.D.
Professor and Executive Vice Chair,
Department of Psychiatry,
University of New Mexico

Clive C. Solomons, Ph.D., F.A.I.C.
Research Director, Scientific
Connections, Denver, CO

Margaret Spinelli, M.D.
Director, Maternal Mental Health
Program,
New York State Psychiatric
Institute

Walter E. Stamm, M.D.
Professor of Medicine
Head, Division of Allergy and
Infectious Diseases,
University of Washington Medical
Center

Felicia H. Stewart, M.D.
Director, Reproductive Health
Programs,
Kaiser Family Foundation

Richard L. Sweet, M.D.
Professor and Chair,
Department of Obstetrics,
Gynecology and Reproductive
Sciences,
University of Pittsburgh/Magee-
Women's Hospital

Cheryl Walker, M.D.
Assistant Professor and Director,
Reproductive Infectious Diseases
and Immunology,
University of California, Irvine

Carol S. Weisman, Ph.D.
Professor of Health Management
and Policy,

University of Michigan School of
Public Health

Ann Colston Wentz, M.D.
President, Society for Gynecologic
Investigation

Jocelyn C. White, M.D.
Assistant Professor of OB/GYN,
Oregon Health Sciences Center

John Willems, M.D.
Scripps Clinic and Research
Foundation, La Jolla, CA

Beverly Winikoff, M.D., M.P.H.
Program Director, Reproductive
Health,
The Population Council, New York

Susan F. Wood, Ph.D.
Acting Deputy Assistant U.S.
Secretary for Women's Health,
U.S. Department of Health and
Human Services

Joanne Yount
Executive Director, Vulvar Pain
Foundation

Jonathan Zenilman, M.D.
Associate Professor of Medicine,
Division of Infectious Diseases,
Johns Hopkins University School of
Medicine, Baltimore, MD

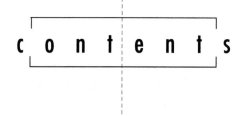

contents

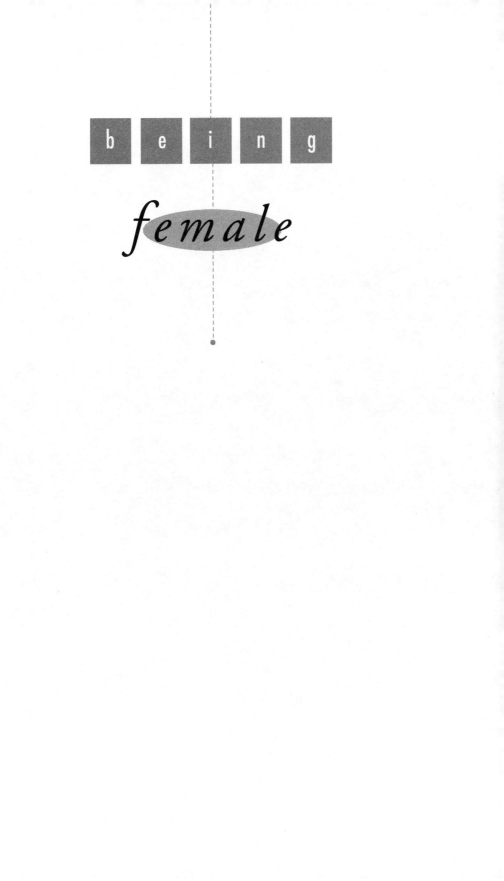

being

female

Your Body/Your Concerns

∞ *R o b i n ' s   S t o r y* ∞

"I don't know about most women, but before I started trying to get pregnant and found out I had endometriosis, I never thought much about my reproductive system. It sounds terrible, but I had only a vague idea what really went on each month. I knew my body produced hormones; I knew I had a vagina, a uterus and two ovaries and that I got periods. I sure never knew my periods went out the other way. But who really thinks about their plumbing unless something goes wrong?"

If, like Robin, you think your female "plumbing" is merely your vagina, uterus and ovaries, think again. A woman's reproductive system is a complex network of specialized tissues, organs, glands, ducts, nerves and muscles.

Contrary to myth, a woman's reproductive organs are not "delicate" but are quite strong. The muscular uterus can expand to hold a baby weighing seven pounds or more, the cervix stretches to allow that baby to pass into the birth canal and the vagina is tough enough to withstand the rigors of childbirth.

But that doesn't mean your reproductive system runs trouble-free, and if a problem arises in one area, it can affect the entire system. Many problems can share common symptoms. For example, abnormal bleeding can be a sign of a hormonal disruption of ovulation, benign fibroid tumors in the uterine wall or cancer. Abnormal discharge can be a sign of simple vaginitis or a fertility-threatening sexually transmitted infection. Fortunately many problems can be easily treated *if* you know the warning signs and act quickly. Unfortunately too few women do.

Vaginitis is responsible for up to 5 million visits to health care providers each year, urinary tract infections prompt an additional 6 million doctor visits and one million women are treated annually for *pelvic inflammatory disease (PID)*, the most common complication of sexually transmitted diseases. A recent study in the journal *Obstetrics and Gynecology* reported that 571,600 women a year were treated in hospitals for benign ovarian cysts, 566,400 for endometriosis, 549,000 for menstrual disorders and 531,200 others for uterine fibroids, yet a major survey conducted for the American Medical Association (AMA) found that more than 40 percent of women don't know very much about PID, fibroids *or* endometriosis.

"It is disturbing that women don't know about some of the early warning signs of things that could threaten their fertility, particularly pelvic inflammatory disease," remarked Anita Nelson, M.D., an associate professor of obstetrics and gynecology at the University of California, Los Angeles School of Medicine and the medical director of the Women's Health Care Clinic at the Harbor-UCLA Medical Center, in releasing the survey. "There are clearly gaps we need to fill with education."

The 1995 survey of more than 2,000 women revealed a number of gaps in women's knowledge about their gynecological health:

• Almost a third of the women admitted not being very knowledgeable about cervical, uterine and ovarian cancer, cancers that will be diagnosed in more than 76,000 women this year.

• While nine out of ten women knew that Pap smears are used to detect cervical cancer, 72 percent mistakenly believed the test *also* detected uterine cancer, and 17 percent thought it could diagnose pregnancy.

• Fewer than half of white and Latina women thought they were very knowledgeable about sexually transmitted diseases, compared with two thirds of African-American women.

• While eight out of every ten women said they were somewhat to very knowledgeable about when ovulation occurs, about a third of Latina and African-American women, and one quarter of women in their twenties, lacked knowledge about the timing of ovulation.

• More than 90 percent of women believed they were very knowledgeable about contraception, but only 25 percent thought birth control pills are very safe, and only 7 percent knew the pill could help lower their risk of gynecologic cancers.

- Nine out of ten women believed that unplanned pregnancies occur only among teenagers. In reality, *two thirds* of unintended pregnancies occur among women well past their teens, and half among women who were using contraception!

- Myths about women's health lingered: More than 10 percent of those surveyed believed breast-feeding mothers cannot become pregnant, 16 percent thought a woman should not exercise during her period and half believed that women who took oral contraceptives needed an occasional "rest period" from the pill.

While most women surveyed were confident in their knowledge about pregnancy and menopause, many others had questions they did not feel comfortable asking physicians. Even though 40 percent of women in their forties have experienced urinary incontinence and 30 percent say they've had discomfort during sex, half were reluctant to discuss these matters with their gynecologists. Women were even less likely to talk about lack of orgasm or unsatisfying sexual partners.

Women in their twenties and those who have never given birth were most concerned about fertility; women in their thirties and forties said cancer was their greatest reproductive health concern. "We need to help women understand that there are things they can do to preserve their fertility, and that there are steps they can take to prevent cervical, endometrial and ovarian cancers," said Dr. Nelson.

▪ How This Book Can Help You ▪

This book is designed to address these issues and fill in gaps in your knowledge, from *menarche* (the time periods begin) to *menopause* (the time periods stop) and beyond. In addition, we will answer questions that you might not ask your doctor.

You'll also learn about common conditions, including fibroids and urinary tract infections, as well as problems less often discussed, such as vulvar pain, urinary and fecal incontinence and pelvic prolapse. We'll look at the complete spectrum of reproductive choices, including sterilization and abortion. We will report the newest scientific studies and treatments for women's top gynecologic health concerns: cancer and infertility. We will also spotlight cutting-edge research into how the immune system interacts with the environment to play a possible role in conditions like endometriosis and infertility.

This book will answer questions you may have about what's "normal" and what isn't, from vaginal discharge to sexual functioning. We will help you gain a better understanding of reproductive organs and how to keep them in good shape.

While scientific knowledge is changing all the time, every effort has been made to keep this book as current as possible. Everything has been prepared under the guidance of the Department of Obstetrics and Gynecology at the New York University School of Medicine and NYU Medical Center and the physicians of NYU's Women's Health Service. Many of the country's leading experts in reproductive health have also been interviewed, along with ordinary women from all backgrounds who share their experiences.

We will also address issues of concern to women of color, lesbian health issues, the health concerns (and questions) of adolescents and elderly and disabled women and will look at the effect of culture on knowledge and behaviors regarding female health.

First, let's look at female reproductive anatomy. We'll begin with the external genitalia; you may want to get a mirror so you can see what we're describing. If you've never taken a good look "down there," now's the time!

▪ Female Anatomy 101 ▪

The VULVA, also known as the *pudendum*, is the term for all of the visible external female genitalia. *Vulva* means "covering" in Latin, and indeed, these folds of skin protectively fold over the openings of the vagina and urethra. The vulvar area is bounded on top by the *mons pubis* and the *clitoris*, the *labia minora* and *labia majora* on each side and the *perineum* to the rear, bordering on the anus. The mons pubis is basically a cushion of fatty tissue over the pubic bone. It's also called the *mons veneris*, which is Latin for "mountain of Venus" (the term *venereal disease* has the same linguistic roots).

The fat beneath the skin of the vulvar area is sensitive to the hormone *estrogen*, just like the fat on the hips and in the breasts. The area becomes enlarged when estrogen is produced in large amounts at puberty (estrogen also triggers breast development), then thins and shrinks after menopause, when estrogen production declines.

At puberty the mons also begins to sprout *pubic hair*, in response to *androgens* (male hormones) produced by the ovary rather than estrogens (androgens also stimulate the growth of underarm, or *axillary*, hair). Pubic hair may spread to the inner thighs. It may or may not match the color of the hair on your head, but it does turn gray, and there's even some hair loss after

┌─────────── **Fig. 1: A WOMAN'S EXTERNAL GENITALIA** ───────────┐

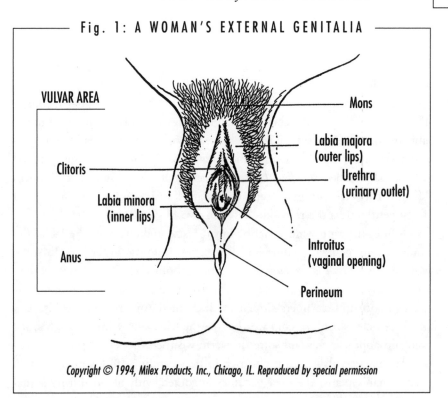

VULVAR AREA

Mons

Labia majora
(outer lips)

Clitoris

Urethra
(urinary outlet)

Labia minora
(inner lips)

Anus

Introitus
(vaginal opening)

Perineum

Copyright © 1994, Milex Products, Inc., Chicago, IL. Reproduced by special permission

menopause. Pubic hair helps protect the inner and outer lips of the vulva in much the same way that eyelashes keep irritants from getting into the eyes.

Pubic hair growth occurs in five stages, which, along with the five stages of breast development (called *Tanner staging*), can indicate to physicians whether a girl is maturing normally. Girls in the U.S. appear to be developing pubic hair and other signs of puberty earlier than ever before, especially African-American girls. A 1997 study of over 17,000 girls across the country reported the average age of puberty for black girls was eight or nine years, and ten years for white girls (with some girls showing signs of puberty as early as age six).

The appearance of the first pubic hairs is followed by a growth spurt when girls start to accumulate fat around the hips. Periods still begin (*menarche*) around age twelve and one-half. However, you may have been a "late bloomer" who didn't get your period until age fourteen. As we'll learn in Chapter Two, that's not "abnormal."

The *LABIA MAJORA* (outer lips) extend from the mons in two folds of skin meeting at the perineum. They contain loose connective tissue and pads of fat under the surface of the skin, covered by pubic hair. The hairless inner surface has many oil-producing (*sebaceous*) and sweat glands, which, along with vaginal secretions, keep the area moist and form a protective layer against irritants.

The *LABIA MINORA* (inner lips) enclose the urethral and vaginal openings. The delicate folds of the labia minora grow downward from the front of the labia majora on each side, joining above and below the clitoris. At the perineum the inner lips blend into the labia majora. There's a slightly raised ridge of skin called the *fourchette* that usually flattens out after childbirth. The inner lips contain many sebaceous glands, which feel like grains of sand if you gently press the thin skin between two fingers.

While there are wide variations in the size and shape of the labia, the outer lips are generally larger and sometimes hide the inner lips. In some women the inner lips are enlarged and project outward. But no two women look exactly alike. The vulva can be sensitive to temperature. The labia contains smooth muscle fibers similar to those in the male scrotum; just as a man's testicles shrink in cold weather, so the labia can wrinkle up when it's cold and appear larger and softer in warm weather.

The entire vulvar area is also rich in nerve endings and is highly erotic. Like a man's penis, the area becomes engorged with blood during sexual excitement, swelling to two to three times its normal size during arousal. That's because the labia contains *erectile tissue* filled with open spaces that fill and swell with blood, darkening the skin when we're sexually excited.

The *CLITORIS* is an exquisitely sensitive bulb of erectile tissue hidden beneath a protective hood, the *prepuce*. The junction of the lips below is called the *frenulum*. The clitoris gets its name from the Greek word for "key," and indeed it is the physical key and nerve center of a woman's sexuality. There are more nerve endings on the clitoris than on any other part of a woman's body. Like a penis, the clitoris responds to stimulation by becoming erect with its spongy tissues becoming engorged with blood.

The *URETHRAL ORIFICE* is about an inch below the clitoris and is shaped like a small, elevated dimple. Inside, the urethra is about three inches long and connected to the neck of the bladder, closed off tightly at the top by *sphincter muscles* and controlled by several sets of nerves. The urethra folds flat and opens only when we're urinating.

Below and on either side of the urethra are two tiny openings from the *paraurethral* or *Skene's glands*. These glands secrete a small amount of mucus and, along with similar mucus-secreting glands in the wall of the urethra, keep the bladder outlet opening moist and lubricated for the passage of urine.

The *VULVAR VESTIBULE* is the area around the vaginal opening, bordered by the inner labia and the perineum. On either side of the vagina are the two tiny ducts of the pea-size *Bartholin's glands* (sometimes called the *greater vestibular glands*), which produce mucus. Occasionally the ducts can become obstructed and form painful cysts. Sometimes the glands, blood vessels and nerves in the area become irritated and inflamed, causing *vulvar vestibulitis*, a condition so painful that even the lightest touch of a cotton swab sends women into agony (see page 111).

The *HYMEN* is a thin membrane of skin just inside the vaginal opening that grows larger at puberty. A great deal of folklore and mythology surround this bit of skin, which has *no known function at all*. It was commonly believed that the hymen, named after Hymen, the Greek god of marriage, covered the vaginal opening and tore during first intercourse, producing a great deal of bleeding. If no bleeding occurred, the woman was assumed not to be a virgin. But that's not always so. Not even a doctor can tell if intercourse has taken place by looking at the hymen (you can tell if a woman has had a baby, though). The hymen may be tough, as wispy as a cobweb or nothing more than a fringe of skin.

"The hymen usually has one or more holes in it to allow for the passage of menstrual blood and vaginal discharge," explains Ilona V. Brandeis, M.D., an assistant professor of clinical obstetrics and gynecology at NYU Medical Center. "The hymen is also quite flexible, so that young girls can use tampons without losing their virginity."

In rare cases, according to Dr. Brandeis, the hymen may remain completely intact, blocking the opening of the vagina, a condition called an *imperforate hymen*. When a girl menstruates, the imperforate hymen causes the vagina and the uterus to fill with blood, which can back up into the fallopian tubes. The problem can be solved by cutting the hymen.

The *VAGINA* is essentially a tube of tissue, comprised of many folds of moist mucous membrane, ascending from the vulva to the uterus. Despite lingering myths, the vagina can stretch to accommodate any size penis (as well as a baby during childbirth). There is no relationship between a woman's body size and shape and the size of her vagina (the same is true of a man's penis).

The vaginal lining, or *epithelium*, consists of layers of scalelike *squamous cells* atop connective tissue, which contains blood vessels and nerves. Since they are closer to blood vessels, the deeper, or *basal*, layer of cells proliferates faster than the cells in the top layer, replacing first the intermediate layer and then the superficial cells, which are constantly being sloughed off. Vaginal

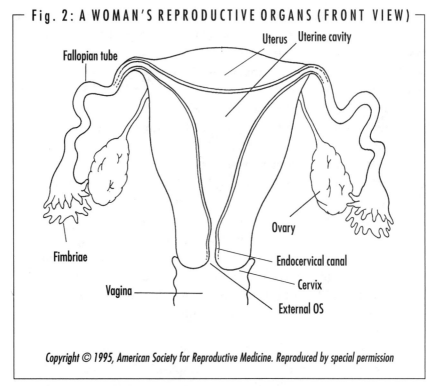

Fig. 2: A WOMAN'S REPRODUCTIVE ORGANS (FRONT VIEW)

Uterus Uterine cavity

Fallopian tube

Fimbriae

Ovary

Endocervical canal

Cervix

Vagina

External OS

Copyright © 1995, American Society for Reproductive Medicine. Reproduced by special permission

Note: The ovaries are depicted as being farther apart from the uterus than they actually are. The ovaries and fallopian tubes usually rest against the sides of the uterus.

discharge, comprised of these dead cells and other secretions, may begin several months to a year before menstruation. "Many young women may run to a doctor to be treated for what they think is a vaginal infection when it is really just normal *leukorrhea*, shedding of cells," says Dr. Brandeis.

This constant turnover of vaginal cells is stimulated by estrogen. Estrogenic activity can actually be measured by the numbers of basal, intermediate or superficial cells in a smear taken from the vaginal lining. Before puberty and after menopause, when little estrogen is present, the vaginal epithelium is thin and almost entirely made up of basal cells. During the reproductive years, when the ovaries produce estrogen, there are large numbers of sloughed-off superficial cells. It's even possible to determine the phases of the menstrual cycle by analyzing the shape and qualities of these cells under a microscope. When estrogen is present and a vaginal smear dries on a glass slide, it produces a pattern called "ferning."

Estrogen activity also determines the *pH*, the acid to alkaline balance, of the vagina. During the childbearing years the vagina is acidic (low pH), because of the rapid growth of basal cells that contain *glycogen* (the stored form of *glucose*, blood sugar, which provides fuel for cell growth). Beneficial bacteria that normally live in the vagina, called *Döderlein's bacilli* or *lactobacilli*, break down this glycogen to form *lactic acid*, and this accounts for the acidity of the vagina, which helps keep the growth of other microorganisms in check. Lactobacillus also produces hydrogen peroxide, which kills bacteria.

If the number of lactobacilli is reduced by antibiotics or douching too often, for example, other harmful bacteria and yeast present in the vagina can multiply and cause infections. Before puberty, when there's little estrogen, the pH is more alkaline (high pH) and less resistant to infection. After the menopause, when estrogen levels fall and the vaginal lining thins, glycogen levels decline and there are less lactobacilli, resulting in a more alkaline pH and an increased vulnerability to infection. During the menstrual period the vagina also has a higher pH.

Normal vaginal discharge is acidic and clear or milky, containing superficial cells, bacteria and other microorganisms, fluids from the vaginal wall and mucus from cervical glands and the uterine cavity. "Vaginal discharge is a kind of self-cleaning mechanism," comments Dr. Brandeis. This discharge, along with a relatively tough vaginal epithelium (it has no glands or hair follicles to provide entry for microorganisms), protects the vagina from infection. Again, when there's less discharge and thinner tissues before puberty and after menopause, the vagina is more vulnerable to irritation and infection.

There is always a certain amount of vaginal discharge, but sexual stimulation produces even more lubrication through increased secretions.

The CERVIX is actually the neck of the womb, which opens into the vagina. The opening of the cervix is called the *external os*; the inch-long canal from the os to the uterine cavity is the *endocervical canal*. The cervix is made of smooth muscle and collagen fibers, which give it the elasticity to accommodate the thirteen-inch head and the body of a full-term infant and then return almost to its prepregnancy contours within three months. However, the cervix becomes softer, and the opening, or os, which looked like a small, round dimple before childbirth, becomes a crosswise slit with irregular edges.

The cervical canal is lined with cells that look different and grow differently from the cells in the vagina and on the outer part of the cervix. The superficial squamous cells in the vagina and outer cervix grow in layers and are shaped like fish scales; the *endocervical cells* lining the canal are columnar-shaped and grow in a single layer. Certain microorganisms target the columnar cells and the area around the os, which has fewer layers of squamous cells, making these areas more vulnerable to infection than the thicker walls of the vagina.

The area in the lower part of the endocervical canal where the squamous cells meet the columnar cells is called the *transition zone (squamocolumnar junction)*. This is where most cervical cancers arise. Cell samples from the transition zone and the external cervix are taken for a *Papanicolaou (Pap) smear* to screen for early, precancerous changes (see Chapter Thirteen). The boundaries of the transition zone change in response to estrogen, appearing outside of the canal during puberty and receding inward at menopause, says Dr. Brandeis.

The *endocervical glands* in the canal secrete a mucus that changes in response to sex hormones. Before and during ovulation cervical mucus is thin and clear with the consistency of egg whites (to help sperm swim up to the uterus) and contains high amounts of estrogen. After ovulation it becomes much thicker and opaque, acting as a barrier to sperm.

The UTERUS, or womb, is a hollow, muscular organ shaped like an upside-down pear. The top portion is called the body or *fundus*; the bottom portion is the neck (or cervix). A normal, nonpregnant uterus is about three inches long and two inches wide at the fundus. During a pelvic exam your gynecologist can feel its entire circumference.

The uterine walls are about one-half inch thick and have three layers. The inner layer, the *endometrium*, is comprised of tissue that contains blood vessels and small glands. The innermost cell layer of the endometrium multiplies in response to hormonal signals each month to prepare for implantation of a fetus. If that does not occur, the extra cells are shed as menstrual flow.

The tough middle layer of uterus, the *myometrium*, is made of smooth muscle and connective tissue. Unlike voluntary muscles, which contract at will, the involuntary muscles of the uterus contract only when stimulated by chemicals produced during labor, false labor or menstruation. During labor, uterine contractions help deliver the fetus. During menstruation, lesser contractions expel blood and tissue. This tough and resilient muscle can expand to many times its normal size during pregnancy and return to its original shape none the worse for wear after delivery. The myometrium is covered by a smooth outer layer, or *serosa*.

The uterus can be slightly "tipped" forward (*anteverted*), backward (*retroverted*) or any angle in between; in most women the uterus is tipped slightly forward. (However, a "tipped" uterus doesn't affect fertility, childbirth or menstrual pain.) The uterus can also shift slightly in place, depending on how full the bladder or the rectum is and how many children a woman has had.

There have been a number of peculiar notions about the uterus. The word *hysteria* is derived from the Greek *hystera*, meaning "womb" and was used 2,000 years ago to describe the mental afflictions allegedly caused by the dysfunctions or the physical "wanderings" of the uterus. The Greek physician Hippocrates even believed the uterus went "wild" unless it was regularly fed male semen! For centuries it was widely believed that women's reproductive organs rendered them psychologically unstable (and inferior to men). In the nineteenth century psychiatric problems were often treated by removal of the uterus and ovaries.

The *fallopian tubes (oviducts)* are named for the sixteenth-century anatomist Gabriele Fallopius. They originate from the top of the uterus and end next to the ovaries, providing a passageway for an egg to reach the uterine cavity. The Greek word for "tube" is *salpinx*, and that prefix often appears in words referring to the fallopian tubes, such as *salpingitis*, inflammation of the tubes, and *salpingectomy*, removal of a tube.

Three to four inches long and less than a third of an inch in diameter (about the diameter of a small pencil), the fallopian tubes have four sections. The *interstitial*, or internal, portion is very short and narrow, buried in the uterine fundus. The *isthmus*, the straight half of the tube, has a thick muscular wall and is the area that is "tied" (actually cut) during *tubal ligation* for sterilization. The *ampulla*, the other half of the tube, has a thinner wall containing many folds. The *infundibulum*, nearest the ovary, flares out in a catcher's mitt shape with fingerlike projections called *fimbriae*, which rest against the ovary. The fimbriae catch the egg expelled each month and bring it into the tube.

"The fimbriae actually move toward the ovarian follicle that is destined to expel an egg," says John R. Quagliarello, M.D., an associate professor of obstetrics and gynecology and infertility specialist at NYU Medical Center. "In fact, the ovaries can be so close together that an egg expelled from the right ovary can be taken up by the fimbriae of the left tube."

The tube walls are rich in blood vessels and contain smooth muscle tissue that, at ovulation, contracts in waves to help move an egg down the tube, explains Dr. Quagliarello. They are also lined with hairlike projections, called *cilia*, that beat thousands of times a minute, creating a current that propels the egg to the uterine cavity. The tubes can generally not be felt during a gynecological exam. "The tubes are thin and delicate and can be easily damaged or scarred by inflammation and infection. Tubal damage caused by sexually transmitted diseases is a very common cause of infertility," Dr. Quagliarello says.

The *OVARIES* are small oval-shaped glands nestled on either side of the uterus that produce eggs (*ova*) and sex hormones, including estrogen and progesterone. The ovaries and fallopian tubes are often referred to as the *adnexa* because they are adjacent or next to the uterus. During a woman's reproductive years the ovaries are about the size and shape of a large almond in its shell; they shrink after menopause.

The ovaries are attached to the uterus by *ovarian ligaments* and by the peritoneal covering over the back of the uterus (the *broad ligament*). They are suspended from the body by *suspensory ligaments*. The ovaries are displaced during pregnancy and may never return to their original spot. They can be felt in most nonobese premenopausal women during pelvic exams.

We are born with a fixed number of *primary ovarian follicles* that will develop into eggs (*oocytes*). At twenty weeks of fetal life, there may be more than 7 million of them! A majority degenerate before birth, leaving perhaps one million eggs. By puberty the number is decreased to about 500,000. Each month, as many as 1,000 follicles are available to be stimulated by ovarian hormones, but only one will become the *dominant follicle* and expel an egg; the rest die away. At menopause a woman may have only a few thousand eggs left. The release of the egg each month actually creates a tiny hole in the ovary surface. Over time the ovaries take on a wrinkled and pockmarked appearance.

OVARIAN HORMONES include three types of estrogen produced by the ovaries—*estradiol, estrone* and *estriol*—as well as male hormones, or androgens, including *testosterone* and *androstenedione*. Almost all estrogens come from the ovaries, but fatty tissues can also produce estrone. The ovaries secrete another female hormone, *progesterone*, from the *corpus luteum*, the shell of a follicle that's left after an egg has been expelled.

The production and proper balance of ovarian hormones are controlled by a feedback loop among the *hypothalamus*, a key structure deep within the brain; the *pituitary gland* (a pea-size gland behind the bridge of the nose) and the ovaries. A glitch in this feedback loop can disrupt ovulation and menstruation or lead to overproduction of androgens, causing excess growth of body hair, acne and other signs of masculinization.

Estrogens stimulate the development of the breasts, the reproductive organs and the bladder and urethra, as well as the monthly proliferation of the uterine endometrium during the reproductive years. Many other cells in the body have *receptors* for estrogen (even muscle in blood vessel walls). Progesterone inhibits the growth-stimulating effects of estrogen on certain tissues. For example, after menopause, replacement estrogen alone ("un-

Fig. 3: A WOMAN'S REPRODUCTIVE ORGANS (SIDE VIEW)

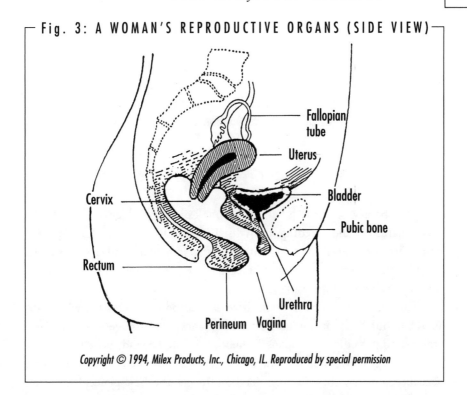

Fallopian tube

Uterus

Cervix

Bladder

Pubic bone

Rectum

Urethra

Perineum   Vagina

Copyright © 1994, Milex Products, Inc., Chicago, IL. Reproduced by special permission

opposed") may cause abnormal growth of endometrial cells; prescribing progesterone along with estrogen prevents that.

The uterus sits atop the bladder, with the colon to the rear. With the organs so close together, it's easy to understand how a problem in one area can affect another and how it may also be hard to tell where pelvic pain is actually coming from. Referred pain may originate in one place but be felt in an area some distance away. "Pelvic pain can stem from many sources; menstruation, problems in the uterus, infections, ovarian cysts and gastrointestinal or urinary pain," says Dr. Brandeis.

The *PELVIC FLOOR MUSCLES* form a hammock that supports the reproductive organs and connects them to the *bony pelvis*. The bony pelvis is a ring-shaped series of bones that support the body in the upright position, distributing the weight evenly between the two round tops of the thighbones within the hip joints. The bottom front of the bony pelvis is the pubic bone; the rear is a triangular structure comprised of the *sacrum* and the *coccyx*, your tailbone. Muscles and ligaments are strung from the front, rear and sides of the bony pelvis.

The most important of these supporting muscles is the *pelvic floor*, or *levator ani*, muscle, which surrounds the urethra, the vagina and the rectum. These muscles can become damaged or stretched during childbirth and weakened from lack of estrogen after menopause, allowing the uterus and other organs to sag (*prolapse*). This can cause a number of problems, ranging from urinary incontinence to the actual slippage of the cervix and uterus to such a degree that they protrude from the vagina, a problem we discuss in Chapter Three.

▪ Now That You Know What's Below ▪

The chapters in the first half of this book discuss problems related to the menstrual cycle and bleeding, growths that arise in the uterus and ovaries, endometriosis, infections and irritations that affect the vulva and vagina, troubles that arise in the urinary tract and the prevention and treatment of sexually transmitted diseases.

The second half of the book discusses reproductive choices, what happens to your body during and after pregnancy, miscarriage, *perimenopause* (the period preceding menopause), menopause and beyond, as well as cancers of the reproductive system. There is also an important chapter on female sexuality. Finally, we will consider how to get the best gynecologic care, including a description of what should take place during a pelvic exam (what your doctor can see and feel and what it may mean) and what screening tests you'll need over the years.

The more you know about your body and your gynecological health, the better able you will be to obtain the best medical care in today's changing health care environment in which many physicians are encouraged to see far more patients in far less time. "We have systems in which physicians are given only a few minutes to talk to patients during an annual visit," comments Dr. Anita Nelson. "If these systems are going to work for women, we need the patient to alert us to warning signs of a problem. We need to know that she is asking the questions she needs to ask and that she is an informed partner in her health care team."

Preventive medicine will be the new frontier of medicine, according to Dr. Nelson, because it simply makes economic sense. That also means women must be informed and involved in maintaining healthy lifestyles and making sure they are regularly screened for cancer and other diseases. We hope this book will help you take charge of this critical area of your health.

Menstruation and Abnormal Bleeding

Alternately called "the curse" and "my friend," menstruation is the subject of many myths, misconceptions and fears. Health historians claim the nickname the curse actually has biblical origins, that menstruation was a curse inflicted on Eve because of her sin, to be passed along to all women thereafter.

In primitive cultures magical powers were attributed to menstruation and menstrual blood. It was variously believed that a menstruating woman could actually blight crops, curdle milk, or even cause natural disasters, like floods! Beliefs that imply menstruation is somehow unclean persist to this day.

Monthly bloodletting was once believed to be the way the body rid itself of poisons. In many cultures, including Native American groups, women during their periods are sequestered, forbidden to cook, touch food or have sex with their husbands. Orthodox Jewish women must make sure there is no trace of menstrual discharge in the vagina before they take a ritual immersion bath (*mikvah*) to "purify" themselves before they can resume sexual relations. (However, studies show most women within these groups do not regard such rituals negatively; many see them as a respite and even a spiritual experience.)

Monthly periods were also once thought to make women weak or sickly. In the nineteenth century many educators believed menstruation made women unfit for the rigors of a college education. Not so long ago the persistent notion of women being "sick" during periods prompted many girls to be excused (or excuse themselves) from physical education classes or sports during their menses.

However, many women do suffer physical and emotional symptoms before and during their periods, such as cramps or *premenstrual syndrome (PMS)*. PMS is often the butt of jokes, compounding some women's negative feelings about periods.

∞ P a t ' s S t o r y ∞

"My mother never told me a thing about menstruation. I was at school when I started to bleed, and I went to the school nurse. She called my mother, and my mother came marching into my eighth-grade classroom with a big box of sanitary napkins. I was so embarrassed! There was a little booklet in the box. That's how I found out about periods."

▪ All About Periods ▪

Even today many women start out like Pat, knowing little about periods. A 1990 survey of college women reported in the journal *Women & Health* found that their basic knowledge of menstruation (and menopause) was mostly incorrect. So let's start at the beginning, with what Mother may never have told you.

The appearance of a girl's first menstrual period is known as menarche. The average age of menarche for North American women is now around twelve. Some girls reach menarche as early as age ten, and some do not have periods until after age sixteen (called *primary amenorrhea*, see page 30). Many women will start periods around the same age as their mothers and grandmothers, says Lisa B. Schwartz, M.D., an assistant professor of obstetrics and gynecology at NYU Medical Center.

Body weight affects puberty. A certain amount of body fat (which produces small amounts of estrogens) is needed to trigger the process that starts menstruation. Overweight girls tend to menstruate earlier, while athletes with very little body fat or girls with the eating disorder *anorexia* (who stop eating or eat very little) may have delayed puberty or stop menstruating.

Puberty and periods are governed by reproductive hormones produced by two of our *endocrine glands*: the pituitary gland (a pea-size extension of the brain located behind the bridge of the nose) and the ovaries. (The other endocrine glands are the *thyroid*, the *parathyroid*, the *adrenals* and the *pancreas*.)

The hormonal process that initiates puberty starts when the *hypothalamus*, a key regulatory structure in the brain, sends to the pituitary gland a chemical messenger called *gonadotropin-releasing hormone (GnRH)* that tells the pituitary to release *follicle-stimulating hormone (FSH)* and *luteinizing hormone (LH)*. These *gonadotropin hormones* signal the ovaries to begin producing estrogen, which triggers development of breasts and enlargement of the genitals and initiates ovarian cycles.

There is a constant feedback loop among the brain, the pituitary and the ovaries (the *hypothalamic-pituitary-gonadal axis*, or *HPG axis*). GnRH is secreted in small pulses every couple of hours, but surges during the menstrual cycle, triggering increases in FSH and LH. They govern production of estrogen and progesterone, which send back signals to regulate release of the gonadatropins. If any part of this delicate balance is upset, it affects ovulation and menstruation. The HPG axis also interacts with other endocrine systems and brain chemicals (including stress and thyroid hormones).

FSH governs the first, or *follicular*, phase of the menstrual cycle, triggering increased estrogen production and stimulating multiple follicles in the ovary. "Only one follicle will progress to the stage where it releases a mature egg. The others undergo *atresia*; they degenerate and are eventually resorbed by the ovary," explains Dr. Schwartz. A woman may ovulate perhaps four hundred to five hundred eggs by menopause. By menopause, the few thousand remaining ovarian follicles have atrophied.

At mid-cycle a surge of luteinizing hormone causes the follicle to burst open and release the mature egg. The egg is then taken up by the fingerlike projections (fimbriae) at the openings of the fallopian tubes and propelled down one of the tubes, where it must be fertilized within six to twelve hours or begin to deteriorate. The "shell" of the follicle becomes the corpus luteum, which produces progesterone. (*Corpus luteum* means "yellow body" in Latin; this shell actually leaves a yellow pockmark on the surface of the ovary.)

Ovulation typically occurs fourteen days before the start of the next menstrual period (day one of your cycle is the first day of menstruation), right after the LH surge. Some women have a slight cramping or other sensations

Fig. 4: THE MENSTRUAL CYCLE

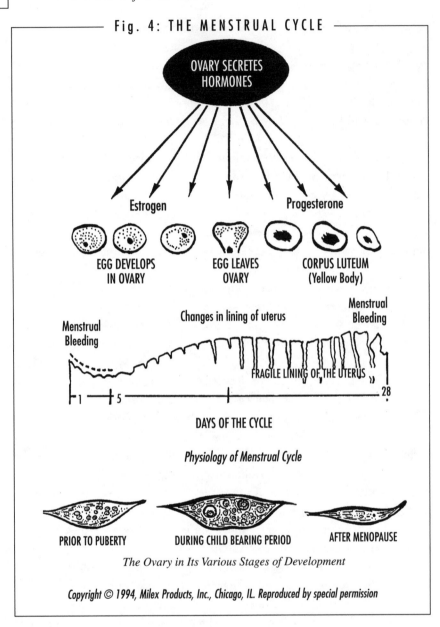

OVARY SECRETES HORMONES

Estrogen

Progesterone

EGG DEVELOPS IN OVARY

EGG LEAVES OVARY

CORPUS LUTEUM (Yellow Body)

Menstrual Bleeding

Changes in lining of uterus

Menstrual Bleeding

FRAGILE LINING OF THE UTERUS

1 — 5 — 28

DAYS OF THE CYCLE

Physiology of Menstrual Cycle

PRIOR TO PUBERTY

DURING CHILD BEARING PERIOD

AFTER MENOPAUSE

The Ovary in Its Various Stages of Development

at ovulation, called *mittelschmerz* (from the German for "middle pain"). "This is a very real sensation produced by the enlargement of the dominant follicle, which grows to about the size of a small cherry. It may produce a slight pressure or irritation in the pelvic area," says Dr. Schwartz.

A visible sign around the time of ovulation is the thinning of cervical

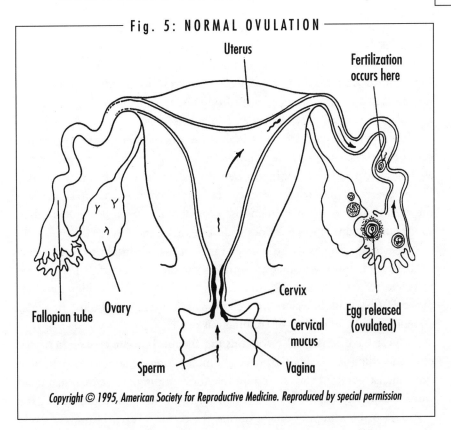

Fig. 5: NORMAL OVULATION

Uterus

Fertilization occurs here

Cervix

Cervical mucus

Egg released (ovulated)

Fallopian tube

Ovary

Sperm

Vagina

mucus, which makes it easier for sperm to swim upstream to the tubes (this can take as long as twenty-four to forty-eight hours). At the same time, basal body temperature (your temperature first thing in the morning) rises slightly, from 98.6° to around 99°, and stays elevated until menstruation. This is due to progesterone's effects on the central nervous system's temperature regulatory center, according to Dr. Schwartz.

Commercial kits that detect the LH surge in urine can predict ovulation within the ensuing forty-eight hours. Tracking basal body temperature may indicate ovulation has already occurred, too late for women trying to conceive (or avoid getting pregnant). New research indicates your most fertile period is from six days before to six hours after ovulation.

During the third, or *luteal*, phase of the cycle, LH levels fall as the corpus luteum produces more progesterone, which, with estrogen, stimulates growth of the top layer of the endometrium, containing tiny veins, arteries and secretory glands. This forms a blanket of blood vessels, tissue and nutrients inside the uterus to prepare for the implantation of a fertilized egg. Progesterone levels peak about seven days after ovulation. If pregnancy occurs, the corpus luteum continues to pump out progesterone, and the cycle is interrupted until after delivery. If pregnancy does not occur, the corpus luteum degenerates and progesterone levels drop. The uterine lining breaks up and is shed as menstrual flow. And the cycle begins anew.

The typical ovulatory-menstrual cycle runs between twenty-six and thirty-two days. But some women have cycles as short as twenty days, others as long as forty days; anything in between is considered "normal," stresses Dr. Schwartz. A menstrual period can last anywhere from two to eight days; the average is five. Most women lose only about three and one-half tablespoons of blood (although it does seem like much more).

The color of menstrual discharge varies; it may be bright red at the start of the period, and it becomes brownish as the flow tapers off. It may appear to be clotted, but in fact, clotting factors normally found in blood are not present. What look like clots are a combination of red blood cells, glandular secretions, mucus and bits of endometrial tissue.

Menstrual discharge also contains the chemical products of endometrial cells, including *prostaglandins*, which stimulate uterine contractions to help expel menstrual fluid and are responsible for cramping. More than half of all women experience some cramps (dysmenorrhea) just before and during the first days of bleeding, especially during the teenage years. However, severe cramps can be a sign of such problems as fibroids and endometriosis (for more on cramps, see page 29).

Menstrual blood is sterile *and is in no way "unclean"* (unless a woman carries such chronic infections as hepatitis or HIV); it develops an odor only after being exposed to air. Use of tampons can avoid odor. Such devices for collecting menstrual blood date back some three thousand years. Women in ancient times used rolls of papyrus or cotton cloth, flannel, soft wool and even grass to absorb their monthly flows. Later on rags were used and re-laundered each month (the origin of the derisive expression *on the rag*). The first disposable menstrual pads, made of gauze and cotton, were manufactured in 1896. The first tampons were sold commercially in 1933.

The old wives' tale that a girl will lose her virginity by using a tampon has now been dispelled by scientific research. A 1994 study of 300 postpubertal girls by Boston Children's Hospital and Harvard Medical School found that complete tearing or stretching of the hymen was common in sexually active girls but *not* in sexually inactive girls who used tampons. That's because the hymen is usually very flexible and will allow insertion of a tampon. In some women the hymen has an opening in the middle (even several small openings) or may be only a narrow fringe of skin around the vagina. (Contrary to popular belief, the Harvard study also found that vigorous sports, gymnastics and horseback riding do not result in tearing of the hymen.)

A normally formed vagina will easily accommodate a tampon, although some women may need a smaller size or a water-based lubricant to ease insertion. However, tampons need to be changed frequently. Bacteria can multiply on tampons left in the vagina too long, leading to *toxic shock syndrome (TSS*, see page 31). Pads should be changed often to avoid odor and bacterial growth.

Menstrual flow is usually heaviest in the first forty-eight hours, gradually tapering off. In some women, flow may be heavy the entire time or fairly light, or it may stop for a day and then begin again. Although the term *heavy bleeding* is relative, it's generally considered to be a 50 percent increase in normal flow or if a woman is soaking through more than ten tampons or pads a day. "If a woman starts to bleed more heavily than usual, and the bleeding persists over a couple of cycles, she should consult her gynecologist," Dr. Schwartz advises. Heavy bleeding can be a sign of fibroids, polyps, a hormonal imbalance or, rarely, cancer.

A woman's cycle is usually established in the first year or two after menarche. During these years a girl may menstruate each month but not always ovulate. If cycles do not become regular within five years, a woman is likely to be irregular throughout her reproductive years. Cycles do change; some women find that their cycles become shorter or longer after pregnancy.

"Since there's so much variation in menstrual periods, I advise women to keep track of their cycles," says Dr. Schwartz. "You can either mark a calendar or use a chart, noting the first and last days of each period and whether bleeding is heavy or light. Any change in your usual pattern, such as spotting or bleeding lasting more than a week when it's usually three or four days, that continues for several cycles can indicate a problem."

Ovulation can be interrupted not only by pregnancy but also by breast-feeding (*lactation*), illness, drastic dieting, thyroid problems and too vigorous athletic training. Birth control pills contain doses of synthetic estrogen and progesterone, which block ovulation, causing lighter endometrial shedding. "Stress can cause a woman to skip a period. Stress hormones like cortisol can interfere with the HPG axis, shutting off GnRH," says Dr. Schwartz.

In the years before menopause, or perimenopause, estrogen production gradually starts to taper off. A woman in her late forties may have irregular and shorter periods, along with some symptoms of menopause (pages 239–

240). When a woman has had no menstrual periods for a year, she is said to be in menopause.

When the ovaries produce low levels of estrogen, the hypothalamus desperately signals the pituitary to pump out extra FSH in an attempt to stimulate the ovaries. Menopause is confirmed by blood tests for elevated FSH. Without enough estrogen, the ovaries and the lining of the uterus atrophy.

∞ *S u e ' s S t o r y* ∞

"My periods were heavy from the day I started having them when I was eleven. I would lose a week to a week and a half each month, either because I was nuts from the PMS or because I was hemorrhaging. I couldn't get off the toilet. I was passing blood constantly. They never did anything about it when I was a teenager. I would stay home, or sometimes the school nurse would feel sorry for me and let me rest in her office. I also had menstrual migraines. I could see why they called it the curse.

"But I had a great doctor who gave me some behavioral suggestions, and I was able to eliminate maybe eighty percent of the PMS. Things like avoiding caffeine, exercising. I have never missed a day of work because of my period or the PMS. On the other hand, I have never missed a period either!"

▪ Common Menstrual Problems ▪
Abnormal Bleeding

More than a million women visit physicians each year complaining of heavy or irregular periods. As with Sue, about 20 percent of abnormal bleeding occurs during puberty, 30 percent during the childbearing years and 50 percent during the peri- and postmenopausal years. The most frequent complaint is prolonged, heavy menstrual bleeding (*menorrhagia*).

"Menorrhagia isn't just heavy bleeding at the start of menses for three or four days, but prolonged bleeding that lasts more than seven days," says June La Valleur, M.D., the director of the General Obstetrics/Gynecology Division at the University of Minnesota. "*Hypermenorrhea* is excessive bleeding, but of normal duration during menses. *Metrorrhagia* is uterine bleeding that occurs at irregular, frequent intervals, usually heavy, but the amount can be variable."

Excessive menstrual bleeding is usually defined as more than 80 milliliters (ml), about five and one-half to six tablespoons, or twice the average amount of blood lost during a typical period. If a woman bleeds heavily for seven to eight days, she may be at risk for iron deficiency and anemia.

Abnormal bleeding can be caused by fibroids, endometrial polyps, *endometrial hyperplasia* (abnormal cell growth in the cells lining the uterus), endometriosis, *adenomyosis* and cancers of the cervix, uterus or vagina, according to Dr. La Valleur. Adenomyosis, growth of endometrial tissue into the muscle layer of the uterus, can cause a sense of fullness in the pelvis and pain during intercourse (see page 52).

"However, if a woman of childbearing age has genital bleeding that is abnormal, she is considered pregnant until proven otherwise," says Dr. La Valleur. Menorrhagia can also be caused by *ectopic pregnancy* (a fertilized egg that implants outside the uterine cavity) or an early miscarriage.

In rare cases abnormal uterine bleeding can be caused by certain leukemias or by kidney or liver dysfunction. Clotting disorders, which prevent blood from coagulating normally, often present themselves as severe menorrhagia.

Dysfunctional uterine bleeding (DUB) is any bleeding that does not stem from anatomic problems like fibroids or medical illnesses, explains Dr. La Valleur. "In eighty-five percent of cases, dysfunctional uterine bleeding is caused by a disruption of normal ovarian function." DUB is usually painless.

Among the problems that can interfere with ovulation are disorders of the thyroid (hypothyroidism or hyperthyroidism), the pituitary, or the adrenal glands (such as *Addison's* or *Cushing's disease*) and *polycystic ovarian syndrome (PCOS)*. Polycystic ovarian syndrome occurs when there is continual disruption of the ovarian cycle by excess amounts of LH, leading to overproduction of androgens (male hormones) by the ovary. Several small follicles develop that do not expel an egg, so ovulation does not take place (anovulation) and irregular bleeding occurs. (For more on PCOS, see page 74.)

Dysfunctional bleeding can also occur as an unusually short menstrual cycle, periods every two or three weeks instead of once a month. The bleeding may not be excessive, but it happens more frequently. This may occur after pregnancy, as a woman's hormonal system returns to its normal rhythms, or during perimenopause.

In another type of DUB a woman has a normal cycle, but the corpus luteum doesn't produce progesterone normally, so the endometrium breaks down erratically, causing heavier, more prolonged periods. This is often called a *persistent corpus luteum*, or a short luteal phase.

In some cases a follicle ripens but doesn't release an egg. The ovary produces estrogen, but no progesterone, because ovulation has not occurred. The uterine lining continues to build until estrogen levels become so low they can no longer maintain the endometrial lining, resulting in heavy bleeding. This is common among perimenopausal women; when ovulation does not occur, the unopposed (but low) estrogenic stimulation of the endometrium can produce spotting in mid-cycle.

Infrequent, unpredictable uterine bleeding (at intervals greater than forty-five days) is termed *oligomenorrhea* and is usually due to ovulatory dysfunction.

■ *Diagnosing Abnormal Bleeding* ■

After pregnancy has been ruled out in younger women with severe episodes of DUB, a gynecologist will screen for a clotting disorder or an endocrine disorder. "As many as 20 percent of teenagers who are having abnormal uterine bleeding will have some sort of coagulation disorder," says Dr. Schwartz. "In addition, we check thyroid function, since low or high levels of thyroid hormone can frequently be associated with irregular periods. We also check *prolactin,* another hormone secreted by the pituitary gland. *Hyperprolactinemia,* high levels of prolactin, can result from a benign pituitary tumor, or adenoma, and can cause irregular bleeding by interfering with normal ovulation."

Although cancers and endometriosis are rare at this age, a young woman would be examined to rule out those possibilities as well. Abnormal bleeding in younger women is frequently associated with anovulatory cycles. In women between twenty and forty (and especially after age forty), it's not uncommon to have one or two anovulatory cycles a year. If a woman is usually regular, is not pregnant, and does not have fibroids or other problems, she may simply be watched more closely by her gynecologist.

The first intervention for young women with abnormal bleeding would be transvaginal ultrasound and, if necessary, an endometrial biopsy to rule out fibroids, polyps, endometrial hyperplasia, or tumors, says Herbert A. Goldfarb, M.D., an assistant clinical professor of obstetrics and gynecology at NYU Medical Center, who specializes in treating women with abnormal bleeding and fibroids. "If the findings reveal anovulatory bleeding, we will use a course of low-dose progesterone to see if we can normalize their bleeding cycle. If the bleeding does not improve, there may be a pathological problem and we will schedule a hysteroscopy," says Dr. Goldfarb.

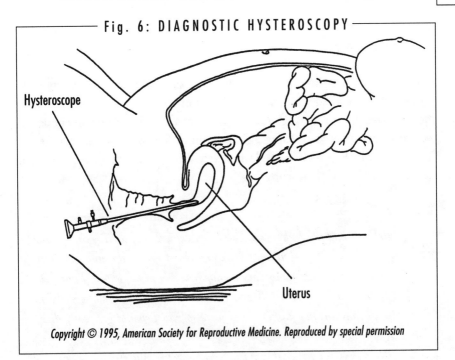

Fig. 6: DIAGNOSTIC HYSTEROSCOPY

Hysteroscope

Uterus

Copyright © 1995, American Society for Reproductive Medicine. Reproduced by special permission

Hysteroscopy is done with a small lighted scope inserted into the uterus to examine the uterine cavity. First, the cervix is slightly dilated or stretched. Then saline solution or carbon dioxide is injected into the uterus through the hysteroscope to expand the uterine cavity and clear away blood and mucus for better viewing. Hysteroscopy can detect endometrial polyps and fibroids that can cause abnormal bleeding. It is done on an outpatient basis under general or local anesthesia, usually right after menstruation. A woman may have cramping, vaginal discharge and some bleeding for several days afterward; sexual intercourse should be avoided for a few days (or for as long as bleeding occurs). The most common complication is a small puncture (*perforation*) of the uterus, which usually heals on its own.

Operative hysteroscopy to treat abnormalities found during the diagnostic procedure can often be done immediately, using a larger hysteroscope to admit surgical instruments or lasers.

Diagnostic laparoscopy may be performed if ovarian cysts or endometriosis are suspected, says Dr. Goldfarb. Under general anesthesia a small lighted telescope is inserted through a small incision near the belly button. The abdominal cavity is lightly inflated with air to view the pelvic organs (see page 88). In *laparoscopic surgery*, additional incisions are made to admit tiny surgical instruments.

Postmenopausal bleeding (other than withdrawal bleeding from hormone replacement therapy) is regarded as a sign of cancer. Approximately 20 percent of women with such bleeding who are not on replacement hormones either have premalignant lesions or cancers. So the postmenopausal woman may undergo transvaginal ultrasound, followed by an endometrial biopsy, in which a tissue sample is taken through a hysteroscope, and, if needed, diagnostic laparoscopy.

⚭ *S u e ' s   S t o r y* ⚭

"Before I had my endometrial ablation (where they destroy the uterine lining), they put me on Lupron for six months to shrink the endometrium. Had I known how bad temporary menopause would be, I would not have taken the Lupron. It was much, much worse than my PMS had ever been, and I had constant hot flashes. They were so bad I would get really dizzy and light-headed.

"I had only a partial ablation with an electric roller ball. They never told me that they ablated only around 75 percent of the endometrium. They just told me I might not have periods again . . . I don't know why they didn't destroy the entire endometrium, but I suspect I had a huge amount of endometrial tissue. They missed some, but what they did worked well. The periods I have had since then have been nice, normal periods."

▪ *Treatments for Abnormal Bleeding* ▪

More than 300,000 hysterectomies, removal of the uterus (*myomectomy*) and/or ovaries (*oophorectomy*), are performed every year to treat abnormal bleeding. (We discuss hysterectomy in Chapter Three.) But there are less drastic treatments.

ORAL CONTRACEPTIVES may be the treatment of choice if no pathological problem is found. A woman may be given a high-progestin (synthetic or natural progesterone) oral contraceptive every eight hours over three to four days. Progestins cause less build-up of the endometrial lining and lighter monthly bleeding. "For some women, a progesterone-only regimen may be advisable, particularly in obese women who are up to ten times at higher risk for endometrial hyperplasia," says Dr. La Valleur. A normal dose of an estrogen-progestin pill may be given for up to six months. Or small doses of the progestin *medroxyprogesterone acetate* (Cycrin, Provera) may be given for the first ten days of a cycle, for three to six months, to achieve a normal bleeding pattern.

Oral contraceptives offer a number of advantages: They provide birth control while correcting abnormal bleeding, and they reduce the risk of ovarian and endometrial cancers as well as iron-deficiency anemia, ectopic pregnancy, premenstrual syndrome and menstrual cramps. They can help regulate periods right up to menopause, if a woman doesn't smoke and if there are no other reasons why she shouldn't take it. (For more on the pill, see Chapter Nine.)

HORMONAL TREATMENTS for heavy bleeding also include low-dose progesterone and androgenic hormones. "A course of 5 mg. *norethinidrone acetate* (Aygestin) usually stops the bleeding immediately," says Dr. Goldfarb. "If abnormal bleeding is due to endometriosis, oral testosterone-derivatives which bring on a temporary menopause, such as *danazol* (Danocrine), can be used, or GnRH agonists, such as *leuprolide* (Lupron), may be used for three to six months to make the endometriosis less active." Lupron is also used to control bleeding as well as shrink fibroids prior to removal of either the fibroids or the uterus. (For details on GnRH agonists, see page 48.)

DILATATION AND CURETTAGE (D&C) has traditionally been used as a treatment for abnormal bleeding by scraping away dysfunctional endometrium. But that is slowly changing. "If the abnormal bleeding is caused by such pathology as fibroids, polyps or tumors it will not help diagnose or treat the problem," says Dr. Goldfarb. "It is really an outdated, ineffective treatment for bleeding. It should be used only with hysteroscopy to obtain a tissue diagnosis."

ENDOMETRIAL ABLATION is a treatment option for women with persistent, recurrent abnormal bleeding who wish to avoid hysterectomy and who do not plan to have more children. The procedure attempts to destroy all or part of the lining of the uterus, resulting in either cessation of periods or infrequent periods, but leaves the uterus and ovaries intact.

Endometrial ablation uses either a roller ball or roller bar device which delivers an electric current, an electrosurgical cutting device or, less commonly, a laser. It is performed through a hysteroscope under general anesthesia, as day surgery. GnRH agonists may be used for a month or two beforehand, to reduce the amount of endometrium that needs to be destroyed.

"At least two thirds of women who present with menorrhagia, who have a normal-size uterus, who undergo hysteroscopic ablation are improved by the treatment," says Robert L. Barbieri, M.D., chairman of the Department of Obstetrics and Gynecology at Harvard Medical School and Brigham and Women's Hospital in Boston. "Fifty to 60 percent of women will have a resolution of their bleeding for at least several years, and 20 percent will have a reduction in the amount of bleeding."

However, there is always the concern that a spot of endometrium may have been missed during ablation and could undergo malignant changes, without the early-warning sign of bleeding, cautions Dr. Barbieri. That is why women need to consult a practitioner who is highly skilled in the procedure.

A new ablation technique called Therma Choice may help solve that problem. The treatment involves inserting a disposable balloon into the uterus through a hysteroscope, inflating the balloon with water to conform to the contours of the uterus, then heating it for eight minutes to destroy the uterine lining. Afterward the balloon is deflated and removed. The procedure can be done under local anesthesia in an outpatient setting. Results from clinical trials found the treatment was 95 percent successful in women with menorrhagia (reducing flow or producing normal periods) after six months of follow-up. "Since the technique does not require surgical skills, it may be possible for physicians to do it as an office procedure," says Dr. Barbieri. Other trials are under way with a device that freezes the endometrium.

∾ E l i s s a ' s S t o r y ∾

"I had bad, bad cramps from the day I got my first period. It would begin as sharp twinges in my lower abdomen a day or two before. Once I got my period, it would feel like someone was twisting my insides. My back would ache too, and I would bleed like crazy. I went through boxes of Kotex. Now people tell me it was because of the aspirin I took for the pain, but who knew? Then the cramps would slowly go away, and I'd feel fine, until next time.

"I'm now in my forties, and the cramps are not as bad. The bleeding got better until I developed fibroids. I dreaded having surgery for my fibroids, but I must tell you that after that I hardly had any cramps for some reason."

Painful Periods/Dysmenorrhea

While more than half of all women experience some discomfort with their periods, up to 15 percent may be incapacitated one to three days a month with severe pain, or dysmenorrhea.

There are two categories of dysmenorrhea. *Primary dysmenorrhea*, which has no associated disorder, may occur shortly after menarche. *Secondary dysmenorrhea* is linked to medical conditions such as fibroids, endometriosis or *cervical stenosis (occlusion)*.

Dysmenorrhea was once thought to occur in a woman's head and not in her pelvis. Now it's known that menstrual cramps are real, caused by the presence of prostaglandins. These chemicals, produced to some degree by every cell in the body, are secreted in large quantities by the uterine lining and stimulate contractions, "squeezing" the blood vessels of the endometrium to limit menstrual bleeding. But when produced in excessive amounts, they cause prolonged and intense contractions, and those blood vessels completely block off, reducing oxygen delivery and resulting in severe pain. Women with dysmenorrhea have higher than normal concentrations of prostaglandins in their menstrual fluid.

Menstrual cramps usually begin just before a period or on the first day and last twenty-four hours or more. Women typically experience cramping in the lower pelvic area, along with backache and, in some women, a "pulling sensation" in the thighs. "The low backache and thigh pain that occur in dysmenorrhea are actually referred pain from the uterus, where there is increased pressure and severe blood vessel constriction," explains Dr. La Valleur. "Severe menstrual cramps may also be associated with sweating, tachycardia, headache, nausea and vomiting and diarrhea. All these are really due to the presence of prostaglandins."

The most effective medications for menstrual cramps are *prostaglandin synthetase inhibitors*, including over-the-counter *nonsteroidal anti-inflammatory drugs (NSAIDs)*, such as *ibuprofen* (Advil, Nuprin, Motrin), *naproxen* (Aleve) and *ketoprofin* (Orudis KT, Actron), or aspirin. *Acetaminophen* has little effect on cramps since it doesn't affect uterine prostaglandin production.

Hot-water bottles, heating pads and soaking in a hot tub can relieve mild dysmenorrhea. That's because heat promotes a decrease in muscle spasm and an increase in blood flow. Prescription-strength NSAIDs, such as *naproxen* (Naprosyn) and *naproxen sodium* (Anaprox), may be needed in severe cases. A newer prostaglandin inhibitor, *bromfenac sodium* (Bromfenac), is also being tested. Other prescription drugs include *mefenamic acid* (Ponstel) and *flufen-amic acid* (Arlef).

Because NSAIDs also block prostaglandins' effects on uterine contractions and impair the function of blood platelets, menstrual bleeding may be prolonged in some women (paradoxically, many women find that NSAIDs decrease the amount of menstrual flow somewhat). Other possible side effects are headaches, dizziness or blurred vision and gastrointestinal distress (NSAIDs should not be taken on an empty stomach).

Dr. La Valleur advises patients to try two or three types of NSAIDs and use each one during at least two menstrual cycles to see which is most effective. "It's really important that the therapy begin at the onset of bleeding, at the very moment that the patient sees the first spot of blood, or even before her period, when she may first feel pain," she says. "It's also important to continue at least through the first two to three days of menstruation."

Since dysmenorrhea usually occurs only with ovulatory cycles, one of the best ways to prevent (or reduce) severe menstrual cramps is to block ovulation with oral contraceptives. "With the birth control pill there is a decrease in endometrial proliferation and prostaglandin secretion. Several studies have shown that with low-dose or even medium-dose birth control pills, menstrual fluid or menstrual flow is diminished by up to fifty percent," explains Dr. La Valleur.

Some women find that menstrual cramps lessen (or disappear) after they've had children. If cramps are due to fibroids or endometriosis, treating these problems often resolves pain.

Many women experience tension and anxiety with menstrual cramps that increase along with the pain. Moderate exercise, such as walking and meditation and yoga, can be helpful. Herbal teas and other soothing drinks may also be relaxing and break the pain-tension cycle.

Amenorrhea

The absence (or cessation) of periods during a woman's reproductive years is known as amenorrhea.

Primary amenorrhea is the failure to menstruate by age sixteen (as well as failure to develop secondary sex characteristics, such as breast buds, by age fourteen). Causes can range from family patterns of late maturation to endocrine problems, especially problems in GnRH secretion by the hypothalamus, pituitary tumors, hypothyroidism or adrenal dysfunction. Physical causes include an imperforate hymen and nonfunctioning ovaries. The treatment for ovarian failure is replacement hormones.

Since a girl will not start periods unless she has a minimum amount of fatty tissue (22 percent seems to be the minimum), eating disorders or extreme dieting can delay menarche, as can vigorous athletic training (which often goes hand in hand with eating disorders in young girls taking part in gymnastics or other sports). Treatment of anorexia and the attainment of higher body weight will often bring about menarche.

Secondary amenorrhea occurs when periods stop at any point after menarche (for reasons other than pregnancy). The most common causes are premature ovarian failure (early menopause), hypothalamic dysfunction, pituitary tumors leading to high prolactin, intrauterine scarring and polycystic ovarian syndrome.

Women who have stopped menstruating because of estrogen deficiency will require some sort of replacement hormones. In younger women this may be birth control pills. For selected women in their thirties and forties, replacement estrogen and progesterone may be given in the same regimen as postmenopausal women, or the birth control pill may be used if the woman is not a smoker.

If a young woman has some ovarian function and wants to become pregnant, she may receive fertility drugs, such as *clomiphene citrate* (Clomid). (For more, see page 220.)

∞ Toxic Shock Syndrome (TSS) ∞

Tampons left in the vagina for more than four hours can provide a place for bacteria that normally reside in the vagina, such as *Staphylococcus aureus*, to grow and multiply. Strains of the bacteria produce a poison (dubbed *toxic shock toxin*) that is absorbed into the bloodstream and causes a body-wide illness called *toxic shock syndrome*. In severe cases this infection can result in liver problems and kidney failure, which causes a rapid drop in blood pressure that leads to shock.

In mild cases toxic shock syndrome is characterized by a rash similar to sunburn, along with high fever (over 102°F/8.9°C), sore throat, body aches, vomiting and diarrhea. In severe cases there can be dangerously low blood pressure as well as kidney, heart, liver and blood-clotting difficulties. Between 2 and 3 percent of patients die of complications resulting from TSS.

Treatment always involves hospitalization, intravenous fluid replacement and other measures to combat shock, and antibiotics. Many strains of *S. aureus* are resistant to penicillin, so synthetic versions, such as *nafcillin* or *oxacillin*, are given. In severe cases intensive care may be needed. TSS can recur in about 30 percent of menstrually related cases.

Although the disease has been recognized since the 1920s, it came to widespread attention in 1979, when cases of TSS were first associated with use of superabsorbent tampons. The tampon involved, Rely, was withdrawn from the market in 1980; all boxes of tampons now contain warnings about TSS. However, TSS continues to affect up to 17 out of 100,000 menstruating women (especially teenagers and women under 30). It can also occur after childbirth or surgery and can result from infections caused by burns or wounds.

To avoid TSS, use less absorbent tampons, and change them frequently. Any tampon, whether superabsorbent or regular, must be changed at least every four hours. Wash your hands with antibacterial soap before inserting a tampon to avoid introducing bacteria from your fingers into the vagina.

If you've had one bout with TSS, it's probably a good idea not to use tampons at all. If you develop fever, nausea and vomiting during or just after your period, contact your doctor right away (if you are using a tampon, remove it immediately).

---

๑ *T i n a ' s   S t o r y* ๑

"I was a late bloomer; I first got my period when I was around fourteen. I had bad cramps, and later on, in my twenties, I also started to have bloating, weight gain and breast tenderness in the week or two before my period. I could gain as much as seven or eight pounds in 'water weight.' But my doctor gave me a diuretic, and that took care of it.

"If I was a little more irritable before my period, I chalked it up to premenstrual tension, but in my thirties I started to have anxiety attacks, feeling totally out of control, panicky, overwhelmed. At first I thought it was because of job pressures. I remember one instance very vividly. I had a business meeting in an area of the city I'd never been in before. I got lost,

and I started to panic. I stood there, right on that street corner and screamed! People were looking at me! I made myself calm down. I went into a coffee shop, calmly asked directions, and finally made it to the meeting.

"My gynecologist suggested the anxiety might be premenstrually related since I had a history of other symptoms. She said that I might have a very severe form of premenstrual syndrome, where some women get very depressed and others get really anxious. She told me to keep track of all my physical and emotional symptoms for three cycles. I was really amazed to see the correlation between the bloating and weight gain and these horrible episodes. Just being aware of that made it easier to handle the anxiety.

"She gave me a prescription for antianxiety medication, and I take it when I start to have anxiety before my period. You can't imagine what a change this has made in my life."

▪ Premenstrual Problems ▪

Premenstrual syndrome (PMS) is now regarded as a constellation of symptoms which arise in the days between ovulation and menstruation. Researchers theorize that some women have a special sensitivity to normal hormonal (or physical) changes in the luteal phases of their cycles that may trigger symptoms. But so far no proof of a biological cause for PMS has been found.

There are more than two hundred symptoms associated with PMS. They include fluid retention, bloating, weight gain, headaches, acne, breast tenderness and cravings for sweets or carbohydrates. Psychological symptoms include depression, anxiety, irritability, mood swings, tearfulness and changes in sexual drive.

Some women have PMS from their first menstrual periods, but most develop it during their thirties and forties, especially after a major interruption of their ovulatory cycles, such as pregnancy or stopping the pill. "It may well be that premenstrual syndrome occurs in the thirties and forties as part of a process of hormonal and endocrine changes leading up to menopause," suggests Sally K. Severino, M.D., professor and executive vice chair of the Department of Psychiatry at the University of New Mexico and a leading PMS researcher. She notes that women who experience PMS are also likely to suffer more severe menopausal symptoms.

Many women who believe they have PMS do not have the severity of symptoms needed for a formal diagnosis. A National Institutes of Health consensus conference stated that symptom intensity must increase by at least 30 percent premenstrually, for at least two consecutive months, and must interfere with normal functioning for a diagnosis of PMS to be made. While around 75 percent of women have occasional premenstrual symptoms, only 20 to 30 percent of women have PMS by the NIH definition.

Perhaps 3 to 7 percent of women experience especially severe emotional symptoms every month, including (but not limited to) depression. The problem is currently classified as *Premenstrual dysphoric disorder (PMDD)*, in the psychiatrist's diagnostic manual, the *Diagnostic and Statistical Manual of Mental Disorders, DSM-IV*. However, PMDD should not be confused with PMS.

"Whereas PMS is mostly characterized by physical symptoms, with some associated mood problems, PMDD is primarily a disorder of mood, not just depression but anxiety as well, with associated physical symptoms," says Dr. Severino. Symptoms of PMDD must be severe enough to interfere with school or work and social or marital relationships and must be confirmed through charts or diaries for at least two cycles. Mood symptoms include:

- A markedly depressed mood, with feelings of hopelessness or self-deprecating thoughts.

- Heightened anxiety, tension, feeling "keyed up," "on edge," overwhelmed or out of control.

- Noticeable mood variability, such as suddenly feeling sad, tearful, irritable or angry.

- Persistent and striking anger or irritability, or increased interpersonal conflicts, or difficulty concentrating.

- Lethargy, easy fatigability or noticeable lack of energy; sleeping too much or being unable to sleep.

- Distinct changes in appetite, such as overeating, or having specific food cravings (such as for sweets).

A number of medical conditions can exacerbate both PMS and PMDD, including migraine headaches, asthma and allergies.

Women suffering from PMS have often been told it's "all in your head." But PMS is real. Women in cultures as diverse as those of Nigeria, Japan and Sweden experience premenstrual symptoms. What differs are the types of symptoms and whether women are distressed by them. For example, recent studies comparing American, Italian and Bahraini women in their twenties and thirties found that a third of them shared five symptoms: breast swelling, breast pain, irritability, mood swings and fatigue. The American women reported more irritability, mood swings and weight gain, while the Italians said they had more breast swelling and pain, and the Bahraini women complained more often of backaches. Interestingly, few women in Italy or Bahrain knew about PMS or "premenstrual tension." In fact, the Italian women reported feelings of energy, well-being and orderliness before their periods!

Studies show that women who have more life stresses seem to have more severe symptoms; women socialized to have negative ideas about menstruation also report more symptoms. On the other hand, premenstrual symptoms may themselves be a source of stress. Women who have better coping skills may also have less PMS.

Treating PMS and PMDD

Before premenstrual problems like PMS or PMDD can be diagnosed or treated, a woman must track her symptoms over several menstrual cycles to note which ones are experienced as well as whether they occur (or worsen) only premenstrually.

"It's very dramatic how the symptoms turn on at a particular phase of the cycle. For some women it's days before menstruation; for others it's eight, nine, ten days before," comments Jean Endicott, Ph.D., chief of the Department of Research Assessment and Training at the New York State Psychiatric Institute, who developed the most widely used symptom rating chart. "The pattern in which these symptoms turn off is also similar in a woman from cycle to cycle. Some women report that within a day or two of starting their periods, they have no symptoms. For others, it's almost the end of the menses before all the symptoms go away."

Daily ratings can help determine when to start or adjust medication or take other measures to minimize symptoms. "We also use the daily ratings to help women identify the *best* days of the month—for most women it's around day six through day ten or eleven—so that they can take advantage of the good days, not just focus on the difficult days," says Dr. Endicott. From 10 to 15 percent of women actually report *positive* changes premenstrually.

Medication is reserved for severe PMS; women with moderate symptoms may be advised to make dietary changes and exercise. A frequent dietary

Fig.7: YOUR SYMPTOM RATING CHART

Make extra copies of this chart so you can track your symptoms for at least three menstrual cycles. Fill in the date on the line under the day of the week when you start your daily ratings; start a new page each Monday. On the line under the date, note whether you are spotting (S) or menstruating (M). If you consistently rate your premenstrual symptoms in the moderate to severe range over several cycles (or if symptoms of depression or anxiety occur to a lesser degree throughout the month), and your ratings in the last three categories indicate symptoms are interfering with your life, it may be advisable to seek professional help.

If you have mild to moderate premenstrual symptoms, this chart may help you better manage those symptoms.

Note the degree to which you experienced each of the problems listed below. Make your ratings each evening. Circle the number which corresponds to the severity as noted here:

1—Not at all,   2—Minimal,   3—Mild,   4—Moderate,   5—Severe,   6—Extreme

Rating under correct day of the week:	MON	TUES	WED	THU	FRI	SAT	SUN **
Note date under day of wk.							**
Note *spotting* or *menses* with S or M:	—	—	—	—	—	—	—
1a. Felt depressed, sad, "down," or blue"	1 2 3 4 5 6	1 2 3 4 5 6	1 2 3 4 5 6	1 2 3 4 5 6	1 2 3 4 5 6	1 2 3 4 5 6	1 2 3 4 5 6
1b. Felt hopeless	1 2 3 4 5 6	1 2 3 4 5 6	1 2 3 4 5 6	1 2 3 4 5 6	1 2 3 4 5 6	1 2 3 4 5 6	1 2 3 4 5 6
1c. Felt worthless or guilty	1 2 3 4 5 6	1 2 3 4 5 6	1 2 3 4 5 6	1 2 3 4 5 6	1 2 3 4 5 6	1 2 3 4 5 6	1 2 3 4 5 6
2. Felt anxious, tense, "keyed up" or "on edge"	1 2 3 4 5 6	1 2 3 4 5 6	1 2 3 4 5 6	1 2 3 4 5 6	1 2 3 4 5 6	1 2 3 4 5 6	1 2 3 4 5 6
3a. Had mood swings (e.g., suddenly felt sad or tearful)	1 2 3 4 5 6	1 2 3 4 5 6	1 2 3 4 5 6	1 2 3 4 5 6	1 2 3 4 5 6	1 2 3 4 5 6	1 2 3 4 5 6
3b. Was more sensitive to rejection or my feelings were easily hurt	1 2 3 4 5 6	1 2 3 4 5 6	1 2 3 4 5 6	1 2 3 4 5 6	1 2 3 4 5 6	1 2 3 4 5 6	1 2 3 4 5 6

——— Fig.7: YOUR SYMPTOM RATING CHART ———

Note the degree to which you experienced each of the problems listed below. Make your ratings each evening. Circle the number which corresponds to the severity as noted here:

1—Not at all,   2—Minimal,   3—Mild,   4—Moderate,   5—Severe,   6—Extreme

Rating under correct day of the week:	MON	TUES	WED	THU	FRI	SAT	SUN **
Note date under day of wk.	__	__	__	__	__	__	__ **
Note *spotting* or *menses* with S or M:	__	__	__	__	__	__	__

4a. Felt angry, irritable	1 2 3 4 5 6	1 2 3 4 5 6	1 2 3 4 5 6	1 2 3 4 5 6	1 2 3 4 5 6	1 2 3 4 5 6	1 2 3 4 5 6
4b. Had conflicts or problems with people	1 2 3 4 5 6	1 2 3 4 5 6	1 2 3 4 5 6	1 2 3 4 5 6	1 2 3 4 5 6	1 2 3 4 5 6	1 2 3 4 5 6
5. Had less interest in usual activities (e.g., work, school, friends, hobbies)	1 2 3 4 5 6	1 2 3 4 5 6	1 2 3 4 5 6	1 2 3 4 5 6	1 2 3 4 5 6	1 2 3 4 5 6	1 2 3 4 5 6
6. Had difficulty concentrating	1 2 3 4 5 6	1 2 3 4 5 6	1 2 3 4 5 6	1 2 3 4 5 6	1 2 3 4 5 6	1 2 3 4 5 6	1 2 3 4 5 6
7. Felt lethargic, tired, fatigued, or had a lack of energy	1 2 3 4 5 6	1 2 3 4 5 6	1 2 3 4 5 6	1 2 3 4 5 6	1 2 3 4 5 6	1 2 3 4 5 6	1 2 3 4 5 6
8a. Had increased appetite or overate	1 2 3 4 5 6	1 2 3 4 5 6	1 2 3 4 5 6	1 2 3 4 5 6	1 2 3 4 5 6	1 2 3 4 5 6	1 2 3 4 5 6

Continued

Fig.7: YOUR SYMPTOM RATING CHART

Note the degree to which you experienced each of the problems listed below. Make your ratings each evening. Circle the number which corresponds to the severity as noted here:

1—Not at all,   2—Minimal,   3—Mild,   4—Moderate,   5—Severe,   6—Extreme

Rating under correct day of the week:	MON	TUES	WED	THU	FRI	SAT	SUN **
Note date under day of wk.	——	——	——	——	——	——	—— **
Note *spotting* or *menses* with S or M:	——	——	——	——	——	——	——
8b. Had cravings for specific foods	1 2 3 4 5 6	1 2 3 4 5 6	1 2 3 4 5 6	1 2 3 4 5 6	1 2 3 4 5 6	1 2 3 4 5 6	1 2 3 4 5 6
9a. Slept more, took naps, found it hard to get up when intended	1 2 3 4 5 6	1 2 3 4 5 6	1 2 3 4 5 6	1 2 3 4 5 6	1 2 3 4 5 6	1 2 3 4 5 6	1 2 3 4 5 6
9b. Had trouble getting to sleep or staying asleep	1 2 3 4 5 6	1 2 3 4 5 6	1 2 3 4 5 6	1 2 3 4 5 6	1 2 3 4 5 6	1 2 3 4 5 6	1 2 3 4 5 6
10a. Felt overhelmed or that I could not cope	1 2 3 4 5 6	1 2 3 4 5 6	1 2 3 4 5 6	1 2 3 4 5 6	1 2 3 4 5 6	1 2 3 4 5 6	1 2 3 4 5 6
10b. Felt out of control	1 2 3 4 5 6	1 2 3 4 5 6	1 2 3 4 5 6	1 2 3 4 5 6	1 2 3 4 5 6	1 2 3 4 5 6	1 2 3 4 5 6
11a. Had breast tenderness	1 2 3 4 5 6	1 2 3 4 5 6	1 2 3 4 5 6	1 2 3 4 5 6	1 2 3 4 5 6	1 2 3 4 5 6	1 2 3 4 5 6

Fig.7: YOUR SYMPTOM RATING CHART

Note the degree to which you experienced each of the problems listed below. Make your ratings each evening.
Circle the number which corresponds to the severity as noted here:

1–Not at all,   2–Minimal,   3–Mild,   4–Moderate,   5–Severe,   6–Extreme

Rating under correct day of the week:	MON	TUES	WED	THU	FRI	SAT	SUN **
Note date under day of wk.							**
Note *spotting* or *menses* with S or M:							

11b. Had breast swelling, felt "bloated," or had weight gain

	MON	TUES	WED	THU	FRI	SAT	SUN
	1	1	1	1	1	1	1
	2	2	2	2	2	2	2
	3	3	3	3	3	3	3
	4	4	4	4	4	4	4
	5	5	5	5	5	5	5
	6	6	6	6	6	6	6

11c. Had headache

1	1	1	1	1	1	1
2	2	2	2	2	2	2
3	3	3	3	3	3	3
4	4	4	4	4	4	4
5	5	5	5	5	5	5
6	6	6	6	6	6	6

11d. Had joint or muscle pain

1	1	1	1	1	1	1
2	2	2	2	2	2	2
3	3	3	3	3	3	3
4	4	4	4	4	4	4
5	5	5	5	5	5	5
6	6	6	6	6	6	6

At work, at school, at home, or in daily routine, at least one of the problems noted above caused reduction of productivity or inefficiency

1	1	1	1	1	1	1
2	2	2	2	2	2	2
3	3	3	3	3	3	3
4	4	4	4	4	4	4
5	5	5	5	5	5	5
6	6	6	6	6	6	6

At least one of the problems noted above interfered with hobbies or social activities (e.g., avoid or do less)

1	1	1	1	1	1	1
2	2	2	2	2	2	2
3	3	3	3	3	3	3
4	4	4	4	4	4	4
5	5	5	5	5	5	5
6	6	6	6	6	6	6

At least one of the problems noted above interfered with relationships with others

1	1	1	1	1	1	1
2	2	2	2	2	2	2
3	3	3	3	3	3	3
4	4	4	4	4	4	4
5	5	5	5	5	5	5
6	6	6	6	6	6	6

Reproduced by permission of Jean Endicott, Ph. D. Director of Research Assessment & Training, New York State Psychiatric Institute.

recommendation is to reduce caffeine intake. Women suffering from PMS-related fatigue often boost their coffee consumption, says Dr. Endicott, but there's good evidence that coffee and other caffeinated beverages can increase anxiety and irritability (and may contribute to breast tenderness). Women are also cautioned to avoid alcohol since they may be more sensitive to its effects (and have higher blood levels) premenstrually.

Among other PMS management strategies:

EXERCISE: While there's no clinical proof that exercise has any effect on PMS symptoms, most physicians recommend it. Exercise can reduce depression and anxiety, boost energy and self-esteem. There's also some evidence that it increases *endorphins,* the body's natural pain reliever and mood elevator. Exercise may help reduce bloating.

DIURETICS: Medications such as *chlorthalidone* (Hygroton), *furosemide* (Lasix) and *hydrochlorothiazide* (Hydro-D) help the kidneys get rid of excess salt and water, reducing premenstrual fluid retention. Your doctor should monitor potassium levels if you take diuretics; you may need potassium supplements.

An over-the-counter product combining *ammonium chloride* and caffeine (AquaBan) has somewhat less diuretic action, but studies show it also relieves premenstrual bloating and acts as a mild stimulant. Other over-the-counter preparations, such as Premensyn, also contain mild diuretics.

BIRTH CONTROL PILLS: Taking oral contraceptives can minimize premenstrual symptoms in many cases, but some women find that PMS symptoms (such as migraines) shift to pill-free days and may worsen because of the drop in hormones. Some experts advocate taking oral contraceptives for six to twelve weeks, without breaks in between for withdrawal bleeding. A small study reported in 1997 in the journal *Obstetrics and Gynecology* found that five to thirteen extended pill cycles reduced menstrual-related symptoms.

PSYCHOTROPIC MEDICATIONS: The antidepressants known as *selective serotonin reuptake inhibitors (SSRIs)* have been found to be clearly effective against both PMS and PMDD. Serotonin is a brain chemical associated with depression and is known to be lower in women with PMS. SSRIs help prevent the quick reabsorption of serotonin in the brain, resulting in higher levels and relief of depression. Recent randomized, controlled clinical trials have shown that the SSRIs *fluoxetine* (Prozac) and *sertraline* (Zoloft) were effective in relieving tension, irritability and depressed mood in women with PMS; fluoxetine has also been shown to be effective in PMDD.

Clinical trials have also shown that the antianxiety drug *alprazolam* (Xanax) helps relieve some PMS-related symptoms as well as PMDD-related anxiety, irritability, severe tension and feelings of being out of control.

A GOOD NIGHT'S SLEEP: Disruptions of the sleep-wake cycle, or *circadian rhythm*, may play a role in both PMS and PMDD. Some preliminary animal studies suggest that sex hormones may help regulate circadian rhythms. PMS researcher Dr. Sally Severino speculates that sleep disruptions might contribute to premenstrual irritability and depression, or vice versa. "Studies have shown that women with PMS have some sleep changes and seem to sleep less efficiently in the premenstrual period. However, increases in tension and arousal during the premenstrual period, rather than hormonal shifts, may account for these problems."

Dr. Severino believes that learning "sleep hygiene" may be an effective nondrug therapy for PMS. Sleep hygiene involves learning good sleep habits: going to bed and waking up at the same time each day, limiting noise and light in the bedroom, avoiding vigorous exercise and caffeine within a few hours of going to bed and developing a soothing routine at bedtime.

CARBOHYDRATES—A "NATURAL" PMS TREATMENT?: Low levels of serotonin not only may produce premenstrual depression but also may trigger the cravings for starches and sweets some women experience before their periods. Research by Richard J. Wurtman, M.D., a professor of neuroscience and specialist in brain chemistry, and Judith Wurtman, Ph.D., a cell biologist and nutritionist, at the Massachusetts Institute of Technology has found that women with PMS consumed five hundred extra calories in such foods as potatoes, rice, cookies, candy and pretzels before their periods, apparently in an unconscious attempt to "medicate" PMS symptoms; controlled studies showed such foods did indeed elevate mood and boost serotonin levels.

The Wurtmans reported in 1995 that women with PMS given a carbohydrate-rich beverage formulated to raise levels of serotonin (now marketed as PMS ESCAPE) had fewer symptoms of depression, improved cognitive function and decreased carbohydrate cravings, compared with women given placebos. This research suggests that giving in to cravings for chocolate and other carbohydrates (in moderation, of course) may well provide a nondrug therapy for PMS for some women.

Fibroids, Uterine Problems and Hysterectomy

The uterus is a tough, elastic organ, mostly made of muscle. It is capable of expanding to accommodate a baby weighing seven (or more) pounds, then shrinking to its original upside-down pear contours within six weeks after a woman has given birth.

But a number of problems can arise within the structure of the uterus. Chief among them are *myomas*, commonly called *fibroids*, benign growths that arise in the half-inch-thick uterine wall (*myometrium*). Myomas occur in up to 30 percent of women over age thirty, but the true incidence may be higher since many women have no symptoms.

The pelvic muscles supporting the uterus can be stretched by childbirth and weakened by lack of estrogen after menopause. These supports may become so lax that the uterus slips down into the vagina, a problem known as *uterine prolapse*. Cancer can also develop in the uterine lining or wall (see Chapter Thirteen).

More than a third of all hysterectomies are performed because of fibroids, 16 percent because of prolapse, 11 percent because of cancer, with many more resulting from abnormal bleeding.

▪ Fibroids ▪
Facts About Fibroids

The proper term for fibroid is *leiomyoma* (*leio* meaning "smooth," *myo* meaning "muscle" and *oma* meaning "growth"); fibroids are often called myomas for short. These whorled balls of smooth muscle and connective tissue sometimes grow larger than a grapefruit, protruding into the uterine or pelvic cavity.

Just what causes myomas to form is not well understood, but estrogen may stimulate their growth. Fibroids may get larger early in pregnancy, when estrogen levels are higher, and often disappear after menopause. Women who start their periods early may be more at risk of developing fibroids, as are women who've never had children or delay childbearing. Two to five times as many African-American women have fibroids as white women, develop them at an earlier age and have more severe symptoms. Myomas are also more common in women of Eastern European or Jewish ancestry, but it's not clear why. Obesity may play a role, but some of these women may have newly discovered "fibroid genes."

According to Cynthia C. Morton, Ph.D., professor of obstetrics, gynecology, reproductive biology, and pathology at Harvard Medical School and director of cytogenetics at Brigham and Women's Hospital in Boston, a gene involved in fibroids, *HMGI-C*, does not appear to be inherited as an abnormal gene. Rather, mutations are somatic, likely occurring during a woman's reproductive years. The DNA of the gene is broken and rearranged, and this may start (or be part of) a cascade of events that leads to formation of fibroids, speculates Dr. Morton. Her research team found an abnormal HMGI-C gene in 10 percent of fibroid samples studied. It's not yet known whether some women might be predisposed to have alterations in the gene or related genes now being studied.

There are three types of fibroid:

- *INTRAMURAL (INTERSTITIAL) FIBROIDS* grow within the uterine wall. They may produce few symptoms other than a heavy, tender, achy uterus. In rare cases an intramural fibroid may enlarge the wall enough to block a fallopian tube, causing infertility.

- *SUBSEROUS (SEROSAL) FIBROIDS* often begin in the uterine wall but push into the outer layer (the serosa) and can become *pedunculated* (attached by a stem). A subserosal fibroid can put pressure on the bladder, causing pain and frequent urination, put pressure on the rec-

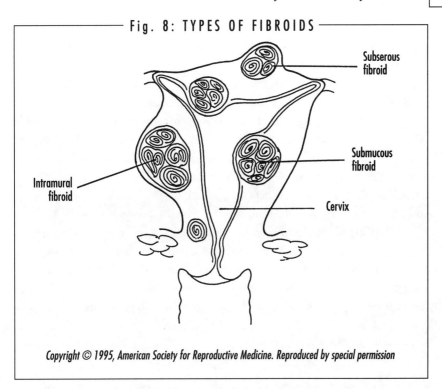

Fig. 8: TYPES OF FIBROIDS

Subserous fibroid

Submucous fibroid

Intramural fibroid

Cervix

Copyright © 1995, American Society for Reproductive Medicine. Reproduced by special permission

tum, causing constipation and pain, or twist on its stalk, provoking severe abdominal pain.

- *SUBMUCOUS FIBROIDS* begin within the middle uterine wall but grow inward, invading the lining of the uterus, or endometrium. They can cause excessive menstrual bleeding and severe cramps, as the uterus contracts to try to push the tumor out. These fibroids can also grow on stalks, dangling into the cervix and beyond, causing painful intercourse. Submucous fibroids may interfere with the implantation of a fertilized egg or prevent the placenta from properly attaching to the womb.

Many women have more than one fibroid, and they can grow so large a woman may look pregnant. "Some women have severe symptoms even with a single small fibroid, while others with several large growths have little or no symptoms," observes Steven R. Goldstein, M.D., professor of obstetrics and gynecology and director of Gynecological Ultrasound at NYU Medical Center.

Between 20 and 50 percent of women with fibroids experience minor abdominal discomfort or "heaviness," frequent urination, constipation and heavy or unpredictable menstrual bleeding. About a third have pelvic pain. Others experience symptoms of pressure caused by a fibroid pressing on the bladder or rectum. This also causes urine retention (leading to urinary tract infections) or urine overflow, or *overflow incontinence.*

The heavy bleeding associated with submucous and intramural fibroids has to do with their disruption of the endometrium and the blood supply that fibroids develop in order to grow. During menstruation these blood vessels open and pour out blood. Bleeding may be so heavy a woman develops *anemia*, with dizziness, weakness and pale skin, says Dr. Goldstein. Fibroids can also cause irregular bleeding, such as spotting between periods.

When a pedunculated fibroid twists on its stem, the blood supply is abruptly cut off, causing sudden and intense pain. The fibroid may also begin to die. The body has an inflammatory response to the dying tissue, causing contractions and cramping. A fibroid pressing on blood vessels supplying the legs can cause pain, as well as varicose veins with prolonged standing.

❧ *E l i s s a ' s   S t o r y ,   C o n t ' d* ❧

"I had had little fibroids for a long time, but I had no problems from them. The symptoms came on gradually. I started to feel bloated. I had to urinate a lot, and I was getting very constipated. When I had intercourse I started to have bad pain. If I lay down, I would have pain. And I started to have much heavier periods.

"My doctor said he would try to get the fibroids out without removing the uterus and ovaries. I remember thinking, What if it's cancer? I was very scared. I'm still in my forties; I might still want to have a child. But I was just so uncomfortable. If it had to be a hysterectomy, then it had to be.

"After the surgery my doctor told me there were eight fibroids. He described their size as grapefruit, cantaloupe and oranges. He said it was like eight separate surgeries. But he saved my uterus and my ovaries, and I'm very grateful for that."

Diagnosing Fibroids

Most fibroids are discovered during a routine pelvic exam. The uterus will feel enlarged, firm and irregular. *Transvaginal* or *endovaginal ultrasound* may be used to confirm the diagnosis, showing the number of fibroids and their location, says Dr. Goldstein. The ultrasound can also show whether the fibroids are impinging on nearby structures, such as the fallopian tubes.

When fibroids are growing within the uterine cavity, hysteroscopy may be done. The fiber-optic hysteroscope is inserted into the uterine cavity, with the patient under light sedation in a physician's office. The procedure may cause some cramping. A biopsy to check for endometrial hyperplasia can be done at the same time, and *polyps* or small submucous fibroids discovered during the exam can be removed immediately using an instrument called a *hysteroscope-resectoscope*, sometimes requiring only a local anesthetic (see page 49).

Submucous fibroids can also be observed with a special X ray called a *hysterosalpingogram*, in which radiopaque dye is injected into the uterine cavity with a catheter; the dye will silhouette the myomas as well as any blockage of the fallopian tubes.

If the fibroids are confined to the inside of the uterine wall, most gynecologists will simply "watch and wait," unless there is pain or severe bleeding. A woman may be asked to return in three or four months for a repeat ultrasound. "If the fibroid is not growing, the interval between follow-up sonograms can be lengthened to every six to twelve months," says Dr. Goldstein. A rapidly enlarging growth raises the possibility of a rare malignancy called *leiomyosarcoma*. However, less than half of one percent of fibroids actually become malignant.

Fibroids can grow rapidly during pregnancy, causing both acute and chronic pain. If the placenta implants over a submucous fibroid, there can be abnormal bleeding or abnormal fetal growth. Other complications include premature rupture of the membranes, separation of the placenta (*placenta previa*), which can cause hemorrhage, difficult childbirth and postpartum hemorrhage. While pregnant women with fibroids need to be watched more carefully, the vast majority have no complications.

Options for Treating Fibroids

Until fairly recently, a woman with troublesome fibroids frequently ended up having her uterus removed, and sometimes the ovaries as well. But there are now treatment options that make hysterectomy for fibroids a last resort.

"It used to be thought that when a fibroid got bigger than twelve-week gestational size, about the size of a good-size orange, it needed to be removed because the gynecologist could no longer evaluate the ovaries," remarks Dr. Goldstein. "With the use of ultrasound that is no longer an issue. In most cases we can easily follow the health of the patient's ovaries with yearly ultrasound, regardless of the size of the fibroid."

A statement by the American College of Obstetricians and Gynecologists (ACOG) advises that "hysterectomy is a treatment of last resort which should only be performed when conservative treatments have failed and fertility is not a consideration."

Since most fibroids are relatively slow-growing, the first line of treatment may be *no* treatment (especially in the absence of symptoms), with periodic ultrasound monitoring.

If you're taking oral contraceptives, your doctor may either advise going off the pill or prescribe an all-progesterone minipill, *norethindrone* (Micronor, Nor-QD) or *norgestrel* (Ovrette). The minipill suppresses estrogen production and ovulation and may help shrink fibroids. A repeat ultrasound within a couple of cycles will show whether they have shrunk.

Mild pelvic discomfort can be relieved with nonsteroidal anti-inflammatory agents like ibuprofen, and mild anemia from heavy bleeding can be treated with iron supplements. "If excessive uterine bleeding results in an anemia that iron pills can't correct, if bleeding is so severe that transfusion becomes an issue, if symptoms are interfering with a woman's quality of life or she wants to become pregnant, then we proceed to other treatments," says Dr. Goldstein. Those treatments depend on a woman's age, how bad her symptoms are and whether she wants to have children. Size alone does not usually dictate treatment unless the fibroid is unusually large or causing severe symptoms.

HORMONAL THERAPY to block estrogen production and shrink fibroids may be the next step for women who want to avoid surgery and preserve their fertility. The hormone produced by the hypothalamus that stimulates estrogen production is gonadotropin-releasing hormone (GnRH). More potent synthetic versions of GnRH interfere with its action and are called GnRH agonists.

The GnRH agonist leuprolide acetate (Lupron), injected once a month, reduces estrogen production to postmenopausal levels. As a result, the blood vessels that supply the fibroid shrink and the size of the fibroid is reduced, sometimes up to 50 to 60 percent within three or four months. Around 95 percent of women show a reduction in fibroid size with leuprolide.

However, fibroids can start growing again once the drug is stopped. Moreover, women on leuprolide often experience such menopausal symptoms as hot flashes, vaginal dryness, decreased sex drive, mood swings and fatigue. Particularly worrisome is the accelerated bone loss caused by lack of estrogen. In one study of women in their forties treated for six months with GnRH agonists to shrink fibroids, bone density in the hip continued to decline after treatment ended. Some women taking GnRH agonists may need to have additional therapy to stem bone loss, such as the newly approved drug *alendronate* (Fosamax), or "add-back" therapy of very low doses of estrogen.

Leuprolide may be used to shrink large fibroids so they can be removed more easily by surgery. In women suffering recurrent miscarriages or infertility, GnRH agonists can be used to shrink fibroids so minimal surgery can be used to spare the uterus.

Danazol (Danocrine), a derivative of the male hormone testosterone, also suppresses normal ovarian-pituitary signaling to decrease estrogen production and induce a temporary, simulated menopause. Danazol is given in tablet form. Because it's a synthetic version of testosterone, danazol has *androgenic* side effects, such as acne, deepening of the voice and hair growth, especially on the face, and adverse effects on cholesterol. The drugs cost an average of $400 to $500 a month, with the average treatment lasting between three and six months.

In the future a more potent, synthetic version of the natural hormone known as *LHRH (luteinizing hormone-releasing hormone)* may be used to shrink fibroids. The anti-progesterone agent *mifepristone* (or RU-486) is also being used experimentally.

Once the hormone therapy has reduced the size of the fibroids, they may be removed in a number of ways.

RESECTOSCOPIC ELECTROCOAGULATION using a hysteroscope-resectoscope may be an option for some women with very small submucous fibroids causing bleeding. The resectoscope is an electrical device that, in this case, is fitted with a cutting tip or a wire loop. It is inserted vaginally via a hysteroscope to shave down a part of the endometrium and cut down (or cut out) the fibroid. The procedure takes about thirty minutes under general anesthesia. Recuperation involves a day or two of bed rest.

Since it does not cause total scarring of the endometrium, a woman can later have a child. However, resectoscopic electrocoagulation doesn't always destroy the entire fibroid or the blood supply that feeds it, so the fibroid may recur.

LAPAROSCOPIC MYOMA COAGULATION (MYOLYSIS) is a new technique that uses either a laser fiber or twin electrocautery needles (*bipolar needles*) guided by laparoscopy to destroy the blood supply within the fibroid. This shrinks the growths and prevents recurrence, explains NYU's Dr. Herbert Goldfarb, author of *The No-Hysterectomy Option* (Wiley), who helped develop the technique.

A small incision is made in the abdomen for the laparoscope and a tiny TV camera attachment provides a picture of the pelvic cavity. Through another incision, a laser fiber or bipolar needles repeatedly pierce the fibroid in a circular pattern destroying it and the tiny blood vessels within the myoma. The remaining tissue atrophies, shrinking the growth an average of 80 percent with no further treatment. The procedure can be done on an outpatient basis (the woman remains for four hours to recover fully from the anesthesia). Complete recovery takes four or five days.

The procedure is not for women who want to have children, stresses Dr. Goldfarb, because it can weaken the muscle of the uterine wall and theoretically cause it to rupture under the pressure of pregnancy. Myoma coagulation is still experimental and is not yet in widespread use.

UTERINE ARTERY EMBOLIZATION is another experimental fibroid treatment being tested. In embolization a small catheter is inserted in an artery in the groin area and threaded through to the uterine arteries. Small plastic particles are then injected into the artery supplying a fibroid until blood flow is blocked. The procedure is done on an outpatient basis, under special X-ray guidance, using local anesthesia and sedation.

A preliminary study in 1996 of ten women at the University of California, Los Angeles Medical Center found most of them had significant improvement in their bleeding and pain after eight months of follow-up. Fibroids were reduced in size an average of 60 percent.

CRYOTHERAPY is also being tested for treating fibroids. A liquid nitrogen probe is inserted into the fibroid, freezing it from the center outward, forming an ice ball and killing the abnormal tissue (which would then shrink away). Cryotherapy is being combined with *magnetic resonance imaging* (*MRI*) to monitor the formation of the ice ball so as not to damage healthy tissue.

∞ *E l i s s a ' s   S t o r y ,   C o n t ' d* ∞

"I was in a tremendous amount of pain after the surgery. My doctor explained that although I had a small 'bikini cut' on the outside of the

abdomen, there was a big incision in the inner layer, cutting through the muscle, which would take time to heal. They said I'd recover in four to six weeks. But it took much longer. Maybe if I hadn't had to go back to work so soon, it might have been easier.

"More than a year later I can still feel the incision scar pulling inside. It doesn't hurt, but if I work out, I can feel a kind of tightness. It took a year for me to start exercising again. I still have a slightly swollen stomach, but swimming has helped tremendously. I'm up to about a half mile every day now, and I started unable to do a lap."

When Fibroid Surgery Is Needed

MYOMECTOMY, removal of the fibroid, by either abdominal surgery or hysteroscopic methods, is recommended for larger fibroids of all three types. Myomectomy preserves the uterus and, for many women, their ability to bear children. "In some cases the fibroids are severe enough to prevent a woman from conceiving, or they have had miscarriages because of fibroids," says Dr. Goldfarb. "These women may be candidates for myomectomy."

However, these women may need special follow-up care. They can develop significant *adhesions*, inflammatory bands of fibrous tissue that stick to the incision sites on the uterus and impair reproductive functioning. A follow-up laparoscopy two weeks after surgery can disconnect the adhesions. Further adhesions may still form, but they may be less significant. Many women who undergo myomectomy may require a scheduled cesarean sections to prevent uterine rupture at the internal incision site during labor.

Abdominal myomectomy is done for larger intramural or subserosal fibroids. It is often performed through a "bikini" incision in the lower abdomen (although the site and size of the incision can vary). There's at least a three-day hospitalization. Full recovery may take four to six weeks.

Vaginal myomectomy can be done for small submucous fibroids and those growing into the uterine cavity on stalks. The day before the surgery one or more small rods of *laminaria* (dried, compressed seaweed) are inserted into the cervix (this may cause some cramping). The laminarias readily absorb secretions and slowly swell to four times their original diameter to gently dilate the cervix overnight. The next day the laminarias are removed and instruments are inserted through a resectoscope into the uterus to remove the fibroids. "This approach causes less bleeding than abdominal surgery, and since it's an outpatient procedure, a woman can be back to work in a couple of days," explains Dr. Goldfarb.

There is a key drawback to myomectomy: Fibroids can recur. Some studies show about 25 percent of myomectomy patients have recurrences and go on to have a hysterectomy within five years. However, a skilled surgeon may be able to remove tiny "seedling" fibroids, preventing them from growing later on. Some women may opt for hysterectomy instead of repeat myomectomies, especially if symptoms are severe (see pages 58–60).

▪ Adenomyosis ▪

Adenomyosis occurs when endometrial tissue lining the uterus invades the muscle wall. It is often referred to as *internal endometriosis* because of the presence of endometrial tissue in an abnormal location. In this case both endometrial tissue and its secretory glands are present; that is why the condition is called adenomyosis (*adeno* meaning "gland"). (For more on endometriosis, see Chapter Five.)

"During menses there is cyclic bleeding inside these small islands of trapped endometrium in the muscle of the uterus, often producing an inflammatory response from the body. Women with adenomyosis usually have pelvic pain and heavy menstrual bleeding," says Dr. Robert Barbieri, chief of OB/GYN at Harvard Medical School and Brigham and Women's Hospital in Boston. A common symptom is a chronic feeling of fullness or pressure; some women experience severe pain with deep penetration during sexual intercourse. But many women with adenomyosis have no symptoms. It may occur in 6 to 8 percent of women forty to fifty years old.

Because of its symptoms, adenomyosis may be mistaken for fibroids. Unlike fibroids, however, the uterus does not become greatly enlarged, notes Dr. Barbieri. The misplaced endometrial tissue leads to slight enlargement of uterine muscle fibers, causing the uterus to become spongy and tender.

Although the uterine enlargement can be felt during a pelvic exam, the condition is often discovered *after* the uterus has been removed for other reasons. Unlike fibroids, adenomyosis is hard to diagnose with ultrasound. Some research is being conducted on ultrasound-guided needle biopsy for diagnosing adenomyosis.

Many women with adenomyosis get relief of symptoms with endometrial ablation, using a roller ball or loop device to remove a deeper layer of cells.

"But if the pain and bleeding are severe, a hysterectomy is the only treatment that will eliminate them," says Dr. Barbieri.

∞ *M i l d r e d ' s   S t o r y* ∞

"I never expected something like this would happen to my privates. You simply do not think one of your organs can fall out. I'm sixty-three. My husband and I have six children and four grandchildren. I had been having some urinary incontinence for a while. My gynecologist said it was not unusual at my age. I went through the change ten years ago, but I didn't like the hormones. I didn't want to bleed anymore, so I stopped taking the pills after a year or so. But the urine leakage had gotten pretty bad, and I had to wear pads again. . . .

"I began feeling this pressure in my vagina. I could feel a weight there, like I had something stuck inside me. Finally I could feel something pro-truding. My doctor said immediately it was prolapse. I was surprised. I thought that only happened to very old ladies. But my doctor said it can happen to women who have large families like I did. He said the muscles in my vagina just gave out . . . but they could be repaired.

"My doctor said I should have a hysterectomy, that it would be easier to make the repairs. He took my ovaries out too, since I had been through menopause. I felt a hundred percent better after the surgery, like a weight had been taken out. He said he tightened up all the muscles in the vagina, and around the bottom of the bladder, so that my incontinence would be better too.

"The first few days after the surgery I was in a lot of discomfort. It's like having a new life. I don't need those uncomfortable incontinence pads. My youngest daughter even went and bought me some fancy underwear! I can do everything now better than before. I have even gone back to my bowling league, which I had to drop out of because the prolapse made it very uncomfortable. I am good as new, maybe better."

▪ Uterine Prolapse ▪

In uterine prolapse the pelvic muscles and ligaments weaken and stretch, losing their ability to support the uterus and the vagina. These structures begin to sag, and the uterus slips down into the vagina, which may invert, turning itself inside out. Uterine prolapse is more common after menopause, especially in women who have had several children, and can interfere with the normal functioning of the vagina, bladder, colon and rectum.

The principal damage usually occurs during labor, as the baby's head pushes against the *levator ani* (muscles surrounding the vagina, uterus and rectum) and other pelvic muscles and ligaments. These tissues may not return to their prepregnancy state, and with each new vaginal delivery, more damage occurs. In some cases the sphincter muscles around the bladder neck weaken, causing urine leakage (see Chapter Seven). Some women have also laxity in the anal sphincter, causing mild fecal incontinence.

"In rare instances prolapse can occur in women who have never been pregnant, suggesting that a structural or constitutional abnormality or even genetics may also play a role," says Robert F. Porges, M.D., professor and vice chairman of OB/GYN and director of the Division of Pelvic Reconstructive Surgery at NYU Medical Center. Uterine prolapse is uncommon among black women. Pelvic support defects are more common among women who have *hyperelastosis,* a condition in which the joints are abnormally flexible, he notes.

Loss of muscle tone can be felt during a pelvic exam when a woman is asked to tighten the pelvic floor muscles around the physician's examining fingers and is unable to do so. "However, this may not be part of a routine pelvic exam. So the initial damage that occurs during childbirth may not be recognized until years later, when a woman has begun to experience symptoms," says Dr. Porges. "Early symptoms may include a vague discomfort in the vagina, a sense of pelvic fullness or pressure. A woman may have low back pain aggravated by walking, being in an erect position. There may also be a change in the sensations during intercourse."

Anything that increases pressure in the abdomen and on the pelvic organs can worsen prolapse, adds Dr. Porges. This includes weight gain, chronic constipation with straining, lifting heavy objects, regular high-intensity exercise and even chronic coughing (such as cough caused by smoking and asthma). There may also be irritation of prolapsed vaginal tissues by underwear or clothing, which may cause bleeding from the genital area. Sometimes bleeding rather than pressure prompts a visit to the doctor.

A woman may also experience changes in bowel and bladder function— that is, a sense of incomplete voiding or constipation—and occasional *stress incontinence,* leakage of urine when pressure increases on the abdomen during a cough or a sneeze (see Chapter Seven). As the bladder's position distorts, it may become difficult to empty it completely. Bacteria multiply in stagnant urine, causing urinary tract infections, or there can be asymptomatic *bacteriuria*, bacteria in the urine without signs of infection (more common in older women and during pregnancy).

Prolapse becomes more noticeable after menopause, when lack of estrogen thins tissues and further weakens the supporting muscles. Incontinence may also worsen. There may be a physical sensation of something dropping down or pressing into the vagina when a woman is standing. The uterus may noticeably descend, sometimes even protrude from the vagina itself.

A woman may see a temporary improvement in urinary incontinence, but what's really happening is that urine is trapped in a pouch formed as the bladder descends, called a *cystocele*. Or feces in the rectum become trapped by sagging muscle tissue, a condition known as *rectocele*, making it difficult to empty the bowel. A common sign is having to insert a finger into the vagina to press down on the rectum in order to void completely. In women who have had hysterectomies, the vaginal vault can prolapse. Occasionally intestinal contents herniate into the vagina in a pouch called an *enterocele*. In each case there may be tissue protruding from the vagina.

Treating Uterine Prolapse

As many as 40 to 50 percent of postmenopausal women have some degree of prolapse, but only 10 to 15 percent have noticeable symptoms. Mild prolapse symptoms usually require no treatment, but as the condition progresses, hormones, support devices or surgery may be needed.

In the early stages women may be able to prevent prolapse from progressing by losing weight, quitting smoking (to relieve a chronic cough) and using fiber supplements to avoid constipation. Estrogen replacement therapy (ERT) and the use of estrogen cream can help prevent further thinning of tissues and improve pelvic muscle tone, but hormones can't reverse muscle damage.

Pelvic floor exercises, known as *Kegel exercises*, can help strengthen pelvic muscles to manage minor prolapse and control mild urinary incontinence. But they may be useful only if a woman learns to engage the proper muscles and performs the exercises regularly (for instructions, see page 137). They will *not* help when the muscle has been so damaged that it cannot be voluntarily contracted sufficiently to interrupt the urinary stream during urination, stresses Dr. Porges.

Support devices called *pessaries* may make some women more comfortable. Similar to a diaphragm, but more rigid, a pessary is inserted into the

Fig. 9: USE OF PESSARY FOR PROLAPSE

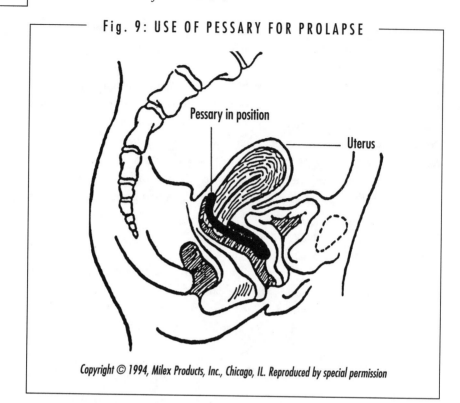

Pessary in position

Uterus

Copyright © 1994, Milex Products, Inc., Chicago, IL. Reproduced by special permission

vagina to hold sagging pelvic structures in place. Pessaries sit beneath the pubic bone and the back of the vagina. They come in various sizes and shapes and are fitted like a diaphragm. The largest size possible must be used to reduce the chances it will slip out of the vagina. Pessaries must be removed every ten to twelve hours for cleaning with soap and water.

Most women can learn how to insert and remove a pessary. In some cases it can cause abrasions when inserted or irritate the vaginal lining, leading to infection. Women may use estrogen cream or protective creams (such as Trimo-San Jel) to help prevent irritation and make it easier to insert pessaries.

Pessaries may be especially helpful in elderly women who have other medical conditions that make them poor candidates for surgery or in women who wish to avoid surgery. Special pessaries are used to minimize stress incontinence (see Chapter Seven).

"Pessaries can be useful in women who are pregnant, who may experience some protrusion of the cervix or bladder and cannot undergo surgery," says Dr. Porges. "They are useful sometimes in women who have had a longstanding protrusion which develops an ulceration. Use of the pessary for three weeks can allow the ulceration to heal prior to surgery."

The only cure for prolapse is reconstructive surgery. Surgical procedures generally involve trimming stretched, sagging tissues, muscles and ligaments and stitching the tightened areas into place. This can be done abdominally or vaginally. Urinary incontinence can also be remedied during the procedure. Hysterectomy may be done as part of the repair process.

One surgical procedure, *sacrospinous fixation*, pulls back prolapsed vaginal tissues into their proper place using sutures attached to the *sacrospinous ligaments*, which stretch from protrusions (*ischial spine*) on each side of the rear pelvic bone to the sacrum, the triangular bone at the base of the spine. This secures the vagina and draws back the *genital hiatus*, the opening in the *levator muscle* surrounding the vagina. The levator muscle and vaginal tissues are trimmed and tightened; repairs may also be done to the bladder or rectum. "The procedure differs with each patient, depending on the nature of the prolapse," says Dr. Porges, one of the country's pioneering gynecologic surgeons. "If the uterus is not removed, it can also be drawn back and fixed in place by attaching it to the sacrospinous ligaments.

"In younger women who still wish to become pregnant, one can repair only the front and back walls of the vagina. Sometimes it is necessary to remove a small portion of the uterine neck. In this case a woman would likely deliver by cesarean section to avoid strain on the uterus and the repaired structures," he adds.

After vaginal surgery most women leave the hospital in a couple of days and resume normal activities in three or four weeks. With abdominal surgery the hospital stay and recovery are longer. During recovery a woman should avoid heavy lifting or straining.

In 5 to 10 percent of women prolapse can recur, especially if the connective tissue atrophies or a new pelvic defect develops, and repeat surgery may be needed.

Nonsurgical interventions are now being tested. "The cutting edge of new research in this area involves electrical stimulation of pelvic floor muscles. This involves the use of vaginal stents where, perhaps for fifteen minutes a day, you stimulate and regenerate the muscle fibers, eventually restoring the normal reflexes," says Dr. Porges. "If electrostimulation is done before prolapse becomes extensive, it may enable some women to undergo less extensive procedures or avoid surgery altogether."

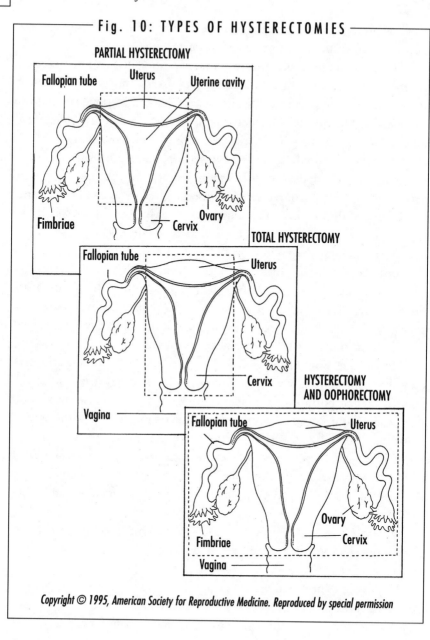

Fig. 10: TYPES OF HYSTERECTOMIES

PARTIAL HYSTERECTOMY

Fallopian tube

Uterus

Uterine cavity

Fimbriae

Cervix

Ovary

TOTAL HYSTERECTOMY

Fallopian tube

Uterus

Cervix

Vagina

HYSTERECTOMY AND OOPHORECTOMY

Fallopian tube

Uterus

Ovary

Cervix

Fimbriae

Vagina

▪ Hysterectomy ▪

There are several types of hysterectomy. In a *total hysterectomy* the uterus and the cervix are removed; in some cases both ovaries are also removed (*total hysterectomy with bilateral oophorectomy*). In a *subtotal,* or partial, hysterectomy, only the top (*fundus*) of the uterus is removed and the cervix is left intact, but the endocervical canal inside the cervix is destroyed or removed. In a radical hysterectomy, the uterus, both ovaries, the fallopian tubes and surrounding connective tissue are removed (*hysterectomy with bilateral salpingo-oophorectomy*).

When the ovaries are removed from a woman who still has periods, it produces a surgical menopause (see page 61). Depending on the woman's age, the degree of menopausal symptoms and her risk factors for heart disease, breast cancer and osteoporosis, she may or may not need treatment with replacement estrogen. Around half the women undergoing the surgery have a total hysterectomy with bilateral oophorectomy, with the highest rates in women older than forty-five, when the risk of ovarian cancer increases and estrogen production by the ovaries is declining.

A total hysterectomy can be done through an abdominal or a vaginal incision. An abdominal incision requires either a four- to six-inch bikini-cut incision near the pubic hairline or, less commonly, a vertical incision; vaginal hysterectomy is done through an incision in the wall of the vagina. Abdominal surgery requires a three- to four-day hospital stay, versus two days for a vaginal hysterectomy. The vaginal approach leaves no external scar, a quicker recovery and fewer complications. Some surgeons are using laparoscopy to assist in vaginal hysterectomy, but a recent study shows there's no major benefit (and the costs are higher).

Hysterectomies for prolapse are best done vaginally to allow for better reconstructive surgery. "Abdominal hysterectomy should be done only if there's a very large fibroid, if there's a malignancy or if one needs to do other things in the pelvic cavity," says Dr. Porges.

For women past menopause, removing the ovaries along with the uterus removes the risk of ovarian cancer, which rises after age forty-five. Younger women with family histories of ovarian cancer who need hysterectomy may opt for oophorectomy. "The risk of ovarian cancer is actually very small, a 1.6 percent lifetime risk. So I would not automatically say that a woman within five years of menopause must have her ovaries removed," comments gynecologic oncologist Joanna M. Cain, M.D., chairman, Department of Obstetrics and Gynecology at the Pennsylvania State University School of Medicine and the Milton S. Hershey Medical Center. (The reported incidence of cancer in ovaries retained after hysterectomy ranges from 1 to 14 percent.)

In cases of severe endometriosis, removing the ovaries takes away the estrogen that might stimulate microscopic endometrial growths. But there's no *medical* reason to remove the ovaries in a woman in her early forties who has fibroids and may be years away from menopause, according to Dr. Cain.

While removing the uterus is necessary in endometrial cancer, "radical hysterectomy may not always be needed in women with early-stage invasive cervical cancers that are not aggressive. In some cases the ovaries can be left in place since there is a low risk of spread to the ovaries, However, careful staging of the cancer is extremely important," Dr. Cain notes.

A woman who has had premalignancies of the cervix or abnormal Pap smears would *not* be a candidate for a subtotal hysterectomy, since her risk for cervical cancer may be greater. On the other hand, a woman with consistently normal Pap smears, who is in a monogamous relationship and is at lower risk for sexually transmitted diseases (including *human papilloma virus, HPV,* which is linked to cervical cancer) could retain her cervix, says Dr. Porges. However, she would still need Pap smears, as would women who have had total hysterectomies and have had abnormal Pap smears or cervical premalignancies in the past.

Opinions are divided on whether a subtotal hysterectomy is more beneficial than a total hysterectomy. Some experts believe that retaining the cervix helps maintain the support system and nerves in the vaginal vault, which may enhance sexual functioning.

Is hysterectomy more effective than *non*surgical treatments for fibroids, endometriosis or abnormal bleeding? A 1994 conference held by the Agency for Health Care Policy and Research (AHCPR) surprisingly concluded that "evidence regarding the effectiveness of hysterectomy and alternative treatments is seriously lacking." The conferees called for more studies comparing hysterectomy with "watchful waiting" and for studies comparing different treatment strategies with follow-ups of at least two years. One federally funded study is following 1,000 Maryland women, to compare the outcomes and costs of vaginal versus abdominal hysterectomy (with or without oophorectomy).

How You May Feel After Hysterectomy

Complications from hysterectomy are rare, but they include hemorrhage, injury to the bladder and ureters, the bowel, nerves and other structures as well as infections and *vaginal vault prolapse.* Postoperative problems include pain, abdominal gas, nausea or fatigue. Mortality is low: approximately twenty deaths per ten thousand hysterectomies for women without cancer.

While a hysterectomy typically requires only a day or two in the hospital, it can take up to six weeks for full recovery. The Maine Women's Health study, the largest prospective clinical study of quality of life among hysterectomy patients, found that women experienced two weeks of pain and about twenty-one days of fatigue after their surgery. A small percentage of the women reported new problems with urinating or constipation after their surgery.

After hysterectomy, menstrual periods and fertility cease. However, if the ovaries were not removed, they continue to secrete estrogen and progesterone, producing some of the same premenstrual symptoms as before surgery, such as breast tenderness, water retention and irritability. But studies suggest that ovarian failure may occur an average of four years earlier in women who've had their uteri removed. (It may be that the uterus is involved with ovarian hormone secretion or that surgery lessens blood supply to the ovaries, shortening their life span.)

Removal of the ovaries causes a surgical menopause, and the onset of symptoms is severe and sudden, explains Gloria A. Bachmann, M.D., professor and chief of the Division of Obstetrics and Gynecology at the University of Medicine and Dentistry of New Jersey, Robert Wood Johnson Medical School. "In a natural menopause symptoms may start out being subtle, increasing and becoming more severe over a period of months or years. But in surgical menopause the onset is acute. Many women are not prepared for the sudden and severe symptoms."

In addition to severe hot flashes, women experience night sweats, vaginal dryness and discomfort. Androgen deficiency causes low energy, insomnia and decreased libido.

Surgical menopause may have more adverse effects on cardiac health than does natural menopause. A recent study of 1,150 hysterectomized women found that those women who had had their ovaries removed had a greater risk for heart disease than those who went through natural menopauses. The 1995 study, from the University of California, San Diego (UCSD), found that among women more than twenty years after menopause, those who had their ovaries removed had higher total cholesterol, more "bad" *low-density lipoprotein* (LDL) cholesterol and higher insulin resistance and blood pressure than naturally menopausal women. Donna Kritz-Silverstein, Ph.D., a coinvestigator in the study and an assistant adjunct professor of family and preventive medicine at USCD, noted that oophorectomy is often recommended to eliminate the risk of ovarian cancer, but that is far less than the risk of heart disease and should be weighed carefully in deciding whether to remove the ovaries.

If a woman chooses estrogen replacement therapy, in either pill or patch form, it should begin immediately after surgery to avoid acute menopausal symptoms (see page 245).

∞ *N a y i d a ' s   S t o r y* ∞

"I was a very sexual woman before my hysterectomy, and it changed nothing. I never for a moment thought that I would be 'less of a woman' after the surgery. For me, sex definitely got better afterward. I wasn't afraid of getting pregnant, I didn't have to worry about the bleeding, and the pain that I sometimes had was gone. I have the same sensations during orgasm.

"I was getting so close to menopause that my symptoms were not that bad after removal of my ovaries, so I chose not to take estrogen. There's no history of heart attacks or osteoporosis in my family. I just didn't want to bother with it."

∞ *C a r o l y n ' s   S t o r y* ∞

"To me, a hysterectomy is castration. I did not want to have my ovaries out. I pleaded with him [the doctor] about it, but he argued that there would be less of a risk of cancer later on and that it would not affect my sex life. So I did it, and now I'm sorry. The best way I can describe what I feel is that it's like going from a wide-screen Technicolor movie to a tiny black-and-white TV. Something is definitely missing. Maybe the nerves were cut, or I felt my orgasms in my uterus. Who knows?

"I am now taking hormones, and though the hot flashes are gone, that hasn't put back the zing. I still have orgasms, but they peak more quickly, and they are much less intense. I feel my vagina is shorter, and sometimes, when we are really into it, I feel as if something is tearing or pulling. I also have a decrease in desire, which is not doing my marriage any good.

"All the literature he [the doctor] gave me to read said after a hysterectomy everything should be fine with sex, that some women even had better sex lives. I'd like to meet them. I think many doctors must believe it's all in our heads. At least they are honest with men getting prostate surgery, that they may become impotent. I feel my doctor didn't know or didn't care."

Hysterectomy and Sexuality

A temporary halt to sexual activity is required during the initial six-week recovery period after hysterectomy. Even after that, however, women may feel easily bruised, and in some cases it may be a few months before sex is completely enjoyable.

Many women like Nayida say sex is much better after hysterectomy since it eliminates the pain and heavy bleeding caused by fibroids. Lubricants can help vaginal dryness if a woman chooses not to take estrogen. However, some women like Carolyn complain of diminished sensation during orgasm after removal of the uterus or lowered libido after oophorectomy. Some experts say there are women who experience orgasms not only from clitoral stimulation but also from pressure on the cervix and uterine contractions, and for those women hysterectomy may have a negative effect on sexual functioning. Some experts believe that removing the cervix may destroy some nerve function in the pelvic floor, and that may have an effect on orgasm. Sexual dysfunction after hysterectomy may also be due to anatomic shortening of the vagina. Subtotal hysterectomy may help prevent such problems.

However, studies of hysterectomy here and in Sweden report that most women find their sex lives were better or did not change. The Maine Women's Health Study compared almost 800 Maine women ages twenty-five to fifty who had either elective hysterectomy or nonsurgical treatment for such nonmalignant conditions as fibroids. The study, published in 1994 in *Obstetrics and Gynecology,* found that only 7 percent of the women who chose hysterectomy reported having less interest in sex after hysterectomy, and only 1 percent found sex less enjoyable.

Resuming a normal sex life can play a role in recovery, in part because intercourse helps vaginal tissue to stretch. More important, experts say, it provides a psychological boost. Removing the possibility of pregnancy may increase spontaneity, frequency and enjoyment.

In fact, many women report a definite boost in their overall quality of life after hysterectomy. The Maine Women's Health Study found a majority of the hysterectomy patients (especially those with severe symptoms) believed they had benefited from the surgery. Of the 418 women who chose to have hysterectomy, most reported significant relief of pelvic and back pain, *dyspareunia* (painful intercourse), abdominal swelling, urinary symptoms and fatigue one year after the surgery. Small percentages of women reported new problems at six and twelve months, including weight gain, hot flashes and feeling depressed or anxious or negative about oneself as a woman.

Results in the Maine study were more mixed for the 380 women who chose nonsurgical therapies over hysterectomy. One quarter of the women with abnormal bleeding were still bothered by the problem a year later, and half of those with chronic pelvic pain still had pain. As a result, 25 percent of this group chose to have hysterectomies later on.

Lead researcher Karen Carlson, M.D., director of Women's Health at Massachusetts General Hospital and a clinical instructor of medicine at Harvard Medical School, stresses that the study does not suggest that hysterectomy should be the preferred treatment, only that it can be an effective option, and that patient preference should be a major deciding factor.

A major factor in quality of life after hysterectomy is having as much information beforehand on the psychological impact and the physical changes they can expect, according to Dr. Bachmann. "Not only do some women feel that the uterus is a major sexual aspect of their being, but there is a sense of finality about the cessation of fertility that some women need to deal with."

A 1995 national survey of 400 surgical menopause patients, sponsored by the National Women's Health Resource Center and the Ciba Pharmaceutical company (which manufactures the estrogen patch Estraderm), found many women did not think they had been adequately informed about the surgery or about the sudden menopausal symptoms afterward. Still, the vast majority said they were "very satisfied" with the outcome.

However, most hysterectomy studies have looked at outcomes and quality of life only at six months and a year after the surgery. It's not clear what effects the passage of time may have. New research should provide a more complete picture.

The Hysterectomy Controversy

There has been a decline in the number of hysterectomies since the peak year of 1975, with 725,000 surgeries, to the current level of about 530,000 hysterectomies a year.

Hysterectomy remains the second most common surgical procedure in the United States behind cesarean sections, with a majority performed on women age thirty to fifty-four. By age sixty-five almost 40 percent of women will have had their uteri removed (90 percent of the time for *noncancerous* conditions). In Sweden, the rate is 17 percent; in Britain it's 20 percent.

"We will not see dramatic drops in the hysterectomy rate because of the aging of the population," observes Dr. Bachmann. "Large numbers of women are reaching an age where they're more likely to have problems that lead to hysterectomy."

Federal health statistics show that fibroids lead to approximately one third of all hysterectomies, with endometriosis accounting for 18 percent of the total. Prolapse accounts for 16 percent of hysterectomies, while dysfunctional uterine bleeding is the primary diagnosis for 5 percent of women who undergo hysterectomy (and a secondary diagnosis for a much larger group). Cancer is involved in 11 percent of hysterectomies, and the remaining 10 percent are performed because of chronic infections, ovarian disease and pregnancy-related disorders.

There is considerable clinical and political debate about the possible overuse of hysterectomy. For example, a 1993 Rand Corporation survey found that 41 percent of hysterectomies in seven large health maintenance organizations (HMOs) weren't needed or were questionable. Dr. Goldfarb and others go even further, contending that *half* of all hysterectomies done in this country are avoidable.

There are also wide and unexplained variations in rates of hysterectomy between different parts of the U.S., and among different ages and racial groups. Recent data show that women living in the South are nearly *twice* as likely as women in the Northeast to undergo hysterectomies. Another study, in the journal *Obstetrics and Gynecology,* found that African-American women were 25 percent more likely than white women to have hysterectomies. The study of 53,000 patients showed that black women were also younger than white women at the time of surgery (forty-two years versus forty-six years) and were more apt to have abdominal rather than vaginal surgery. The study also reported that black women were twice as likely to have hysterectomies for fibroids, while white women were more likely to undergo the procedure for prolapse, endometriosis, cancer or menstrual disorders.

Hysterectomy rates have also been correlated with nonclinical factors, such as socioeconomic status. One study found women twenty-five to fifty-four years of age who had not completed high school had twice the rate of hysterectomy of women who had graduated from college. Women with annual household incomes of less than $10,000 had the highest hysterectomy rate.

Another recent study suggests that women who see male gynecologists are more likely to have hysterectomies than those treated by female doctors. According to the 1994 report in the *American Journal of Public Health (AJPH),* male gynecologists are 60 percent more likely than their female counterparts to choose hysterectomy to treat dysplasia and bleeding or painful fibroids.

One possible explanation may be that male physicians in the study tended to be older and had completed their medical training at a time when attitudes toward hysterectomy were different. "Some physicians are still fixated in the fifties, in the old thinking and the old techniques. Many are not up to speed with new treatments and new technology," asserts Dr. Goldfarb. "They see a woman in her forties with heavy bleeding or fibroids, she's had her kids, and they say, 'What does she need her uterus for?' "

The *AJPH* study found that recently trained doctors had lower hysterectomy rates, regardless of their sex. These physicians tended to believe that medication may be better than surgery and that a uterus contributes to a woman's sexual functioning. "In my experience the sex of the gynecologist is not a major factor. If there is an indication for a hysterectomy, a woman gynecologist will be just as likely to recommend hysterectomy as a man," counters Dr. Robert Porges. "Younger doctors also tend to see younger patients, who may be more easily treated with medication and are less likely to need hysterectomies. Older physicians tend to have older patients, women who have been with him or her since they had their first child. And a sixty-year-old woman is more likely to be a candidate for a hysterectomy than a thirty-year-old."

Experts do agree that a woman should always seek a second, or even third, opinion before proceeding with a hysterectomy. "If after careful consideration of all her options, a woman *chooses* to have a hysterectomy, she should not feel as if she has somehow compromised herself or her femininity," says Dr. Steven Goldstein. "No one can dictate what's best for you. While hysterectomy is the last option in most cases, there are times when it can dramatically change a woman's life for the better."

chapter 4

Ovarian Cysts and Other Disorders

For such important organs the ovaries are surprisingly small. In premenopausal women the ovaries normally measure less than an inch in diameter and under two inches in length, and weigh a quarter of an ounce each. Within a space the size of a large unshelled almond, there are tens of thousands of egg-producing follicles and cells that pump out female hormones and small amounts of androgens. The ovaries can be felt during a pelvic exam and can be clearly seen on ultrasound, right down to which follicle has ovulated!

Problems may arise from disruptions in the hormonal feedback loop between the ovaries and the brain that controls ovulation. In up to 10 percent of women, several follicles may be stimulated each month but none ovulate, leading to irregular periods and excessive male hormone production, a condition called polycystic ovarian syndrome. In 1 percent of women the ovaries shut down prematurely. More than 571,000 women are hospitalized each year for treatment of benign cysts and growths. Countless others are diagnosed with functional ovarian cysts.

▪ Ovarian Cysts ▪
Functional Ovarian Cysts

Actually the very *function* of the ovary is "cystic." That is, the follicle that develops in response to a hormonal signal each month becomes a little sac filled with fluid, which collapses after an egg is released. The word *cyst* simply means "fluid-filled," according to Dr. Steven Goldstein, director of gynecologic ultrasound at NYU Medical Center. "Every month in an ovulating woman the dominant follicle enlarges to about two and a half centimeters, about the size of a ripe cherry, and protrudes from the surface of the ovary. When you look at this follicle on ultrasound, you see a cyst. But this is nothing to be alarmed about."

During ovulation this cyst erupts and releases an egg in a gush of follicular fluid, propelling it to the fallopian tube. The fluid is absorbed by the body. The shell left by the dominant follicle becomes the corpus luteum, and other follicle cysts that did not mature die away and are resorbed by the ovary.

Sometimes extra fluid becomes trapped in a follicle, or the dominant follicle fails to ovulate and continues to grow, accumulating more fluid and producing excess estrogen. This is called a *follicular cyst*. Occasionally after ovulation, fluid or blood remains in the corpus luteum, or the corpus luteum does not regress but continues to grow, forming a *corpus luteum cyst*. The ovary can enlarge up to three inches in diameter as a result of these functional cysts, cysts that result from normal ovarian function.

An ovarian cyst can cause bleeding and abdominal pain as a result of pressure by it on the ovarian capsule. Women may experience twinges during exercise, intercourse or defecation. But often such cysts produce no symptoms and are felt during a routine pelvic examination and diagnosed with ultrasound.

Functional cysts typically resolve over the course of one or two menstrual cycles, stresses Dr. Goldstein. "Depending on its size and appearance, follow-up ultrasound examination is almost always indicated. But the vast majority of these cysts will go away by themselves, with no intervention whatsoever," he says.

Sometimes fluid-filled cysts can rupture, causing pain and bleeding into the pelvic cavity. The source of the bleeding can be diagnosed through laparoscopy, and surgery may be needed to repair the ovary. Birth control pills, which suppress ovulation, may help prevent cysts in some women.

In postmenopausal women the ovary is no longer functioning and should be shrunken and *atrophic*, says Dr. Goldstein. Studies indicate that between 10 and 17 percent of postmenopausal women have small fluid-filled cystic structures in their ovaries, but the overwhelming number of these are totally innocuous. However, an enlarged ovary after menopause is a red flag for possible cancer and should be investigated.

Benign Ovarian Cysts and Tumors

A number of benign cysts and growths can arise in the ovaries, sometimes becoming quite large. They all can cause pelvic pain, pressure and bloating—symptoms also associated with ovarian cancer—and should be checked out immediately. These growths are rarely malignant, but they can cause pelvic inflammation and pain if they rupture or twist the ovary.

Benign cystic teratomas, dermoid cysts may account for up to 25 percent of benign ovarian growths among reproductive-age women. Comprised of different types of tissue originating from *embryonic cells* containing *germ cells* (primitive cells programmed to form various organs and tissues in the fetus, including eggs), "dermoid cysts are freaks of nature. They may actually contain hair, teeth, thyroid tissue, bits of cartilage or even bone," remarks Dr. Goldstein.

Dermoid cysts can be tiny or grow to more than ten centimeters (cm) in size (between two and four inches). They are prone to rupture, and their oily contents can cause severe inflammation in the peritoneum. Only 1 to 2 percent are malignant. (However, much rarer germ cell tumors, including *dysgerminomas, endodermal sinus tumors* and *immature teratomas*, are cancerous.)

Cystadenomas are benign fluid-filled growths that take different forms. *Benign serous cystadenomas* account for between 20 and 25 percent of benign ovarian tumors. They range from five to fifteen centimeters (from under two inches to almost six inches). A subtype called *papillary serous cystadenoma* is potentially malignant. *Mucinous cystadenomas* are filled with a thick, gelatinous fluid (*mucin*) and can grow to enormous size; rare cases of mucinous cystadenomas almost twenty inches in size and weighing two hundred pounds have been reported! Mucinous cystadenomas are very common, occurring most often between the ages of thirty and fifty, usually in one ovary, and may become malignant. *Parovarian cysts* grow within the *broad ligament* that suspends the ovaries within the pelvic cavity.

Non-fluid-filled benign ovarian tumors include *Brenner tumors, fibromas* and *thecomas*. Half the time Brenner tumors are found in postmenopausal women and can range from microscopic to as large as 30 cm (around ten inches). Thecomas can lead to excess male or female hormone production, causing a resumption of periods in postmenopausal women or irregular bleeding in younger women and excess facial hair or acne. Fibromas are commonly found in women over age forty, usually in one ovary.

Ovarian inclusion cysts are benign microscopic cysts found in older women as a result of a folding inward (*invagination*) of the ovary that allows cysts to form inside.

Sertoli-Leydig cell tumors are rare and benign 90 percent of the time, but the cells can become malignant. They are found most often in women age twenty to thirty and often secrete so much androgen that women undergo virilization, including male pattern baldness, acne and growth of facial and chest hair.

∽ R o b i n ' s S t o r y , C o n t ' d ∽

"I was still in my twenties when I decided to try to get pregnant, but nothing happened. When I read that endometriosis was a common cause of infertility, I said, "I bet I have that," since I had always had painful periods. But my gynecologist never mentioned the word. He agreed to do a laparoscopy, but when the time came, he said he could give me a pill to help me get pregnant rather than go through a procedure. The first cycle I took Clomid, I got pregnant. So I figured it wasn't endometriosis, and I forgot about it.

"About three years later we decided to try to have another child. Nothing happened. I figured I would get Clomid again. But my doctor felt an enlarged ovary and sent me for other tests. It looked like there were cysts on my ovaries. One was very large. I was worried it was cancer. I asked how soon I could have surgery. I just wanted it out.

"Looking back, I realize I had been having symptoms: I had lost some weight, but it didn't seem like my pants were any looser, I had felt bloated all the time and, with a three-year-old daughter at home at the time, I felt tired and sluggish. When he did the surgery, it turned out to be a thirteen centimeter endometrioma cyst. I was really amazed: How could I have a thing that BIG in my body and never know it? It was like five inches! He said the ovary was nonfunctional tissue and couldn't be saved. The other cyst he was able to remove and save the ovary. We are hoping to have another child, but it hasn't happened yet."

Endometriomas are ovarian cysts that occur in 50 percent of women with endometriosis (see Chapter Five). In this case the endometrial tissue that flows backward through the fallopian tube during menstruation invades the ovary, producing blood-filled cysts. In time the accumulated blood darkens; an unruptured endometrioma is often called a "chocolate cyst." These cysts can range from pea to grapefruit size. Rupture can cause pain, inflammation in the abdominal cavity and scarring, which may form weblike adhesions on the ovary and the fallopian tube.

Theca lutein cysts are caused by fertility drugs that hyperstimulate the ovaries. They generally go away when the medication is discontinued, but if the ovaries grow very large, the ovaries can move or twist, producing severe pain.

Although a woman's lifetime risk of malignant ovarian tumors is relatively low (about 1.5 percent), they can be deadly. The problem is that such symptoms as abdominal bloating, weight loss and constipation usually appear when the cancer is advanced. But new treatment advances have increased survival. (For more on ovarian cancer, see Chapter Thirteen.)

Diagnosing and Treating Cysts

Most cysts can be felt during a pelvic exam. Functional cysts tend to be smaller than five centimeters (around two inches) and nontender to the touch and can be moved slightly when palpated. Since the ovaries cannot usually be felt after menopause, an enlarged ovary in an older woman can be a worrisome sign.

Transvaginal ultrasound can help distinguish between functional fluid-filled cysts and solid, possibly malignant growths because the fluid in a cyst enhances the ultrasound picture, according to Dr. Goldstein. Magnetic resonance imaging (MRI) can also help identify ovarian malignancies.

In a premenopausal woman a functional cyst (depending on its size and whether there's discomfort) will usually be monitored over one to two menstrual cycles to see if it resolves on its own. If it does not resolve or if it enlarges, further imaging will be done to determine whether laparoscopy or *exploratory laparotomy* (abdominal surgery) should be performed. Rapid growth of a solid cyst in a younger woman accompanied by pain can suggest a germ cell tumor; some germ cell tumors can be malignant.

Women at low suspicion of malignancy may undergo diagnostic laparoscopies; cysts have characteristic appearances and colors that help in the diagnosis. Biopsy is not done for cysts or benign ovarian masses, but the fluid may occasionally be drained from some cysts and analyzed.

Exploratory laparotomy is usually reserved for patients with cysts larger than five centimeters (especially after menopause), in whom there's a high suspicion of malignancy or an increased chance of a rupture or other complication. If ultrasound raises a suspicion of malignancy (such as solid features in a cyst or fluid in the abdomen, called *ascites*), blood tests may be done for tumor "markers," including *CA-125* (which can indicate ovarian cancer or, more often, its recurrence). Testing for this marker is most useful in postmenopausal women, according to Dr. Goldstein.

Dermoid cysts have a high risk of rupture or torsion and must be removed surgically (*cystectomy.*) "In most cases the cyst can be shelled out of the normal ovarian tissue and the ovary reconstructed to preserve normal function," says Dr. Goldstein. Assisted by laparoscopy, the capsule of the ovary is opened and the cyst is removed as if it were a pea in a pod, using a laser or electrocautery to stop the bleeding. The ovary is closed, and a patch made of woven cellulose is wrapped around it to help healing and prevent adhesions (the cellulose is eventually absorbed by the body). All benign cysts can be removed this way.

To prevent possibly malignant cells from being shed when a suspicious cyst is removed, a small plastic Ziploc bag is inserted through a laparoscopic incision, or *port*. The ovary is moved into the bag, the cyst is removed inside it, the ovary is washed and the bag is sealed and withdrawn through the port.

For mucinous cystadenomas, the treatment is usually removal of the ovary or, in a woman over forty, a total hysterectomy with removal of both tubes and ovaries. If this type of cyst ruptures, the spilled cells can stimulate the growth of other mucin-secreting cells, which may form clumps in the peritoneal or abdominal cavity that need to be removed. Radiation therapy or chemotherapy may be given after surgery to kill any remaining cells (even though it's not a cancerous condition).

In cases of Brenner cysts and Sertoli-Leydig tumors, the affected ovary must be removed since these growths have malignant potentials. In most cases hysterectomy with removal of the ovaries and tubes is done. However, since Sertoli-Leydig tumors are more common in women in their twenties and thirties, the single affected ovary and its tube may be removed to preserve fertility.

Some women undergoing removal of an ovary for benign conditions are often advised to have the other ovary taken out to reduce their future chance of ovarian cancer (*prophylactic oophorectomy*). But younger women should carefully weigh the risks of surgical menopause against the benefits of the procedure.

∞ *Sandy's Story* ∞

"I'd been having lower abdominal pains off and on, sort of cramps, for several weeks. I thought it was gas or indigestion or stress. I had just started a new job. I was busy, so I just kept taking ibuprofen and didn't think about it much.

"I was on my way to the office when the pain hit again. This time it was ten times worse, and it was all on one side. It was so bad I was doubled over. I was afraid I had appendicitis. I called my gynecologist. I used her as my primary doctor. She said to meet her at the emergency room right away. I could barely function at this point.

"It turned out that I had two huge ovarian cysts! My gynecologist was afraid one of the cysts was about to rupture, so she made arrangements for surgery that afternoon. I was in the hospital for three days, and it took me a couple of weeks to recover fully once I got home. I went back to work full speed after that, but it took awhile to get back to myself.

"My doctor told me the cysts were dermoid cysts, with hair and teeth, which I thought was really bizarre. I'm just glad they got them out! They didn't have to remove my ovary, which was a great relief, since I want to have children someday."

Ruptured Cysts

Any nonsolid ovarian cyst or growth can rupture, spilling its contents into the peritoneal cavity, causing inflammation. Most cases are mid-cycle ruptures of follicular cysts or ruptures of dermoid cysts. Some cysts, particularly corpus luteum cysts of pregnancy (the corpus luteum, which continues to produce progesterone needed to maintain pregnancy), can also hemorrhage.

As in Sandy's case, a ruptured cyst produces sudden, severe lower abdominal pain, which may begin in one area but will gradually spread. A woman may also have low-grade fever. Since abdominal pain can also occur in torsion (see page 78), appendicitis and ectopic pregnancy as well as kidney or gastrointestinal problems, a diagnostic workup will include blood tests, ultrasound and sometimes a sampling of fluid from the peritoneal cavity.

Ultrasound may reveal a mass and fluid in the *cul-de-sac*, the area behind the uterus. Fluid sampling with *culdocentesis* involves inserting a fine needle through the rear wall of the vagina into the peritoneal cavity and drawing out fluid. Yellowish fluid may indicate a leaking corpus luteum cyst; bloody fluid can signal a ruptured cyst or an ectopic pregnancy (page 206).

A ruptured cyst is usually managed with medication to control the pain of irritation and inflammation, which usually eases within forty-eight hours, as the cyst fluid is absorbed by the body. If pain persists, diagnostic laparoscopy will be performed. Surgery is required only in cases of severe hemorrhage.

■ Polycystic Ovarian Syndrome ■

Polycystic ovarian syndrome (PCOS), also known as *Stein-Leventhal syndrome*, occurs when the ovaries enlarge and produce many small cysts. PCOS may affect 5 to 10 percent of women.

Contrary to what the name implies, PCOS is caused not by an ovarian problem but by a disruption in the hormonal feedback among the ovaries, the pituitary gland and the hypothalamus that regulates ovulation. As explained in Chapter Two, during the first phase of a normal ovulatory cycle, the hypothalamus sends a signal to the pituitary to produce follicle-stimulating hormone (FSH), which stimulates estrogen production by the ovary and the maturation of several follicles. At mid-cycle the pituitary is told to send out a surge of luteinizing hormone (LH), which causes one dominant follicle to release a mature egg. The follicle then becomes the corpus luteum, which produces the progesterone needed to maintain a pregnancy, and LH levels fall. If pregnancy does not occur, the corpus luteum degenerates, progesterone levels decline and a woman menstruates.

In polycystic ovarian syndrome, instead of a mid-cycle surge, the pituitary constantly pumps out LH. "In women with PCOS there is too much LH and normal or low levels of FSH. As a result, the ovary doesn't make normal follicles, and because there is no LH surge, women don't ovulate," explains NYU's Dr. John R. Quagliarello. "Because ovulation doesn't take place, the endometrial lining builds up. Since there's no hormonal signal to menstruate, there can be irregular or heavy bleeding."

Since FSH production is only partially suppressed, there is continued

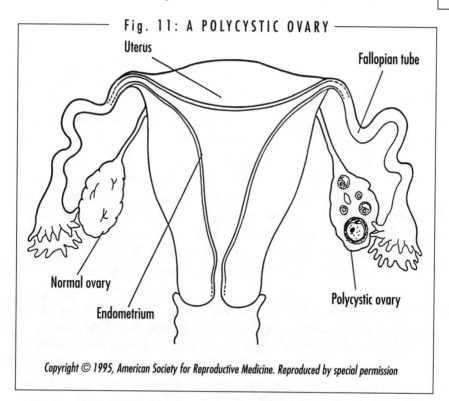

Fig. 11: A POLYCYSTIC OVARY

Uterus

Fallopian tube

Normal ovary

Polycystic ovary

Endometrium

Copyright © 1995, American Society for Reproductive Medicine. Reproduced by special permission

stimulation of ovarian follicles, which continue to grow over several months but never fully mature. High levels of LH cause the ovary to produce more male hormones, principally androstenedione. There's also a reduction in a substance in the blood called *sex hormone–binding globulin (SHBG),* which keeps blood levels of sex hormones in check. Higher levels of circulating androgens cause excess hair growth (*hirsutism*), oily skin, acne and weight gain (principally around the abdomen). The extra fat cells convert androgens to estrone, one of the three forms of the body's natural estrogen. Elevated estrone further disturbs the hormonal feedback system, leading to even more LH production and increased androgens, creating a vicious cycle.

What sets off this hormonal disruption isn't clear. Some women with PCOS have defects in enzymes that play a critical role in sex hormone production and metabolism. PCOS is more common in obese women, especially women with "male pattern" body fat distribution, excess fat around the upper body or middle rather than on the hips, as is usually the pattern in women.

Obese women are also more likely to be insulin-resistant, a condition in which the body does not respond to *insulin* (the hormone that converts food to energy that can be used by cells). Insulin resistance often accompanies PCOS. "There's a theory that insulin resistance, which leads to high insulin levels, can stimulate the ovaries to make excess amounts of androgens," says Dr. Robert Barbieri, who heads the Department of OB/GYN at Brigham and Women's Hospital in Boston. "This could work together with LH to promote anovulation and perpetuate polycystic ovarian syndrome."

While the multiple ovarian cysts of PCOS do not produce symptoms and usually are not felt during a pelvic exam, hirsutism, acne and irregular periods should raise a red flag. "However, PCOS is a diagnosis of exclusion. The tiny cysts can be seen on ultrasound, but an evaluation must include blood tests to measure the ratio of LH to FSH and levels of androgens, including testosterone," Dr. Barbieri says. He points out that testosterone is also elevated in such adrenal problems as Cushing's syndrome or in the presence of certain ovarian tumors (such as Sertoli-Leydig cell tumors), both of which can cause hirsutism. (However, the onset of hirsutism in adrenal or ovarian tumors can be rapid; it is usually gradual in PCOS.)

Other problems that can interfere with normal ovulation include diabetes, *hypothyroidism* (an underactive thyroid gland), and hyperprolactinemia (overproduction of the hormone prolactin, which normally triggers lactation), all of which disrupt the normal release of gonadotropin-releasing hormone (GnRH). All these conditions must be ruled out for a diagnosis of PCOS.

The mainstay of treatment is oral contraceptives along with an antiandrogen. "Oral contraceptives lower the LH, which will lower the androgens," says Dr. Barbieri. Birth control pills regulate the hormonal cycle and expose a woman to progesterone several days a month, reducing the risk of endometrial hyperplasia and endometrial cancer. Antiandrogens, such as *spironolactone* (Aldactone), dampen the effect of male hormones on hair growth and acne. It may also help reduce levels of "bad" low-density lipoprotein (LDL) cholesterol, which can be elevated in women with PCOS, increasing their risk of heart disease.

If a woman with PCOS wants to become pregnant, she will be given fertility drugs like *clomiphene citrate* (Clomid) for five days each month to stimulate ovulation. In cases where ovulation is not induced by hormones, surgical treatment may be needed.

A normal ovary is "pockmarked" where each follicle has erupted and ovulated an egg. "In women with PCOS the ovarian capsule becomes smooth and thickened, and even with hormone stimulation it is difficult for the egg to be released," explains Dr. Quagliarello. "This thickening also makes it difficult for the normal conversion of androgens into estrogens, which takes place in the *cortex*, the area just under the ovarian capsule." So a laser beam is used during laparoscopy to drill deep holes in the capsule, draining the multiple follicular cysts and reducing the amount of tissue inside the ovary producing excess androgens and estrogen. Once the levels of these two hormones drop, the normal hormonal feedback can resume and ovulation will occur once more.

PCOS is a chronic condition, and women prone to it need to take preventive measures. Losing weight can prevent insulin resistance and possibly some of the hormonal changes associated with upper body fat. Exercise appears to make muscle tissue more sensitive to insulin, minimizing insulin resistance.

■ Anovulation and Premature Ovarian Failure ■

Stress, illness, medications: Many factors can disrupt the normal ovulatory feedback loop. A woman may stop ovulating for a few months. "This can be a temporary situation that corrects itself," says Dr. Quagliarello. "But if a woman remains chronically anovulatory, she will start producing higher amounts of androgens and develop polycystic ovarian syndrome."

In some women the pituitary is functioning normally, releasing FSH and LH, but the ovaries don't respond. In natural menopause, ovarian follicles gradually become resistant to FSH and LH over a period of years, producing irregular periods and anovulation before menstruation actually stops. In premature ovarian failure, periods stop before the age of thirty; premature menopause is ovarian failure before age thirty-five. In both cases the pituitary pumps out FSH in an attempt to get things going again; elevated FSH is a telltale sign of ovarian failure. Premature ovarian failure affects about 1 percent of women.

"In some women we can find a genetic cause. There may be a family history of premature menopause," Dr. Quagliarello points out. "In other cases a woman may have developed autoimmune antibodies that may have damaged the ovaries. This is often seen in association with other immunological disorders, such as *Hashimoto's thyroiditis* (a form of hypothyroidism), or *lupus*. But for many cases of premature menopause we can't find a cause."

There have been reports of viruses (like mumps) that can cause transient ovarian failure, or *acute viral oophoritis*. Chemotherapy for cancer is a common cause of premature ovarian failure. Depending on the drugs used, around 50 percent of women under age thirty-five may resume normal menstruation after chemotherapy but may not ovulate. The closer a woman is to natural menopause, the more likely chemotherapy will speed the onset of menopause.

Sometimes premature ovarian failure is temporary. A few women may resume normal cycles, ovulate and even become pregnant. "One possibility is that the immunological problem was minor and corrected itself before the follicles atrophied," speculates Dr. Quagliarello. However, he adds, fertility drugs will not help women with premature ovarian failure as they do women with PCOS.

▪ Other Ovarian Problems ▪

Adnexal torsion literally means "a twisting of the ovary"; the ovary twists on the ligament containing its blood supply. Blood flow may be obstructed, causing swelling, distension and (if not treated) tissue death. Torsion usually occurs because of a large ovarian mass or cyst or during pregnancy, when the expanding uterus pushes the ovary out of position. The fallopian tubes can also become twisted. There can be bleeding into the cyst and into the ovary itself.

The most common symptom of torsion is sharp lower abdominal pain on the side of the torsion, sometimes accompanied by nausea, vomiting and low-grade fever. Some women may have had prior episodes of such pain that went away, suggesting a previous adnexal torsion that spontaneously resolved (*detorsion*).

Torsion is considered a medical emergency. Laparoscopy or laparotomy is required to untwist the ovary or tube and remove any cyst or growth. If there has been tissue death, the ovary is removed. Women who have had torsion are at risk for a repeat episode and should seek medical attention quickly if pain recurs.

Ovarian varicoceles can also cause pelvic pain. A varicocele is a distended, or varicose, vein in the ovary. This fairly uncommon condition is caused by the stretching or distension of the vein by blood pooling downward. A woman who has varicose veins in the vulva or legs may be more prone to this condition. Symptoms include pelvic pain that worsens at the end of the day or after prolonged periods of standing and pain during intercourse.

Ovarian varicoceles can be diagnosed by a *venogram*, a special X-ray study of the affected veins, performed by a radiologist, and are treated surgically. A new outpatient procedure called *ovarian vein embolization* under development in Canada uses clot-forming substances injected into the site to block blood flow to the varicocele.

■ When There's Trouble in the Tubes ■

A number of problems can affect both the ovaries and the nearby fallopian tubes. The pencil-thin tubes can be damaged by sexually transmitted infections such as *chlamydia,* by a ruptured appendix or by endometriosis, causing scarring and blockages. The frondlike fimbriae at the ends of the tubes, which take up the egg released each month, can be immobilized by scar tissue and adhesions from endometriosis or infections. The fallopian tubes can also be damaged by ectopic pregnancy, the implantation of a fertilized embryo in the tube.

Small, fluid-filled cysts that form within the fallopian tubes or the fimbriae are called *paratubal cysts.* They are always benign, but they can rupture or cause torsion. Cancer of the fallopian tubes is extremely rare and generally found in older women who have never had children.

A major problem affecting the tubes results from *salpingo-oophoritis*, pelvic inflammatory disease (PID), caused by sexually transmitted diseases (STDs; see page 147). Conditions related to PID include *hydrosalpinx*, the presence of pus in the tubes because of infection, which damages the lining. According to Dr. Quagliarello, severe PID can result in a *tubo-ovarian abscess*, a pus-filled abscess formed by an inflamed tube that gets stuck to an inflamed ovary that also sticks to the wall of the bowel. Women with PID can have high fever and severe pain and must be admitted to the hospital for intravenous antibiotic therapy.

Diagnosing and Treating Tubal Problems

There are two ways of diagnosing tubal damage: diagnostic laparoscopy and a hysterosalpingogram.

A hysterosalpingogram is a special X ray that uses a dyelike solution that is injected into the uterus and tubes and appears opaque on an X-ray film. The procedure is performed while the patient is awake. Pain relievers or sedation may be used since the procedure can cause cramping; a woman may also be pretreated with oral antibiotics to reduce the risk of pelvic infection. (The procedure usually cannot be done in women with histories of PID since it may cause a recurrent infection.)

The hysterosalpingogram reveals whether the tubes are open or damaged

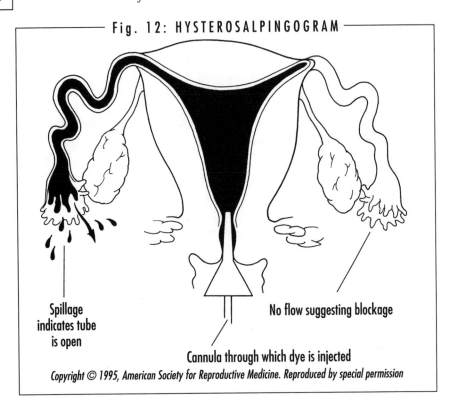

Fig. 12: HYSTEROSALPINGOGRAM

Spillage indicates tube is open

No flow suggesting blockage

Cannula through which dye is injected

Copyright © 1995, American Society for Reproductive Medicine. Reproduced by special permission

and whether the uterine cavity is normal. Often done as part of an infertility workup, it's even believed to be helpful because it "flushes out" the tubes. It is done before ovulation to avoid X-ray exposure to a potentially fertilized egg.

Diagnostic laparoscopy can determine the outer condition of the tubes, revealing adhesions and scar tissue from endometriosis or STDs. Dye injected through the cervix during laparoscopy will indicate that the tubes are open by spilling out the ends. It's an outpatient procedure performed under general anesthesia.

In some cases a *salpingoscope*, a tiny fiber-optic instrument, is passed into the tubes through the uterus or through the opening near the fimbriae to examine the inside of the tubes and the cilia (hairlike projections that move an egg through the tubes) under magnification. "These are instruments that are relatively new, and people are just starting to become familiar with their use, so it's unclear what's normal and what's not or how clinically useful this is," cautions Dr. Quagliarello. "We do know that most pelvic infections destroy the fimbriae, and if the fimbriae are destroyed, the cilia are likely to be as well."

Laparoscopy or laparotomy is usually performed to repair damage and blockages in the *distal* end of the tubes, the wider section outside the uterus near the ovaries. Microsurgery can repair the tubes, and a thin wire or tube can be used to remove blockages or mucus plugs (a common cause of noninfection-related blockages). Adhesions can also be removed, freeing the fimbriae.

Blockages in the *proximal* portion of the tube nearest to and inside the uterus are removed using delicate wires inserted through a hysteroscope, a thin, lighted telescope inserted through the cervix into the uterus.

The success of tubal surgery depends on the extent of the damage and its location; pregnancy rates after the removal of blockages at the proximal end are lower than for blockages at the distal end of the tube. Scar tissue frequently returns even after the most skilled surgery. Repeat procedures have low success rates.

"Although we can remove blockages, the tubes will still be abnormal. Maybe 25 to 50 percent of patients become pregnant after the surgery. But about 20 percent of the pregnancies may be tubal pregnancies," says Dr. Quagliarello. Even if a woman opts for in vitro fertilization, chances of another ectopic pregnancy are greater, so a badly damaged tube may have to be removed.

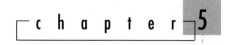

Endometriosis

Endometriosis is a painful, chronic condition that affects around 5 million American women of reproductive age. The problem occurs when the endometrial tissue which normally lines the uterus is found in the pelvis, growing in response to estrogen. These implants swell and bleed during the menstrual cycle, causing pain and irritating the pelvic cavity, tubes, ovaries or bowel. As the inflammation heals, scar tissue forms weblike growths called adhesions. Endometriosis can invade the ovary and form blood-filled cysts called endometriomas.

The most common symptom is severe pain before and during periods, caused in part by chemicals produced by the endometrial tissue. (In adolescents, menstrual pain may increase over time.) However, small numbers of women may have no symptoms at all and are diagnosed only when they find they can't conceive, sometimes due to scars or adhesions that prevent the release of eggs from the ovaries or their uptake by the fallopian tubes. Women with untreated endometriosis also have increased risk of miscarriage.

Once called the career women's disease, because of its high incidence among women who delayed childbearing, endometriosis is now known to occur in adolescents and women who've had children, especially those whose mothers or sisters had the disease.

Researchers believe endometriosis may be partly due to immune system dysfunction. New research has also linked the disease to the chemical *dioxin* and possibly other hormonally active pollutants (see box on page 89). A 1997 study of 20,686 women in Sweden also found that women with endometriosis may have up to a 20 percent increase in the risk of ovarian cancer and a higher risk of breast and thyroid cancers and non-Hodgkin's lymphoma.

๏๏ *M a r y L o u ' s S t o r y* ๏๏

"My endo story really started when I was sixteen and began having bad pain with my periods. Over time the pain became really severe. When I was nineteen, I was put on birth control pills to try to control the pain.

"I had a number of ovarian cyst ruptures during my twenties, but I thought it was more of the same pain. And I had a lot of gastrointestinal problems. I went through a number of gastrointestinal workups, but they found nothing. So I became a health nut, trying everything I could to improve my diet, exercising, and for a while everything got better.

"But in the fall of 1978 I was exposed to very heavy doses of flea spray. By the end of that year I had developed a constant sore throat, swollen lymph glands, was extremely fatigued—what we now call chronic fatigue syndrome—and the pain came back, worse than ever. They did all kinds of tests. But when everything came out normal, they told me it was all in my head.

"I went to the library. The only thing that seemed similar to the pain I was experiencing was endometriosis. And we did find I had endometriosis. My gynecologist put me back on the pill (I'd been on and off for many years), and for a while I was fine. But then two and a half months later I had a near stroke and was told I could never go back on the pill again.

"So I started reading everything I could find and trying to find other women who had it. At first I had a very hard time finding other women. They were everywhere but wouldn't talk about it. I mean, we are talking about menstruation, painful sex, bowel problems, pain with defecation and urination. These are all taboo subjects. When we first started our group in 1980, we had eight women. Now we are a worldwide organization, and

I think we have helped to break down some of the taboos and get this issue out into the open."

Mary Lou Ballweg is the president and executive director of the Endometriosis Association, in Milwaukee, Wisconsin, which she co-founded in 1980. It now has member groups in sixty-six countries and has established endometriosis research programs at a number of academic institutions and funds scientific research. Ms. Ballweg has published two books, *Overcoming Endometriosis* (Contemporary Books) and *The Endometriosis Sourcebook* (Contemporary Books). The above remarks are taken from an interview and printed with her permission.

• A Lingering Mystery •

Despite decades of research, the exact cause of endometriosis remains unclear. The main theory links endometriosis to "retrograde menstruation," the backward flow of menstrual discharge through the fallopian tubes into the pelvic cavity. This discharge contains live endometrial tissue, which has its own blood supply, giving it the ability to grow.

Some experts believe that excessive backward flow into the tubes may be due to increased pressure in the uterus during menstruation. This pressure may be more common in women who have stronger menstrual cramps (indicating stronger uterine contractions) and women without children, whose cervical opening is smaller, perhaps causing backward menstrual flow.

"A number of studies indicate as many as ninety percent of women have some degree of retrograde flow. We think there is some sort of immune system deficit in some women that allows those fragments of endometrial cells to implant themselves," says Lyle J. Brietkopf, M.D., clinical assistant professor of OB/GYN at NYU Medical Center and director of the Endometriosis Clinic at the NYU-affiliated New York Downtown Hospital.

Some researchers believe endometriosis is an immunological disorder. Normally the immune system gets rid of foreign cells and bacteria with scavenger cells called *macrophages*. "When blood is present in the peritoneal cavity, the immune system sends in these scavenger cells to eat up the blood and endometrial cell fragments," explains Dr. Brietkopf. "In some women these immune system scavengers may not be doing their job properly. As a result, endometrial cell fragments remain in the area and are able to implant and grow."

New research at Yale University Medical School focuses on a growth factor, or *cytokine*, called *interleuken-8*, produced by immune cells that may cause an inflammation that itself contributes to endometriosis. "Abnormal amounts of this or other substances produced by immune cells, coupled with excessive retrograde flow, may overwhelm the immune system's ability to get rid of wayward endometrial cells," says David L. Olive, M.D., chief of Reproductive Endocrinology and Infertility at Yale. "Add estrogen further fueling the growth of endometriosis, and you have a vicious cycle."

Endometrial growths produce the same chemicals as the uterine endometrium, including prostaglandins, which cause uterine contractions and menstrual cramps. "Pelvic tissues appear to be very sensitive to prostaglandins, which may also sensitize pain receptors on nerves in the pelvis," Dr. Olive explains. This may be why endometriosis can cause such severe menstrual pain.

Scientists also believe that abnormal immune cell responses triggered by the presence of endometrial implants lead to production of other substances that may cause malaise, fever and other symptoms experienced by women with endometriosis. In fact, some researchers believe that endometriosis may be linked to autoimmune diseases (in which the immune system attacks normal cells in the body), such as lupus. Researchers are currently studying possible immune therapies for endometriosis.

▪ The Effects of Endometriosis ▪

Some women may have a few implants that never spread or grow; others may have widespread, deeply penetrating disease. Common implantation sites include the outer surface of the uterus, the supporting ligaments, the cul-de-sac (the space between the uterus and the rectum), the ovaries and the membrane lining the pelvic cavity. Seen on laparoscopy, tiny, early implants look like small flecks of red paint that will either grow larger or spontaneously disappear. Once the implanted tissue begins to grow under the influence of estrogen, it can invade the walls of the intestine, the tissue that separates the vagina and the rectum, or grow into the bladder wall and the ureters (the tubes from the kidneys), causing bladder or bowel problems. However, while experts stress that endometriosis is *not* a cancer, according to a recent study it is associated with a greater risk of breast and ovarian cancer and non-Hodgkin's lymphoma.

According to the Endometriosis Association, 44 percent of women with

---
Fig. 13: ENDOMETRIOSIS

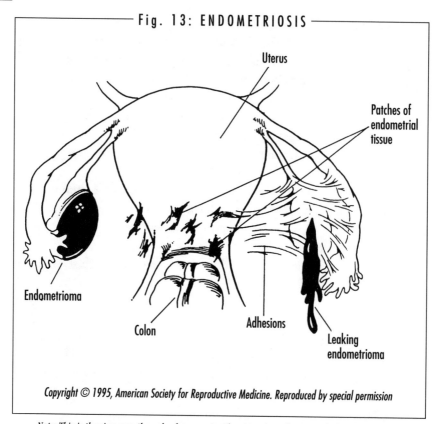

Uterus

Patches of
endometrial
tissue

Endometrioma

Colon

Adhesions

Leaking
endometrioma

Note: This is the view seen through a laparoscope; the uterus is at the top, with the tubes and ovaries on each side.

endometriosis may have fertility problems. There is also a high rate of ectopic, or tubal, pregnancy and an increased risk of miscarriage. Research presented to a conference co-sponsored by the association in 1995 suggests that immune system antibodies triggered by the presence of endometriosis may interfere with the implantation of a fetus, contributing to miscarriage.

In a survey of more than 3,000 endometriosis patients, the association found that almost 60 percent of women experienced pain with sex. A knot (or nodule) of endometriosis in the back of the pelvis near the lower spine can cause backache or *sciatica* (back pain that travels down the thigh). Endometriosis that invades the colon or rectum can cause painful bowel movements, irritable bowel symptoms, diarrhea and/or constipation and intestinal upsets during menstruation.

More than 80 percent of the surveyed women felt lethargic and fatigued, a majority were unable to carry out normal activities one to two days a month and 57 percent had constant pain throughout the month. Almost 40 percent of the women reported low resistance to infection, and around 30 percent low-grade fever. Others reported allergies and related problems, including *candidiasis*, body-wide symptoms due to yeast sensitivities.

Interestingly, the degree of pain is not always related to the extent or the size of endometrial implants. Some research suggests that tiny growths (*petechiae*) produce more prostaglandins than larger ones. Other studies indicate that deeply penetrating growths cause more pelvic pain and that the location is important.

As with Mary Lou Ballweg, symptoms can begin in the teens; one quarter of the women surveyed by the association said their symptoms began between ages fifteen and nineteen. Endometriosis is found in 47 to 65 percent of women under twenty who have chronic pelvic pain or painful periods. (Note: If your teenage daughter is complaining of severe menstrual cramps and heavy periods, have her examined for endometriosis.)

Pregnancy may bring temporary relief from endometriosis, while menopause generally ends cycle-related symptoms of moderate disease. Dr. Brietkopf notes that estrogen replacement can occasionally reactivate endometriosis even if a woman has had a hysterectomy. However, most women with histories of endometriosis can receive hormone replacement without recurrent symptoms.

▪ Making the Diagnosis ▪

There are some telltale signs of endometriosis that can be felt during a pelvic exam. One is hard or tender-to-the-touch or painful nodules along the *uterosacral ligaments* (above the rectum and behind the vagina). A cyst on the ovary or an enlarged ovary can also indicate endometriosis (especially if the ovary is immobile, suggesting adhesions). If endometriomas (see page 71) are suspected, transvaginal ultrasound may be used to view the ovaries or, in some cases, magnetic resonance imaging (MRI).

"While laparoscopy provides a definitive diagnosis, it involves general anesthesia and is expensive. If your index of suspicion is raised by a careful medical history, by definite signs and symptoms, you might proceed to birth control pills in certain patients without laparoscopy to see if you can help their pain," says Yale's Dr. David Olive. "However, laparoscopy and biopsy are the only means of conclusive diagnosis, and the extent of the disease needs to be gauged before one proceeds to strong hormonal treatments."

Diagnostic laparoscopy, performed under general anesthesia, uses a thin,

Fig. 14: DIAGNOSTIC LAPAROSCOPY

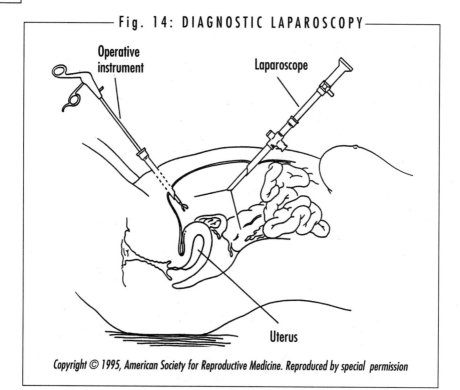

Operative instrument

Laparoscope

Uterus

Copyright © 1995, American Society for Reproductive Medicine. Reproduced by special permission

lighted telescope to look inside the pelvis and inspect the reproductive organs. First, a small incision around ten millimeters wide (about the diameter of two standard pencils) is made in or near the navel. The abdomen is gently inflated with carbon dioxide to make viewing easier and avoid injury. The laparoscope is then inserted through the incision to inspect the surface of the pelvic organs under magnification. A small probe may be inserted through an incision around the bikini line to move organs gently into view. The fallopian tubes can also be checked during laparoscopy for scarring or blockages that can impair fertility.

Since other cysts or pelvic abnormalities can be mistaken for endometriosis, a small piece of tissue may be removed for biopsy. Following laparoscopy, the incisions (closed with tiny Band-Aids) are usually tender, the abdomen is bruised and there may be some discomfort from the gas used to distend the abdomen. However, normal activities can usually be resumed in a few days.

Researchers at Yale and elsewhere have developed a *microlaparoscopy* that could potentially allow *both* diagnostic laparoscopy and treatment to be done in a physician's office rather than in an operating room. The procedure uses only local anesthesia and a laparoscope one fifth the size of a conventional model. Right now it is being used as a diagnostic tool, allowing patients to remain awake and help a physician "map" areas of pain. "If we find specific, localized areas of pain, she would be a better candidate for surgery than a woman who has generalized pelvic pain," says Dr. Olive. The new procedure would not only reduce costs ($1,700 versus up to $10,000 for traditional laparoscopy) but use smaller incisions that allow more rapid recovery. Microlaparoscopy could be in widespread use within five years.

The amount of endometriosis seen on laparoscopy is assigned a numerical score, or stage. The staging system divides endometriosis into minimal (stage I), mild (stage II), moderate (stage III) and severe (stage IV). A score of 1 to 15 indicates minimal or mild endometriosis, and a score of 15 or greater indicates moderate to severe disease. Treatment decisions are usually based on the stage of the disease, age, fertility considerations, and a woman's wishes.

In some cases implants may be eradicated during the initial laparoscopy using a carbon dioxide laser or electrocautery instruments, which vaporize, cut away or burn away lesions (see page 94).

Some women undergo tests for a chemical marker called CA-125. Recent studies indicate that some women with endometriosis may have increased amounts of CA-125 in their blood; the more severe the disease, the higher the CA-125. An elevated CA-125 itself cannot diagnose endometriosis—it can also be elevated in ovarian cancer, fibroids, infections or even after recent pelvic surgery—but it can be useful in deciding whether or not to proceed to diagnostic laparoscopy. "If someone has an elevated CA-125 and you do surgery, it may be helpful to see whether the CA-125 returns to normal," comments Dr. Olive. A new, more sensitive test for CA-125 used in Europe may soon be approved here, perhaps increasing the usefulness of CA-125 as a marker for endometriosis.

The Dioxin Connection

Endometriosis has been tentatively linked to pollutants, including dioxins and related compounds. There are seventy-five varieties of dioxin, one of which *TCDD*, is known to cause immune suppression, cancer and birth defects in animals.

In the late 1970s researchers at the University of Wisconsin first uncovered the connection between TCDD and endometriosis among a colony of twenty-four rhesus monkeys, sixteen of which were fed dioxin to study its effects on reproduction. The four-year trial produced a host of reproductive problems in the monkeys. More than a decade after the study began, three of the animals died of endometriosis that had invaded the intestines and also caused kidney failure. A team of experts assembled by the Endometriosis Association examined the remaining animals and found that 79 percent of the female monkeys exposed to dioxin had developed endometriosis, compared with about 30 percent of the unexposed monkeys. The more dioxin exposure, the more severe the endometriosis.

Animal studies to unlock the dioxin connection currently continue at Dartmouth Medical School. One key may lie in the interface between the immune system and the endocrine system, which produces reproductive hormones, says immunologist Sherry Rier, Ph.D., the Tracy H. Dickinson Research Chair of the Endometriosis Association at Dartmouth, who heads the study. "In animals dioxin causes immune suppression or stimulation, as well as changes in immune cells and the factors they produce. It also acts as a hormone disrupter, interfering with estrogen's ability to lock onto its own receptor sites on cells. The immune and endocrine systems are intertwined; changes in one will affect the other," explains Rier.

Rier speculates that dioxin may affect not only the growth of uterine endometrium but also the ability of immune cells to control endometrial cell growth outside the uterus. Her preliminary research revealed immunologic changes in dioxin-exposed monkeys similar to those in women with endometriosis. Dioxin may disrupt the normal regulation by estrogen of growth factors called cytokines, leading to abnormal growth of the uterine lining and endometrial implants, and causing inflammation that may also spur endometrosis. "This may be another way dioxin, the immune system and female hormones influence one another," Rier suggests.

The Program in Cancer Epidemiology and Prevention at NYU Medical Center will be conducting studies in heavily polluted areas of Russia to look at the effects of dioxin on endometriosis and possible links to cancer.

Other research in Germany has found that women with high blood levels of the pollutant *polychlorinated biphenyls (PCBs)* also have a higher incidence of endometriosis. Dioxin and PCBs are among chemical compounds, called *organochlorines*, that appear to have "estrogenic" effects in the body. Some, like DDT and PCBs, have been banned in this country. But they are highly resistant to breakdown and remain in the food chain for decades, accumulating in fatty tissues of both animals and humans. Some studies have also linked DDT and PCBs to breast cancer.

▪ Hormonal Therapy ▪

The goal of medical treatment is to dampen female hormones and prevent or reduce menstruation using various hormones.

ORAL CONTRACEPTIVES, the most commonly prescribed initial treatment, are given to 43 percent of women with endometriosis. Continuous doses of estrogen and progesterone prevent ovulation, and the progestins in the pill suppress activity of the endometrium and endometrial implants, producing lighter bleeding rather than regular menses. Oral contraceptives also reduce formation of prostaglandins and reduce pain. (For more about birth control pills, see Chapter Nine.)

"The pill is simple, inexpensive, easy to take and works in a large number of patients with moderate symptoms," says Dr. Olive. "A patient can remain on the pill for long periods. It does not have strong side effects, and it has other benefits, providing birth control and regulating cycles." Despite the widespread use of the pill to treat endometriosis, there are little long-term data on its efficacy compared with other treatments. But studies do indicate the pill relieves pain over the short term in around 80 percent of women, according to Dr. Olive.

If birth control pills don't control pain, hormones may be used to halt periods. Currently there are only two classes of drug approved by the FDA for the hormonal treatment of endometriosis: danazol and GnRH agonists.

DANAZOL (DANOCRINE, CYCLOMEN), a male hormone derivative, is usually prescribed for six months to reduce estrogen levels to menopausal levels. A six-month regimen of danazol reduces the size and extent of endometrial lesions by 30 to 50 percent but has little effect on adhesions. More than 80 percent of treated women report pain relief, including less painful intercourse, and 70 to 100 percent of patients go into remission. Endometriomas are usually resistant.

As mentioned in Chapter Three, danazol can have androgenic side effects, including acne, deepened voice, facial hair growth, reduced breast size, water retention and weight gain. It can also raise levels of the "bad" LDL cholesterol.

GnRH agonists mimic GnRH produced by the body but are many times more potent. As agonists they stimulate, then suppress natural pituitary hormones and fool the body into menopause, reducing the symptoms of endometriosis. They are usually given for six months, as a daily or monthly injection of leuprolide (Lupron), as a nasal spray *nafarelin acetate* (Synarel) or *buserelin acetate* (Suprefact) or as an implant form of *goserelin acetate* (Zoladex), placed under the skin of the abdomen.

GnRH agonists relieve pain in 90 percent of patients and cause a 60 to 90 percent regression of endometriosis implants. Large ovarian endometriomas are usually resistant, and GnRH agonists have no effect on adhesions or scarring.

GnRH agonists cause menopausal side effects, including hot flashes, vaginal dryness, headaches, decreased sex drive, mood swings and fatigue, but they may boost the "good" HDL cholesterol.

The main adverse side effect of GnRH agonists is accelerated bone loss, which increases the risk of osteoporosis. A review of recent studies presented at the 1995 international conference on endometriosis showed that average bone loss from six months of GnRH agonist treatment is about 6 percent, twice the rate normally occurring in the first *year* or so of menopause. This is why GnRH agonist therapy is now limited to six months. However, studies suggest that add-back therapies using very small doses of estrogen and progestin can minimize menopausal symptoms and bone loss. New studies show that three-month regimens produce less bone loss, with no need for add-back therapy. New, nonhormonal osteoporosis drugs, such as alendronate (Fosamax) and *etidronate* (Didronol), may stem bone loss during prolonged GnRH treatment.

Other hormonal treatments for endometriosis include:

PROGESTOGENS produce progesteronelike effects on endometrial tissue, inhibiting estrogen's effects and shrinking implants. These include Provera and Depo-Provera, which like danazol relieve pain and shrink implants. The side effects of the prescribed pills or injections can include breakthrough bleeding, water retention, mood swings and clinical depression as well as adverse effects on cholesterol.

ETHYLNORGESTRIENONE (GESTRINONE) is an antiprogestational hormone used extensively in Europe. It appears to work by rapidly decreasing estrogen in endometrial tissues, enhancing the breakdown of cells. Its success with reducing pain and endometrial implants is comparable to danazol, with similar side effects. It may be available soon in the United States.

MIFEPRISTONE (RU-486) is an antiprogesterone (see page 183) that inhibits ovulation and disrupts the normal structure of the endometrium, causing regression of endometrial lesions. Preliminary studies suggest RU-486 may reduce pain with fewer side effects than other hormonal therapies.

GNRH ANTAGONISTS are new drugs that work faster than GnRH agonists, acting directly on the pituitary to produce an immediate blocking of gonadotropins. The major side effect seems to be an "allergic" reaction at the injection site. Clinical trials are now under way, and GnRH antagonists may become available for treating endometriosis within the next few years.

Most experts agree that medical therapy does not *cure* endometriosis. Since some endometrial implants have no receptors for either estrogen or progesterone, they may not be responsive to hormonal treatment, according to Mary Lou Ballweg. For danazol and GnRH agonists, recurrence rates range from 30 to 60 percent within a year after treatment stops, although some women report less pain with recurrence. Also, clinical trials do not show that hormonal treatments help infertility, and there are no studies comparing medical therapy with surgery for endometriosis.

∞ *M a r y   L o u ' s   S t o r y ,   C o n t ' d* ∞

"I had five surgeries for the endometriosis; I'd had one ovary removed because it was so damaged. I had a hysterectomy and my remaining ovary removed six months after my daughter was born. She was a miracle. I decided to have the surgery because I didn't want to miss out on any part of my daughter's childhood.

"After my hysterectomy I did not want to take hormones for a while. I had seen too many women have recurrences of endometriosis after they had hysterectomies and started hormones. But I finally started taking estrogen eight months later because I was having severe menopausal symptoms. Eight years later after we doubled the dose, I started getting joint pain and symptoms of bowel obstruction, and sure enough there was endometriosis

on my bowel and the cul-de-sac. They probably were left behind when I had surgery years before. Even now all too many doctors leave some disease because they think the hysterectomy takes care of it.

"I have a lot of other immune-related problems which women with endo are prone to: extreme sensitivity to candida, Hashimoto's thyroiditis. Moreover, I seem to develop new allergies every six to eight months. . . . I also developed severe osteoporosis because of hormonal treatments. The low dose of estrogen I was taking wasn't enough to prevent it.

"When I convinced my doctor to give me a bone density test, they found my bone mineral density was 5 percent of what women my age should have, but after I was put on a special diet with lots of mineral supplements and natural progesterone, I was able to build back some bone. Thank heaven the endometriosis did not flare up again."

▪ Surgical Options ▪

When medical therapy fails to control symptoms, or if hormone treatments are undesirable, surgery is usually the next step. Surgery is generally done laparoscopically, making small incisions to admit special surgical instruments, lasers or electrocautery devices that remove or destroy implants.

Laparoscopic surgery is done as day surgery under general anesthesia. Laparoscopic surgery causes far less pain than open abdominal surgery, and recovery is faster; most women return to work within a week. There are several techniques in current use.

LASER VAPORIZATION uses a concentrated high-energy beam to vaporize or cut endometriosis implants; the laser heat instantly boils the water contained in cells, destroying them. The most widely used laser in endometriosis treatment is the *carbon dioxide (CO_2) laser*, which cuts and vaporizes tissue. The shallow penetration of the CO_2 laser makes it ideal for destroying endometriosis implants on the surface of the pelvic organs. The laser also causes little heat damage to surrounding tissue, believed to minimize the formation of adhesions.

ELECTROSURGERY passes an electric current through special surgical instruments to cut, coagulate or vaporize implants. Among the newest instruments are electric scissors, which seal small blood vessels as they cut lesions.

SURGICAL EXCISION cuts away endometrial implants with a scalpel, small surgical scissors or forceps (or laser). Cysts larger than two centimeters (around an inch) are usually removed surgically. Deeper implants in and around the bladder, ureter or bowel may need laparotomy (open abdominal surgery).

In severe, invasive endometriosis, sections of the bowel may have to be removed. David Redwine, M.D., director of the Endometriosis Institute of Oregon, has helped pioneer a new transvaginal technique for bowel resection that allows selected patients to avoid open abdominal surgery. An incision is made in the rear vaginal wall, and the diseased portion of the intestines is pulled through, resected and sutured. Adhesions are also excised.

However, this scar tissue can re-form within days after any type of surgery. A *second-look laparoscopy* may be done a week or so after an initial procedure in order to loosen and cut away newly formed adhesions. New materials can also be applied to the excision site to reduce adhesion formation. One is a patch of Gore-Tex, which is left in place after surgery, and another is Interceed, a woven patch of cellulose that is eventually absorbed by the body. Studies show most women who receive Interceed are free of adhesions twelve to fourteen weeks after the initial surgery.

Many surgeons combine several techniques: vaporization or electrocautery for small lesions and excision for large implants. However, some experts believe that excision produces better results because it removes the entire lesion, while vaporization may remove only part of the implant, obscuring the rest.

Surgery may improve fertility by removing adhesions or blockages that interfere with the release and uptake of an egg; a 1997 Canadian study found that treating even mild cases of endometriosis can nearly double the chances of becoming pregnant. If a woman with endometriosis fails to conceive after treatment, she may be a candidate for in vitro fertilization, though some fertility drugs may stimulate endometriosis.

While many women show improvement with therapy, 20 to 50 percent of patients show signs of recurrence five to ten years after their initial therapy. Pain may return within five years in half of patients taking medication and in 40 percent who underwent laparoscopic surgery.

The skill and knowledge of the surgeon are extremely important. A colorectal surgeon may need to work with a gynecologic surgeon to remove endometriosis from the bowel. There are a growing number of specialists in this field. Look for a board-certified surgeon who is a member of professional organizations, such as the American Association of Gynecologic Laparoscopists, the Society of Reproductive Surgeons or the American Board of Laser

Surgery; physicians with a special interest in this area often belong to the Endometriosis Association (see Appendix I).

However, Dr. Brietkopf stresses that even the most skilled surgeon can remove only visible endometrial implants. Even with magnification laparoscopy there may be microscopic lesions left behind. So an additional six months of low-dose hormonal therapy may be needed, especially with severe disease.

HYSTERECTOMY may be the last resort for women with severe (Stage 4) endometriosis who have been unsuccessful with hormones or laparoscopic surgery and have completed their families. However, experts stress that implants must also be removed from all other sites, or pain will return.

Some younger women may choose to retain their ovaries to avoid an abrupt surgical menopause. However, for lasting relief in severe cases, most studies say that (when appropriate), the ovaries should be removed to prevent hormonal stimulation of any microscopic lesions. A recent study following 138 women with endometriosis who had hysterectomies at Johns Hopkins from 1979 to 1991 found 62 percent of those who kept their ovaries had recurrent symptoms and 31 percent required further surgery. Among women whose ovaries had been removed, only 10 percent had continued symptoms and 4 percent needed more surgery. A 1995 multicenter study came to similar conclusions.

If the ovaries are removed, low-dose estrogen replacement therapy (ERT) is often recommended to prevent menopausal symptoms, osteoporosis and heart disease. Even though ERT can cause a flare-up of symptoms in some women, the Johns Hopkins study suggested there was no advantage to avoiding or delaying ERT. Ninety percent of the women on ERT had no recurrent symptoms, probably because the dose of estrogen was lower than natural levels. However, the exact dose of ERT that will relieve menopausal symptoms and prevent recurrent pain of endometriosis has yet to be determined.

For most women the benefits of estrogen therapy after hysterectomy usually outweigh the potential risks (see page 254). Women with severe endometriosis may do well to avoid ERT and find nonhormonal treatments if they are at risk for osteoporosis, according to Dr. Brietkopf. Women taking small doses of estrogen may need additional measures to prevent osteoporosis.

Shindi's Story

"I have had endometriosis for twenty-one years out of the thirty-four years of my life. When I started having pain at age thirteen, I was diagnosed with pelvic inflammatory disease. I had one doctor tell me at sixteen that

I should have a hysterectomy! I wasn't diagnosed as having endometriosis until I was nineteen and I was embarrassed. I didn't want anyone to know. I've had ten laparoscopies. I've taken every drug that's out there. I have been in remission now for several years.

"The biggest thing is to put the word out, to make people aware, especially black women, that it is a disease that is very prevalent and has a lot of different symptoms."

▪ Women of Color and Endometriosis ▪

We now know that endometriosis, once thought to affect only white women, can strike women of all racial and ethnic groups. All too often African-American women like Shindi who complain of pelvic pain are misdiagnosed with pelvic inflammatory disease (PID), says Donald L. Chatman, M.D., clinical associate professor of OB/GYN at Northwestern University School of Medicine who lectures on health issues affecting African-American women. "Because of public health statistics showing a higher prevalence of sexually transmitted diseases in African-Americans, which is largely based on data collected from public clinics and emergency rooms, a bias is created that leads physicians to make that diagnosis." In 1976 Dr. Chatman conducted a study that found up to 40 percent of black women told they had PID actually had endometriosis—a number he says still holds true.

"Unfortunately I still see black women who were only diagnosed after ten years and a dozen physicians; rarely do they get a correct diagnosis on the first visit. What they get is Motrin, birth control pills or ampicillin for PID when they complain of pelvic pain," says Dr. Chatman. "Without laparoscopy you cannot have an accurate diagnosis."

Other problems that may interfere with diagnoses for women of color include the lingering stereotype of endometriosis as a white career women's disease, as a disease of women who have no children, as well as the common belief among black women that monthly pain goes along with being a woman, he adds.

If you are having pelvic pain, painful periods, pain with intercourse or other symptoms, and your physician does not suggest laparoscopy, seek a second opinion, Dr. Chatman advises. He notes that many health maintenance organizations (HMOs) or managed care plans may not pay for laparoscopy, so women may have to pay out of pocket to get proper diagnosis.

▪ Support for Women with Endometriosis ▪

Endometriosis can affect a woman's personal and professional life. The pain can be so debilitating that they cannot maintain normal working lives or relationships. Some lose interest in sex because of painful intercourse. In addition, the hormonal treatments for endometriosis that produce menopausal symptoms can cause depression and inhibit sexual desire. The understanding and support of a partner, family and friends are vital. The Endometriosis Association has chapters around the country and abroad (see Appendix I).

"Women no longer have to suffer in silence. There are treatments for endometriosis, and we are making some progress on finding the causes of this disease, even though we have a long way to go. But you *can* get help," stresses Mary Lou Ballweg.

Vaginal and Vulvar Irritations and Infections

Almost every woman has had *vaginitis* or a yeast infection. These problems are common because of the dozens of microorganisms living on the skin and in the body that can overgrow and cause an infection. Although the vagina has built-in defenses—an acidic environment and a fairly resistant, thick lining—certain conditions make the vulvar and vaginal area vulnerable to irritation and infection.

Inflammation of the vulva (*vulvitis*) may result from skin conditions or reactions to anything from soap to latex condoms. Tissues and muscle irritation in the area can result in a chronic burning pain called *vulvodynia*.

Vaginitis, or *inflammation* of the vagina, is usually an infection by one of three organisms: the fungus *Monilia*, the protozoan *Trichomonas vaginalis* and the bacterium *Gardnerella vaginalis*; Trichomonas and Gardnerella are spread sexually. Another *sexually transmitted disease (STD)* that affects the vulvo-vaginal area is *genital herpes*. (Other STDs are discussed in Chapter Eight.)

▪ Vaginal Discharge ▪

A common sign of a vaginal infection is abnormal discharge (leukorrhea), which may have an unpleasant smell, an unusual color and may irritate the vulvar area.

Some milky or clear discharge from your vagina is normal. It consists of sloughed-off cells from the vaginal lining, cervical mucus and other fluids arising from the capillaries within the vaginal wall. "Vaginal secretions keep the vagina moist and rids the area of debris and bacteria," explains Leonard Wolf, M.D., associate clinical professor of OB/GYN at NYU Medical Center. Secretions from labial sweat glands, the Bartholin's glands at the opening of the vagina, and Skene's glands around the urethra also form a protective layer against urine and other irritants.

While normal vaginal discharge is slightly acidic (keeping microorganisms in check), it does not usually irritate the vulva. *Normal* changes in vaginal discharge occur around ovulation (it's clear, thin and more copious) and after ovulation (it lessens, becoming white and opaque). Hormonal changes during pregnancy may increase vaginal discharge, according to Dr. Wolf. During sexual arousal lubrication increases in the vagina. In some women discharge may not be bothersome, while for others it may soak through underwear, requiring a panty liner. This wetness can cause slight irritation but does not indicate disease.

"Normal vaginal discharge has little odor. But when bacteria or other organisms are present, it may develop an unpleasant, 'fishy' smell," says Dr. Wolf. "Abnormal discharge may be greenish, appear like curds of cottage cheese or be blood-streaked." Abnormal discharge can cause inflammation and redness (erythema) of the vagina and vulva. Other symptoms include itching, painful sexual intercourse, burning during urination and local swelling. Proper treatment will clear up the symptoms and their source.

Before puberty and after menopause there is little vaginal discharge, and the vaginal lining is very thin and particularly susceptible to infection and irritation. In postmenopausal women irritation caused by thinning of vaginal tissue and lack of moisture is called *atrophic vaginitis* (which can be helped by estrogen cream, see page 249). Some vaginal dryness is also normal right after pregnancy, during breast-feeding and at the end of the menstrual cycle (due to low estrogen). Antidepressants, some oral contraceptives and blood pressure drugs may also cause vaginal dryness. Radiation treatment can thin the vagina, cause abnormal discharge and make the area vulnerable to irritation and infection.

▪ Yeast Infections ▪

Monilia or "yeast" infections are the most common cause of vaginitis, affecting 75 percent of women at some point during their lifetimes. Approximately 5 percent of women suffer recurrent yeast infections. The most common culprit is *Monilia*, or *Candida albicans*, one of several types of *Candida* that live normally on the skin, in the digestive system and in the vagina. *Candida* is usually kept in check by a beneficial vaginal bacterium called lactobacillus. But when the pH of the vagina changes, because of hormonal changes, such as those in pregnancy, or when lactobacillus is killed off by antibiotics, *Candida* can multiply rapidly. Moisture trapped by synthetic-fiber panty hose, underwear or wet swimsuits also aids the growth of yeast. Not surprisingly more women get yeast infections in warmer weather.

Diabetic women are more susceptible to yeast infections. "Lactobacilli can't entirely break down the increased glucose in blood and extra glycogen in vaginal cells, which make the vaginal environment 'sweeter' and less acidic," explains Dr. Wolf. Yeast can overgrow in women taking corticosteroids, who are run-down or who douche too often (flushing away lactobacilli). Women with impaired immunity or HIV may have recurrent yeast infections.

Some women with *no* apparent health problems are prone to yeast infections, and until recently no one knew why. The first population-based study to evaluate risk factors for *Monilia* infections, conducted among 691 women at the University of Michigan, came up with a surprising risk factor. The 1996 study found that having receptive oral sex twice or more in the previous two weeks tripled the risk of a yeast infection; the authors note that one third of adults carry yeast in their oral cavities. The study also found that use of oral contraceptive doubled the risk, while spermicides tripled the risk; both can disrupt the normal vaginal environment. Women under age twenty-four had a 75 percent higher risk of yeast infection.

Another study suggests that some women may have a genetic predisposition to repeat infections. The report, in the *Journal of Infectious Diseases,* links recurrent *Candida* infections to the inheritance of certain blood group antigens, previously associated with susceptibility to recurrent urinary tract infections (see page 122). The researchers speculate that these antigens, when present in vaginal tissues, may enhance adhesion of *Candida* organisms.

Typical symptoms of *Monilia* infection are severe itching in the vaginal and vulvar area, redness, irritation, small cracks in the sensitive mucous membrane, which cause pain, and a thick, white, curdish discharge. The discharge is generally odorless. In severe cases itching and redness can spread to the upper thighs. These symptoms may be due to the infection itself or to an "allergic" response to the fungus, which can be severe.

The diagnosis is simple: A drop of vaginal secretion is placed in an alkaline solution that dissolves all cells except the fungus, which is then identified under a microscope. This test, called a *wet prep,* takes a few minutes. However, wet preps can miss some yeast infections, and do not detect all species of *candida,* so a culture is needed to confirm a diagnosis.

Treatment consists of antifungal agents in the form of vaginal suppositories, creams or oral medication. Over-the-counter creams and suppositories include *miconazole* (Monistat 7, Monistat 3), *clotrimazole* (Gyne-Lotrimin, Mycelex) and generic versions; all but Monistat 3 are used for seven days. *Butoconazole* (Femstat), a three-day cream, is now available without prescription; studies involving 600 women showed it worked as well as seven days of miconazole. A one-dose ointment, *tioconazole* (Vagistat-1), is now sold over the counter. Non–*C. albicans* infections, or those resistant to "azole" drugs, may be treated with intravaginal boric acid capsules.

However, women with recurrent infections (or complicating diseases) may need a seven-day regimen. The usual dose of 100 milligrams (mg) of clotrimazole daily for seven days or 100 mg twice a day for three days will clear up most yeast infections. Some preparations include both suppositories to be used at night and topical cream to relieve discomfort during the day. "Anti-itch" creams containing benzocaine do not cure yeast infections but can help relieve external symptoms. In some recurrent cases three weeks of topical therapy may be given.

Stronger, prescription-only vaginal creams include *terconazole* (Terazol), *nystatin* (Mycostatin, Nilstat, Nystex) and nystatin plus *triamcinolone* (Mycolog), which contains both a fungicide and a steroid. Single-dose oral prescription antifungal medications, *ketoconazole* (Nizoral) and *fluconazole* (Diflucan), are most often used for recurrent yeast infections. A recent study of 419 women at the University of Minnesota found a single 150 mg dose of oral ketoconazole slightly more effective than a seven-day course of vaginal clotrimazole. However, oral medications can take several days to relieve symptoms, while creams and suppositories start acting directly on fungal infections and ease discomfort more quickly. Fluconazole can also cause side effects, including nausea, stomach pain and headaches. It should not be taken by pregnant or nursing women or those with kidney or liver disorders. Fluconazole can interact with other medications.

Although all these antifungal agents are between 80 and 85 percent effective, they will not eliminate underlying conditions, including allergic responses, that promote yeast infections. In such cases antihistamines or other drugs may be used.

Women who've had uncomplicated yeast infections before and know the symptoms can generally use over-the-counter creams and suppositories without consulting a physician. But if you've never had symptoms before or they are especially severe, it's wise to see your gynecologist. "Irritation and itching can be a sign of other conditions. Using antifungal medications may irritate things further and delay an accurate diagnosis," notes Dr. Wolf. In fact, a 1997 Temple University study found that only 28 percent of women who thought they had yeast infections actually had them, and in 15 percent over-the-counter medications acted as an irritant. If these preparations don't bring relief in a few days, call your physician.

A vaginal suppository or cream, used days five through ten of the menstrual cycle, or oral medication for days one through five for three to four months, may be given as preventive regimen for recurrent yeast vaginitis. Women susceptible to yeast infections may be advised to use antifungal vaginal cream when they take antibiotics.

Although yeast infections are not usually transmitted sexually, a male partner (especially if he's uncircumcised) may develop a rash and itching on his penis and scrotum as well as urethral inflammation. A woman's partner may also need treatment to prevent her from being reinfected; men can use a little antifungal vaginal cream on the affected areas. Women should avoid sexual intercourse, even with condoms, while being treated for a yeast infection. Some vaginal antiyeast creams and suppositories, including butoconazole, miconozole, tioconazole and terconazole, are oil-based and can weaken latex condoms.

▪ Preventing Problems ▪

There are commonsense precautions that may help avoid yeast infections or prevent recurrences. Gynecologist Susan Klugman, M.D., calls this *peri-care.* The perineal area should *always* be wiped front to back. "In addition to bacteria that can cause urinary tract infections, stool contains yeast, which can get into the vagina and cause infection," says Dr. Klugman, an assistant clinical professor of OB/GYN at the Albert Einstein College of Medicine in New York City. "I also suggest women use fragrance-free nonalcohol baby wipes or moistened adult wipes to clean the perineal area. I have seen an improvement in women with recurrent yeast infections who regularly use wipes."

External hemorrhoids can also harbor yeast and bacteria and require extra cleansing. Hemorrhoid pads contain witch hazel, which can be soothing to irritated tissues.

Gentle cleansing of the vulva and vaginal area with mild soap and water every day is important, as is keeping the area dry since excess moisture is a perfect breeding ground for yeast. Powdering can help, but stick with cornstarch baby powder.

Wearing panty hose and panties with cotton crotches is recommended. Nylon and other synthetics do not "breathe," so the fabric retains moisture and traps heat, creating an ideal environment for yeast to grow. Also, follow the advice your mother gave you about not sitting around in a wet bathing suit. If you've had a yeast infection, wash your panties in very hot water, since *Candida* may survive laundering in cold or warm water. To keep air circulating in the genital area at night, wear nightgowns or nightshirts instead of pajamas (no panties in bed).

The age-old remedy of eating yogurt with active cultures of *Lactobacillus acidophilus* (a slightly different type of lactobacillus) may work. A small 1996 study from Israel found that eating yogurt with live *L. acidophilus* cultures every day not only cut down the number of yeast infections but also reduced episodes of bacterial vaginosis (see below). Some experts believe *L. acidophilus* increases regrowth of vaginal lactobacillus. Studies also suggest that reducing sugar and complex carbohydrates in the diet may help control yeast infections.

Women should generally avoid douching since that flushes away friendly lactobacillus and it can be harmful during an active infection. (A 1997 study suggests douching may increase the risk of ectopic pregnancy.) "When there's an abnormal vaginal discharge, douching can actually help the bacteria or yeast reach the upper genital tract, through the cervix, into the uterus and even into the tubes, causing an ascending infection," cautions Dr. Klugman. An advisory committee to the U.S. Food and Drug Administration issued a statement in 1997 saying that douching may increase the risk of pelvic inflammatory disease (PID) and ectopic, or tubal, pregnancy. So, if you wish to douche, do so infrequently and use a vinegar and water preparation.

▪ Bacterial Vaginosis ▪

Bacterial vaginosis (BV), the second most common cause of vaginitis, is something of a medical mystery. BV was once thought to be caused by the bacterium *Gardnerella vaginalis*. But *Gardnerella* is found in normal vaginal secretions in up to 50 percent of women with no signs of infection and in *higher* concentrations in women with BV, which often has no symptoms.

"It's now generally accepted that some change in the vaginal ecology leading to a decline in lactobacillus may allow *Gardnerella* to multiply. But it is not clear *how* bacterial vaginosis actually develops," says Barbara J. Berger, M.D., an infectious disease specialist and assistant professor of clinical medicine at the Albert Einstein College of Medicine. Frequent douching may predispose a woman to BV because it flushes out lactobacillus. Several other types of bacterium, including *Mycoplasma hominus*, are also associated with BV. Between 10 and 64 percent of women have bacterial vaginosis at some time, many of them with no symptoms.

The most common symptom is a thin gray-white discharge that can irritate the vagina and the vulva and has an unpleasant fishy odor. The discharge can be profuse. There may be burning with urination and painful intercourse.

BV is diagnosed by assessing the pH of the vagina (greater than 4.5 indicates risk), then by adding a drop of alkali solution to a sample of vaginal secretion; the fishy odor will be intensified. This is aptly called a "Whiff test." Finally, when examined under a microscope, vaginal cells may appear covered with polka dots (these are bacteria) and are termed "clue cells."

Bacterial vaginosis is usually treated with 500 mg of oral metronidazole (Flagyl) or 300 mg of *clindamycin* (Cleocin), twice a day for a week. Oral metronidazole can also be given in a single 2-gram dose. Metronidazole topical gel (Metrogel-Vaginal) is inserted into the vagina once or twice a day for five days; clindamycin cream is used at bedtime for seven days. A 1995 study found equal cure rates for oral metronidazole, its topical gel and clindamycin cream.

Topical medications need to be inserted high into the vagina and used for the full prescribed time to prevent recurrence. Treatment can be carried out during the menstrual period, but tampons should be avoided since they may soak up the medication. Because the bacteria associated with BV are present in vaginal secretions, it's theoretically possible to pass them along sexually. Similar organisms have been cultured from male partners of women with BV, but there's no male equivalent. Recent randomized trials have shown no benefit in treating the male partner of a woman with BV. Moreover, treating partners does not prevent recurrence.

A small study performed by Dr. Berger and colleagues among lesbians suggests that bacterial vaginosis *can* be sexually transmitted, through contact with vaginal secretions. "Previous studies also show women who have a higher number of sexual partners are more likely to have bacterial vaginosis. BV is also increased in the presence of other sexually transmitted diseases, suggesting the associated bacteria may be sexually transmitted," Dr. Berger says.

Women with bacterial vaginosis are also more prone to infection by sexually transmitted pathogens because of the disruption in the normally protective vaginal environment. So when a woman is diagnosed with bacterial vaginosis, she is usually tested for the presence of other STDs.

Women who are *not* sexually active can sometimes have BV, since *Gardnerella* is so common. BV is associated with a number of gynecological problems, including pelvic inflammatory disease. But the most common complication involves pregnancy.

▪ *Bacterial Vaginosis and Preterm Delivery* ▪

Between 12 and 22 percent of pregnant women have bacterial vaginosis. If you're one of them, you may be at sharply increased risk of late miscarriage, preterm delivery or delivering a low-birth-weight baby.

A 1995 study published in the *New England Journal of Medicine* said that BV may be responsible for about 6 percent of the 440,000 premature births that occur each year in the United States. The collaborative study by seven medical centers followed more than 10,000 pregnant women and found that women with vaginal infections were 40 percent more likely to deliver premature, low-birth-weight babies than were noninfected women. BV was found more often in black women, women over thirty-five and women who had previously experienced preterm deliveries. British researchers found that women diagnosed in the first sixteen weeks of pregnancy were most at risk for preterm labor.

How BV may trigger these problems is not clear. Evidence suggests that it causes infections of the upper genital tract and that bacteria linked to it may somehow get into the membranes surrounding the fetus or the amniotic fluid itself. One prominent researcher in the field, David A. Eschenbach, M.D., a professor of obstetrics and gynecology at the University of

Washington in Seattle, theorizes that premature labor may result from the presence of toxic proteins produced by the bacteria.

A randomized trial among 624 pregnant women at the University of Alabama, Birmingham found that treating BV with antibiotics substantially cut the risk of preterm delivery. Since most women don't know they have BV, the researchers say screening all pregnant women could prevent many preterm deliveries.

▪ *Trichomonas* ("Trich") Infections ▪

A "trich infection" is caused by a one-celled, sexually transmitted protozoan, *Trichomonas vaginalis*, that travels rapidly up the vagina, propelled by its tiny whiplike appendages. Trich infections cause 10 to 25 percent of all vaginitis, affecting as many as three million women a year.

Symptoms include a profuse yellow-green or grayish discharge (which can have a bad odor), severe itching, irritation and swelling of the vulvovaginal mucous membranes. There may also be frequent urination and pain on intercourse. (Men may have no symptoms or may experience discharge, irritation or burning with urination.) A diagnosis is made by examining the vaginal discharge in a drop of dilute salt solution under a microscope, so the organisms can be clearly seen, explains Dr. Leonard Wolf.

Between 15 and 25 percent of women may carry the organism for years without symptoms and are diagnosed only with a routine Pap smear. *Trichomonas* can remain dormant for years, with an asymptomatic woman developing an infection at any time. Up to 10 percent of men carry trich without any symptoms. *Trichomonas* is found more often in sexually active women, particularly those with multiple partners. "If you have a trich infection, tests should be done for other STDs, such as chlamydia and *gonorrhea*," cautions Dr. Wolf.

Trich infections are treated with oral metronidazole (Flagyl, Metryl, Protostat), either 500 mg twice a day for seven days or a single dose of 1.5 to 2 grams. Both partners are treated, regardless of which is infected. In resistant cases both oral and topical metronidazole (250 gm) for five days is effective.

Drinking alcohol while being treated with metronidazole can cause severe nausea. Other side effects can include diarrhea, dry mouth, a metallic taste in the mouth and a decreased white blood cell count. Experts say metronidazole should be avoided during the first trimester of pregnancy but can safely be given after twenty weeks.

∞ *C h e l s e a ' s   S t o r y* ∞

"I was very sexually active in the 1970s, and I had several STDs. Genital herpes was really awful. I had this huge sore on my labia. It was so bad I couldn't go the bathroom.

"It seemed like I was having outbreaks every six weeks. It was painful, and it was embarrassing. I had one boyfriend who, after I told him, I never heard from again. As scrupulous as I tried to be, I know I gave it to at least four men.

"The worst was that my husband got it from me. And he had it really bad. There were times we both had outbreaks and couldn't even make love. Thankfully, oral acyclovir really helped him."

▪ Genital Herpes ▪

At least 170,000 people contract genital herpes each year. Herpes viruses attack the moist skin surfaces and mucous membranes of the body, such as the mouth and vulva, and are mostly spread by skin-to-skin contact with an active lesion that is "shedding" virus. However, asymptomatic viral shedding can also take place. Though less dangerous than syphilis or AIDS, herpes is painful and can pose some risks to a fetus during delivery.

Eighty percent of genital herpes infections are caused by *herpes simplex-2 (HSV-2)*, and the remainder are caused by *herpes simplex-1 (HSV-1)*, which also causes sores around the mouth and nose. "Around 70 percent of the adult U.S. population have antibodies to HSV-1, about 20 percent of American adults have antibodies to HSV-2, which means they have been infected and are potentially infectious," says William M. McCormack, M.D., chief of Infectious Diseases at the State University of New York (SUNY) Health Sciences Center in Brooklyn. "Most people infected with HSV-2 don't even know it and in fact, most transmission occurs between people who are unaware they've been infected."

There's a high risk of contracting genital herpes from sexual intercourse with an individual who has active herpes lesions. Kissing a person with cold sores or lesions can also transmit herpes; oral-genital sex can also transmit virus from the lips to the genitals or vice versa. (You can infect the membranes around the eyes by touching sores with your hands, then rubbing your eyes.)

Symptoms typically appear within two to seven days following exposure. The infected area first tingles, then itches. Multiple tiny blisters begin to appear on the vagina, vulva, clitoris and even cervix as well as the anal area and the buttocks. They rupture within a day or two and can be painful; if they become infected, they can form large ulcers.

From 10 to 20 percent of people may have extra-genital symptoms during the initial outbreak, including headache, aches and fever and tender, swollen lymph nodes in the groin. Women have more severe symptoms than men, along with profuse vaginal discharge and painful urination. Herpes sores usually heal within a week to three weeks with no scars (infected lesions may take longer). Recurrences are frequent with both types of genital herpes.

There's no cure for herpes, but symptoms and outbreaks can be treated by antiviral agents, most commonly *acyclovir* (Zovirax). Acyclovir is used most often and comes as a topical ointment or an oral or intravenous medication. It attacks the virus's ability to replicate, eliminating it everywhere but in the central nervous system (in *sensory ganglia*) where it hides between outbreaks.

Oral acyclovir is usually given in a 200 mg dose five times a day for a week to ten days (or until symptoms are resolved) during a first episode. It is taken two to five times a day (depending on the dose) for recurrences; it can cut in half the time a person is contagious and reduce healing time. Side effects include nausea, headaches and diarrhea.

Newer oral antiviral drugs—*famciclovir* (Famvir) and *valaciclovir* (Valtrex)—are absorbed into the body and then convert to active medication. They both are taken twice a day and have been approved by the FDA for recurrent herpes; Famvir has been approved for initial episodes.

Prophylactic treatment is usually given to people who have six or more herpes outbreaks a year. Taken preventively twice a day, acyclovir can reduce the number of outbreaks and their duration and prevents viral shedding when there are no lesions.

Topical acyclovir is effective in reducing the length of an outbreak but has no effect on the incidence of recurrent herpes.

Other new drugs include the topical *edoxudine* (Virostat) and *alpha-interferon* (Exovir), which reduced viral shedding and relieved symptoms of recurrent herpes in Canadian trials.

Secondary bacterial infections of open genital herpes sores can be prevented by keeping the area clean and dry: Wash gently with mild soap and water, and dry with a blow dryer set on "cool," rather than a towel, which can spread the virus. Local anesthetics, such as *lidocaine* and *xylocaine*, can help lessen pain.

Tests are being conducted into a potential vaccine for HSV-2. But until there's a vaccine, prevention is vital. Remember, herpes can be passed along when there's just itching or tingling. If a person has a mouth or genital sore, there should be no kissing, no oral to genital contact and no intercourse until the sore is healed. Contraceptive jellies or condoms *don't* prevent HSV transmission during an outbreak, Condoms must be put on before *any* genital contact.

▪ Complications During Pregnancy ▪

Active herpes can cause complications during pregnancy. An initial attack in the first trimester may increase miscarriage risk; later in pregnancy it may elevate the risk of premature delivery.

Herpes doesn't cross the placenta, but it can be transmitted during vaginal delivery; women with active lesions should undergo cesarean section. It has been suggested that even asymptomatic women can transmit infection; one study showed that 39 of 56 women who delivered HSV-infected infants had no signs of herpes at the time of birth. Herpes can overpower a newborn's undeveloped immune system; one in six babies with herpes dies, and others suffer brain damage. A 1997 study of more than 8,500 women by the University of Washington, Seattle, found that women who acquire herpes infections late in pregnancy are more likely to pass infections along to their newborns, because there's not enough time for antibodies against the virus to be formed and passed along to the fetus, giving it some degree of protection. Asymptomatic shedding in women with longstanding HSV infections (or viral antibodies) rarely results in newborn infections. But many obstetricians perform C-sections on women with herpes as a precaution.

∞ *D a n a ' s   S t o r y* ∞

"It felt like my vulva and vagina had been dipped in a vat of acid. The pain came on slowly after a yeast infection about five years ago. The pain became unrelenting. I saw seventeen different doctors over a two-year period. I went through horrible pain with biopsies, which took forever to heal, and they turned up nothing. Doctors gave me steroid creams, lotions, gels, douches, and absolutely nothing worked. My intimate life with my husband virtually died. You don't even want someone to touch you, to hold you. Forget about sex.

"I finally found a doctor who said, 'Let's try estrogen cream before we consider surgery.' I put it on twice a day, not inside but outside the vagina.

I did that for months. Amazingly it helped. It didn't get better overnight, but it's been quite remarkable. My vaginal area is normal now. And my sex life is now back to what it was. I regard this as no less than a miracle!"

▪ Vulvodynia ▪

As many as 150,000 to 200,000 women suffer from vulvodynia, a chronic irritation, rawness and pain in the vulva, the labia or the *vulvar vestibule* (a crescent-shaped area around the vaginal opening). The constant burning pain often makes it difficult to sit, work at a desk, exercise or even wear panty hose. Some women experience severe pain externally; others have deep pain during intercourse. Some women may have a tender redness visible in the vulvar area (erythema). According to the National Vulvodynia Association (NVA), about half the women with the disorder are under forty; 15 percent are sixteen or older. Moreover, 40 percent consulted an average of five doctors before being correctly diagnosed.

Pain in the vulvar area can have many causes, including dermatological conditions and genital herpes, according to Dr. Leonard Wolf. Lupus and *Crohn's disease* can also trigger lesions on the vulvar and vaginal mucosa. The Skene's or Bartholin's glands may be inflamed or blocked, causing pain. Many vulvodynia patients have tiny *vascular lesions,* patches of inflamed surface blood vessels, or inflammation of the glands and nerve endings in the vestibule area. However, many cases appear to have no discernible medical cause (*essential vulvodynia*).

Some of these women have a condition called *vulvar vestibulitis syndrome (VVS),* in which there is extreme pain when the area is even touched lightly with a cotton swab and pain with sexual intercourse. Some experts believe VVS may be associated with *pudendal neuralgia,* an irritation of the pudendal nerve or its branches. The theory is that chronic low-level irritation of pudendal nerves or *nocireceptor* nerve fibers in skin or mucosa (which transmit burning and itching) may make them extremely sensitive, eventually causing abnormal "firing" and excruciating pain. "Irritation of nerves in the vestibule may result from laser surgery, injury or treatments to remove genital warts," says Stanley C. Marinoff, M.D., director of the Center for Vulvovaginal Disorders, Washington, D.C. However, he points out that human papilloma virus (while associated with VVS) does *not* cause vulvar vestibulitis.

Nerve or muscle fiber irritation may also occur in other chronic pain syndromes, to which vulvodynia may be linked, according to Dr. Marinoff. Preliminary data from a patient survey by the NVA found 35 percent of women with vulvodynia also had symptoms of *fibromyalgia* (generalized muscle pain), 50 percent had *irritable bowel syndrome* and many had interstitial cystitis (page 130).

A recent report in the *Journal of Women's Health* found vulvar vestibulitis was more common among white women and among women with recurrent yeast infections. But yeast infections don't *cause* vestibulitis, stresses John Willems, M.D., a gynecologist at the Scripps Clinic and Research Foundation in La Jolla, California, who specializes in treating vulvar pain. "It may well be that women with certain skin types, thinner fair skin that is easily irritated, who have chronic exposure to an irritant like *Candida* or stronger medications for recurrent yeast infections, may become sensitized and eventually develop chronic pain," Dr. Willems says.

Some women with VVS also develop pelvic floor muscle tension and pain. "Once you have inflammation of the vestibule that causes pain with intercourse, your muscles contract in self-defense. The contraction becomes constant and can produce a chronic burning pain in the muscles," explains Dr. Willems. The pain may lead to *vaginismus*, a recurrent, *involuntary* spasm and constriction of the muscles surrounding the vagina. These muscle contractions can be severe and can prevent penetration. A 1996 study at the Oregon Health Sciences University's Vulvar Pain Clinic of women treated the previous year found that vaginismus was a primary or secondary factor in almost half the cases.

Other researchers say vulvodynia may be linked to a sensitivity to *oxalate*, a chemical related to vitamin C that is known to stimulate pain fibers. Clive C. Solomons, Ph.D., an independent biomedical researcher in Denver, Colorado, believes that an oxalate imbalance can lead to vulvodynia or urinary tract irritation in some women, perhaps leaching into tissues and irritating the nerves. "In interstitial cystitis the irritation may occur in the bladder; in vulvodynia the chronic irritation is in the vulvar area," he says. Many women with vulvodynia also have *irritable bowel syndrome* and sensitive skin.

Oxalate is found in many fruits and vegetables, so diet may be related to this chemical sensitivity. Foods like rhubarb, parsley, spinach and peanuts (see list on page 127) may add to oxalate already present in the body. "Antibiotics and oral antifungal agents, which are often prescribed for women with vulvar pain, can kill a bacterium in the intestine, which normally destroys oxalate," says Dr. Solomons.

Since 1991 Dr. Solomons has been conducting studies among large numbers of women with vulvar vestibulitis using a low-oxalate diet, timed doses of *calcium citrate* and Oxabsorb, a gel capsule that's believed to absorb oxalate so it is excreted in feces rather than urine. The newest phase of the study uses a topical preparation (N-Acetylglucosamine) to help maintain moisture in the skin, improving its resilience and perhaps reducing nerve irritation. He reports that over 70 percent of the more than 1,000 women on the treatment regimen experienced sustained relief of vulvar pain and increased functioning. However, the therapy takes four to nine months on average, and some women do have treatable recurrences. There have been no large, double-blinded, clinical trials of the therapy.

▪ Diagnosis and Treatments ▪

A workup for vulvodynia may include examination of the vulva with *colposcopy,* a biopsy of any lesion to rule out malignancy, an examination of the Bartholin's glands and the levator ani muscles for problems, says Dr. Wolf. Finding painful hypersensitivity (*allodynia*) to light touch in the vestibule area, redness and inflammation indicates vulvar vestibulitis. Some practitioners have begun measuring oxalate levels in urine samples over a twenty-four-hour period in patients with vestibulitis.

Conservative treatments for vulvar pain include small doses of the antidepressants *amitriptyline* (Elavil) or fluoxetine (Prozac), which may work by preventing fast reabsorption of brain chemicals thought to mediate pain. Injections of *alpha-2-B interferon* around the vestibule three times a week for four weeks may also help 30 to 40 percent of women with vulvar vestibulitis, according to Dr. Marinoff. Long-term topical use of 0.01 percent estrogen cream can help some women with vulvar vestibulitis. A dab applied to the vulvar vestibule twice a day thickens epithelial tissue, rebuilds connective tissue and appears to make it more resistant to irritants, notes Dr. Willems. Biofeedback-directed exercises and physical therapy to relax and rehabilitate the vulvar area muscles are also helpful for women with muscle tension and pain. Dr. Willems has followed patients with vulvar vestibulitis for more than thirty months and found an 88 percent success rate with topical estrogen, pelvic floor exercises and a reduced oxalate diet.

Occasionally patients with vulvar vestibulitis can be helped by *perineoplasty* or *vestibulectomy,* surgery to remove a small amount of tissue (and sometimes tiny glands) around the vulvar vestibule, pulling some of the vaginal skin over the area, which eventually toughens. A 1995 Johns Hopkins study of 93 patients who had failed previous therapies found that more than half the women had complete relief of symptoms two years after perineoplasty surgery, 30 percent had partial relief, 4 percent reported worsening of pain and 7 percent found no change.

Surgery is undertaken *only* as a last resort, and complete healing can take months, cautions Dr. Wolf. Laser treatments for vulvar vestibulitis are extremely controversial. While lasers have helped some women, many others have suffered damage and disfigurement, and such treatments are generally not recommended. "Try conservative medical therapy first, for eighteen months at least. Surgery or laser treatments often produce more pain than they cure," advises Dr. Willems.

The Vulvar Pain Foundation (VPF), a patient support and advocacy group, reports that many of its members who have failed such medical treatments have been helped by the low–oxalate-calcium citrate therapy or biofeedback-directed pelvic floor exercises and physical therapy. Practical measures from the VPF include: wearing thigh-high or Scanty Hose (hip-high stockings attached to a garter belt), to avoid the moisture and heat accumulation in the crotch caused by panty hose; sitting slightly forward when urinating to avoid urine contact with the vulva; using a squeeze bottle of warm water to rinse the area after urination; taking oatmeal or tea sitz baths and using soft, absorbent cotton for menstrual pads.

▪ Vulvar Dermatoses/Skin Problems ▪

Common skin disorders that cause redness, itching and lesions elsewhere in the body can also affect the vulvar area.

CONTACT DERMATITIS is caused by direct irritation or an allergic reaction from a variety of substances, even genital care products, such as vaginal creams, says Robin Ashinoff, M.D., an assistant professor of clinical dermatology at NYU Medical Center. Major culprits for contact dermatitis include alcohol, contained in many cleansing products; *propylene glycol,* an ingredient in many creams, and laundry detergents and fabric softeners, which can leave residues on underwear. "Body washes" containing *alpha hydroxy acids* can dry and irritate skin in the genital area. Chronic contact with urine caused by incontinence can also cause vulvar irritation.

Potential *allergens* include fragrances, formaldehyde in nail polishes and fabric softeners, topical Benadryl and, in rare cases, benzocaine (often used to stop itching) as well as the latex used in condoms. Reactions may appear two to three days after the first exposure as the body becomes sensitized to the substance. If you develop a rash or irritation, make a list of products that may have come in contact with the area, and stop using any potential offender. Allergic dermatitis can take up to three weeks to clear up.

Sitz baths or using compresses soaked in *Burows solution*, aluminum acetate tablets or powder combined with cool water, several times a day can provide symptomatic relief. Use of a squeeze bottle and warm water to rinse the vulva after urinating may also help, as can short-term use of *corticosteroid* creams.

PSORIASIS, a common skin condition characterized by redness, scaling and itching, can erupt on the mons, the labia and the anal area. Although men can get psoriasis on their penises, it is not infectious. It is a chronic (sometimes inherited) condition that can be controlled but not cured. Treatment usually consists of soaks and topical corticosteroids.

ECZEMA, or *atopic dermatitis*, is another common skin condition that can occur in the vulvar area. Symptoms include redness, burning, itching and dryness of the vulva. Low-dose topical corticosteroids are the treatment of choice, but avoid long-term use in the vaginal area. "Because these are mucosal tissues, without the protective *stratum corneum* layer that skin has, much more of the steroids are absorbed. This can lead to thinning of the tissue, making it more prone to irritation," cautions Dr. Ashinoff.

LICHEN SIMPLEX CHRONICUS is a skin condition provoked by chronic itching, perhaps caused by an irritant or a yeast infection. "What happens is called the itch-scratch cycle. The more you scratch it, the more it itches, and the more you scratch, the more irritation you cause," explains Dr. Ashinoff. "Eventually the skin thickens, taking on an almost leathery appearance." There may also be whitish patches or tiny nodules. To treat lichen simplex and break the itch-scratch cycle, topical corticosteroids and sometimes antihistamines are used.

LICHEN PLANUS is a disease of skin and mucosal tissues, producing severe itching, white, pimplelike lesions in the vulva and vagina and white, flat-topped lesions in the perineal area (sometimes discharge streaked with blood) and sometimes even lesions in the mouth. "Lichen planus can become erosive and very painful. As it heals, it can cause scarring and even closure of the lips, when two erosive areas adhere to each other. It can be very difficult to treat," says Dr. Ashinoff. Initial complaints may be chronic burning and itching in the vulvar area. Most often seen in women over forty, lichen planus is treated with medium- or high-potency topical steroids and, sometimes, systemic corticosteroids or injections.

LICHEN SCLEROSUS is a chronic skin disorder that affects mostly postmenopausal women. It usually appears in a classic hourglass pattern from the clitoris into the labia, then outward around the anus, producing ivory-colored patches and pink erosions in the anal area. The earliest symptom is usually itching, which worsens as the disease progresses (some women have no early symptoms). The skin becomes fragile and vulnerable to trauma, which can result in areas of hemorrhage and abrasions. Treatment includes emollients, topical steroids, low-dose progesterone or testosterone creams and lubricants during intercourse. Usually chronic, in rare cases the disease can develop into *squamous cell carcinoma*, so long-term follow-up is needed.

HIDRADENITIS SUPPURATIVA is a severe acnelike condition that arises when an *apocrine* gland (a sweat gland) or a hair follicle is blocked and produces a cyst in the *axilla* (the fold between the arm and the body), the *gluteal* skin (your buttocks), the vulva and perineum. Rupture of this painful nodule causes inflammation, and bacteria in the area may infect the inflamed or broken skin. Like severe acne, it can cause abscesses and scarring. The condition begins after puberty and can continue well into the thirties. As in severe acne, oral *retinoids*, such as *isotretinoin* (Accutane), and corticosteroids may be helpful. Careful cleansing of the broken skin is important to avoid bacterial "superinfection." When medication fails, surgical removal of nodules may be needed.

PEMPHIGUS VULGARIS is an autoimmune blistering disorder that mostly affects women of Mediterranean or Jewish origin. "In this case the body is attacking the intercellular cement, the area that holds cells together," explains Dr. Ashinoff. "The cells separate and fall apart, causing open blisters and open wounds."

Pemphigus may first appear as oral blisters, followed by blisters elsewhere on the skin and mucosa, including the vulva. Diagnosed with a skin biopsy, it's usually treated with *prednisone*, an oral steroid, in combination with low-dose *methotrexate*, a chemotherapy drug with anti-inflammatory properties, and *azathioprine* (Imuran), an immunosuppressant.

SCABIES AND PUBIC LICE are two tiny insects that can infest the groin and pubic area and cause itching. The mite *Sarcoptes scabiei* is transmitted by skin-to-skin or sexual contact. The tiny female mite lays eggs and deposits feces in the skin, producing a reaction. *Phthirus pubis*, similar to head lice, lays its eggs in the skin, causing itching. The area shows tiny dark lice and dandrufflike nits. Lice can be treated with a *permethrin* cream (Elimite); scabies is also treated with *lindane* (Scabene). Clothing and bed linen should be laundered in hot water and dried on a hot setting to kill any remaining pests.

SKIN CANCERS, including *basal cell* and squamous cell *carcinomas*, can occur in the genital area. Some women have pigmented areas and moles on the vulva and perineum that can develop into *melanoma*. Such areas should be examined during your regular gynecologic exam. If there's any change in size or color or any bleeding or itching, a biopsy should be done.

Bowenoid papulosis is a genital skin cancer, caused by type 16 and 18 human papilloma virus (HPV, see page 151). Bowenoid lesions look like genital warts but are actually squamous cell carcinoma in situ. It's not an invasive cancer, and it does not metastasize, but it has a high rate of recurrence. Bowenoid papulosis lesions are destroyed with a laser or by freezing and treated with low-dose fluorouracil (5-FU) cream once a week for six months. Even in low doses the cream can cause severe irritation. "Since these subsets of HPV also cause cervical cancer, these woman also need more frequent Pap smears," says Dr. Ashinoff.

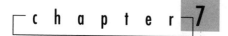

Trouble in the Urinary Tract

Most of us don't think much about urinating until there's trouble in the urinary tract, but such problems are incredibly common. Every year perhaps 24 million women suffer *lower urinary tract infections (UTIs)*, or *cystitis*. Many others have *urinary tract irritability* or *hypersensitivity syndrome*, which triggers many of the symptoms of a UTI but without an infection.

Between 200,000 and 500,000 women suffer from an inflammatory condition called *interstitial cystitis* (IC), which damages the lining of the bladder, triggering urination as often as fifty to sixty times a day, causing pelvic pain and painful intercourse.

More than 11 million women in North America suffer from *incontinence*, or loss of bladder control, and it's not always a consequence of older age. According to the Bladder Health Council, around 30 percent of women experience incontinence before the age of thirty-five because of disease or nerve damage. Unlike UTIs, which usually send women to the doctor, more than half of women with incontinence keep it secret and suffer in silence. Many are embarrassed and don't know that they can be treated.

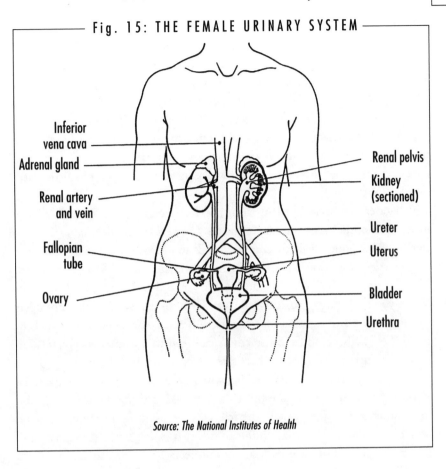

Fig. 15: THE FEMALE URINARY SYSTEM

Inferior vena cava
Adrenal gland
Renal artery and vein
Fallopian tube
Ovary

Renal pelvis
Kidney (sectioned)
Ureter
Uterus
Bladder
Urethra

Source: The National Institutes of Health

▪ How Your Urinary System Works ▪

The *urinary tract* consists of the *kidneys*, which filter waste and water from the blood as urine; the *bladder*, a muscular, balloonlike chamber that stores urine; the *ureters*, two tubes that transport urine from the kidneys to the bladder, and the *urethra*, a flat tube of smooth muscle that is connected to the *bladder neck* and carries urine outside the body. The bladder and urethra (and nearby reproductive organs) are held firmly in place by a hammock of muscles and supporting tissues, strung from the pubic bone to the tailbone, forming the *pelvic floor*.

Urination is a *voluntary* process, controlled by the sphincter muscles and several sets of nerves. Most of the time these sphincters tightly close off the neck of the bladder and urethra, sealing in urine, explains Victor W. Nitti, M.D., an assistant professor of urology and director of Female Urology at

NYU Medical Center. The kidneys constantly produce urine, filling the bladder slowly, until it fully distends. When the bladder is full, sensory nerves send a message to the spinal cord, which transmits the signal to the brain. The brain then sends a message back down the spinal cord and out through the *pudendal nerve* (which serves the genital area) to the *external sphincter*, a "voluntary" muscle, which we can "tell" to relax or tighten. If you're not near a bathroom, you tell the sphincter muscle to contract and hold in the urine. When you do urinate, "you allow the external sphincter to relax and open. At the same time, the bladder wall contracts to help force urine out," says Dr. Nitti.

Bladder contractions stem from another set of nerves. The bladder is made of smooth "nonvoluntary" muscle. The *para-sympathetic nervous system* signals the bladder wall to contract, and another set of signals from the *sympathetic nerve system* tells the internal sphincter of the bladder to open. When it does, it pulls the bladder neck open and urine is pushed through. When you're through urinating, the bladder stops contracting, the sphincters squeeze closed and the urethra folds flat. All this must be perfectly synchronized. Overactive bladder contractions can lead to a *voiding dysfunction*, an urgency to urinate even when there's very little in the bladder (see page 126).

Normally urine is slightly acidic, which inhibits the growth of bacteria. Various problems can tip the pH balance, making urine more alkaline and more amenable to the growth of bacteria. Leaving urine in the bladder too long or not taking in enough fluids to dilute it causes urine to stagnate and fosters the growth of bacteria, leading to infections or inflammation.

Cystitis means inflammation of the urinary tract. The most frequent cause is *acute uncomplicated bacterial cystitis*, an infection of the *lower* urinary tract, the urethra and bladder. Inflammation of the urethra alone is called *urethritis*.

By age thirty half of all women will have suffered at least one UTI. While they are bothersome, UTIs are usually easily treated with antibiotics. About 20 percent of women who've had one UTI will suffer infections four or five times a year. African-American women are more than five times more likely to suffer UTIs than white women.

Left untreated, bladder infections can spread to the kidneys, causing *pyelonephritis*, which can have serious consequences. With repeated infections the kidneys gradually lose their ability to function, and waste products build up in the body. This can be fatal if unchecked. Women suffer 250,000 cases of pyelonephritis each year.

▪ Urinary Tract Infections ▪

Women are especially prone to lower UTIs by virtue of their anatomy. For one thing, a woman's urethra is only three inches and is straight. "The genital area is very rich in all kinds of bacteria. So it's a short, easy trip for bacteria up the urethra into the bladder," remarks Dr. Nitti. "Bacteria may be present normally in urine; infection occurs when they adhere to the bladder wall."

Because the vaginal walls are so close to the urethra and the base of the bladder, they can become swollen and irritated as a result of repeated intercourse (hence "honeymoon cystitis"). Bacteria can also be forced into the urethra by thrusting of the penis during intercourse. Lower UTIs have also been linked with use of diaphragms and the spermicide *nonoxynol-9*. A diaphragm that's too big may temporarily constrict urine flow by squeezing the bladder neck, so the bladder may not empty fully. Spermicide can attack lactobacillus in the vagina, allowing bacteria to grow and enter the urethra. The result: a UTI after making love. Not surprisingly a recent study found that the more frequently you have intercourse, the more acute UTIs you're likely to have.

The outlet of the urethra (the *external urethral orifice*), is located just above the vagina, exposing it to discharge from infections like *Candida*, which can cause urethritis. Vaginitis can cause "external" burning during urination, as urine touches the inflamed vulva. Sexually transmitted diseases like chlamydia can inflame, damage and scar the urethral lining just as they do reproductive organs, causing "internal" burning on urination. STDs need to be treated with appropriate antibiotics (see Chapter Eight).

A 1995 study of federal health statistics in the *Journal of Women's Health* reported that women with diabetes were almost twice as likely to have UTIs as women without diabetes, due to underlying kidney disease and high blood sugar, which is linked to impaired immunity. Pregnant women are more prone to bladder infections because of hormonal changes and obstruction of the bladder by the expanding uterus. Even with the increase in urine output, many women are unable to empty their bladders completely.

Ninety percent of UTIs are caused by *Escherichia coli (E. coli)* or *Staphylococcus saprophyticus*, two types of bacterium that live in the gastrointestinal tract. These bacteria can colonize the perineum and the vulva, migrating up the urethra, when a woman wipes back to front. Once in the bladder, bacteria reproduce rapidly and inflame the usually sterile environment. This causes abnormal contractions, which triggers the feeling of having to pass urine immediately (often right after having gone to the bathroom) and irritates the urethra, causing a burning sensation during urination, or *dysuria*.

Other symptoms include a dull, aching pain just above the pubic bone; *hematuria*, blood in the urine, or *pyuria*, pus in the urine. The urine may appear pink or bloody or cloudy and dark.

Up to 5 percent of young, sexually active women and between 10 and 15 percent of women over age sixty have *no* physical symptoms of infection but have bacteria in their urine (*asymptomatic bacteriuria, ASB*). As many as 40 percent of women over sixty-five may also have blood (hematuria) or pus (pyuria) in their urine without symptoms. It's especially important to treat ASB during pregnancy since kidney infection can trigger premature labor (one reason urine is tested during prenatal visits). Between 20 and 40 percent of pregnant women with untreated ASB develop kidney infections. Symptoms of kidney infection include chills and fever above 101 degrees, pain and tenderness in the flanks (the area of the back just above the waist), nausea and vomiting.

Research presented at a 1994 conference on Women's Urological Health Research, sponsored by the National Institute of Diabetes and Digestive and Kidney Diseases (NIDDK), shed some light on why some women are prone to recurrent UTIs. When estrogen declines (either during the luteal phase of the menstrual cycle or after menopause) so do lactobacilli, which normally keep *E. coli* in check, said Walter E. Stamm, M.D., head of the Division of Allergy and Infectious Diseases at the University of Washington School of Medicine in Seattle. Lack of estrogen increases the vaginal pH, making it prone to colonization by *E. coli*. In fact, after menopause there's a "10-fold increase in acute uncomplicated cystitis," Dr. Stamm reported to the conference. (Replacement estrogen was found to help combat UTIs. See page 253.)

Among the 20 percent of women who suffer recurrent UTIs, repeated infections may result from a single strain of *E. coli*. "In that circumstance, treatment likely eradicates the strain of *E. coli* from the urinary tract, but not from the vaginal or fecal reservoir," Dr. Stamm noted. In such women the cells lining the urinary tract and the vagina may also be especially prone to enhanced bacterial attachment, contributing to their risk of recurrent infection. Other research presented at the conference indicated that some women belonging to blood groups (or secretor types) are at increased risk of UTIs.

This research has led to creation of a potential vaccine against UTIs. The vaccine creates immune system antibodies that block a protein *E. coli* uses to attach itself to the bladder wall. Instead of causing infection, the disabled bacteria are flushed out as the bladder empties. Animal tests found the vaccine effective against most strains of *E. coli*. It's now being tested in humans.

Treating Bacterial Cystitis

The initial burning pain and urgency of cystitis can often be relieved by drinking lots of water. But when a UTI takes hold or if there's blood in the urine (indicating the bladder is inflamed), medication is needed.

To diagnose a UTI, doctors culture a small sample of urine to grow and identify bacteria, to help them choose the most effective antibiotic. Among the antibiotics commonly used to treat *E. coli* bladder infections are *amoxicillin, ampicillin, cephalexin* (often used for UTIs during pregnancy), *nitrofurantoin* (Macrodantin) and sulfa drugs (for women allergic to penicillin or using oral contraceptives), such as *sulfisoxazole* (Gantrisin).

A new single-dose medication *fosfomycin tromethamine* (Monurol) was approved in 1997. It begins killing *E. coli* in two to four hours and remains highly concentrated in urine for more than three days. Research indicates that when bacteria on the bladder wall are continuously bathed in highly concentrated antibiotics, they're killed much more quickly.

Other antibiotics are now given for one to three days, instead of seven to ten days. However, experts say amoxicillin and *cephalosporins* appear to be *less* effective in single doses since they are rapidly excreted by the body. One- to three-day regimens are more effective using drugs like *trimethoprim-sulfamethoxazole* (Bactrim, Septra). If the infection is uncomplicated and confined to the lower urinary tract, shorter regimens can produce excellent cure rates without the side effects of longer treatment, such as vaginal yeast infections, says Dr. Nitti. Seven-day regimens are usually reserved for diabetic or pregnant women; longer courses are required to clear up bacterial kidney infections.

The anesthetic medication *phenazopyridine hydrochloride* (Pyridium), now in over-the-counter strength (Uristat), makes the urine less irritating (it also turns it orange), relieving both the urgency and burning, and is often given with antibiotics.

The Cranberry Connection

Recent research confirms that the old standby of cranberry juice *does* indeed help clear up a UTI. A trial at Brigham and Women's Hospital and

Harvard Medical School (funded by the Ocean Spray company) involved 153 women over sixty-five, randomly assigned to either a daily ten-ounce glass of cranberry juice or a taste-alike drink. Each woman gave a urine sample before the study began and once a month for the six-month study. The results: Cranberry juice *did* reduce the amount of bacteria and pus in the urine.

But it was not a cure-all; 15 percent of the monthly urine samples collected from the cranberry juice group contained bacteria and white blood cells, compared with over 28 percent of the women in the placebo group. Still, women drinking cranberry juice did have a 42 percent lower chance of contracting bacteriuria with pyuria than did the controls.

However, the study also found that the popular wisdom that cranberry juice makes urine more acidic and less hospitable to bacteria was *not* true. Instead the cranberry juice appears to act as an antiadhesive agent, preventing tiny, threadlike protrusions on the surface of *E. coli* (called *pili*) from sticking to the cells of the bladder wall. It should also be noted that for some women, cranberry juice can be a bladder *irritant* (page 127).

Preventing Cystitis

Simply drinking at least six to eight 8-ounce glasses of water each day is an effective way to prevent UTIs because it keeps urine diluted and causes more frequent urination, which flushes out any bacteria in the bladder. If you are getting adequate fluids, your urine will be pale yellow; concentrated urine is darker.

Women prone to UTIs should always try to empty their bladders completely when urinating, not allowing even a small amount of urine to pool in the bladder, where bacteria can grow, advises Dr. Nitti. Women should always wipe front to back. Always urinate after intercourse to flush out any bacteria that may have been pushed into the urethra. Women with recurrent UTIs are advised not to use diaphragms and spermicide. Experts say tampons are preferable to pads during menstruation since pads can provide an area where bacteria from the rectum can thrive. Women who use pads should change them frequently.

When UTIs Are Chronic

Chronic, recurrent UTIs may be caused by antibiotic-resistant bacteria; urinary stones in the kidney or bladder (formed by crystallization of substances in urine), which can harbor bacteria; a structural abnormality of the urinary tract or a kidney infection, says Dr. Nitti.

The workup usually includes a pelvic examination to make sure structures are normal, urinalysis, urine culture and ultrasound to look for residual urine in the bladder or the presence of stones. Sometimes cystoscopy, using a scope passed through the urethra to look at the bladder, may be part of the workup. An *intravenous pyelogram* uses an injected contrast dye that shows up on kidney X rays, to help identify congenital obstructions, stones or other abnormalities. Contrast dye may also reveal *diverticula*, tiny pockets that form in the wall of the urethra, which can harbor *E. coli* and other bacteria, leading to reinfection. These can be removed by surgery. Diverticula can also form in the bladder, as a result of a voiding dysfunction or blockage that increases pressure on the bladder, and may require more extensive surgery.

A common problem that's often overlooked in treating recurrent UTIs is infection of the paraurethral or Skene's glands, at the end of the urethral opening near the vagina, notes Dr. Nitti. Skene's glands secrete a small amount of mucus (along with other mucus-secreting glands), which helps keep the opening moist and lubricated for the passage of urine. These glands tend to become infected and filled with pus. "That pus can cause local pain and inflammation and can form a reservoir for bacteria to reinfect the urethra," says Dr. Nitti. Antibiotics can often clear up the infection, but in some women removal of Skene's glands may help prevent recurrent UTIs.

Voiding dysfunctions (see page 126) can also cause recurrent UTIs. However, when the urinary system is structurally normal and cystitis frequently recurs, there's no one preferred therapy. Some clinicians treat each recurrence with antibiotics, while others prescribe drugs such as Bactrim or Macrodantin in a low dose for six to eight weeks preventively. For younger women with recurrent bacterial cystitis, a number of studies have found that a preventive dose of antibiotic after intercourse could help deter recurrent UTIs.

The drawback to taking antibiotics frequently is the risk of yeast infections (since antibiotics can kill lactobacillus and allow *Candida* to overgrow). In rare cases drug-resistant infections can develop. In addition to a potential UTI vaccine, scientists are testing a vaginal suppository to "immunize" women with repeated UTIs against a variety of infection-causing organisms. Studies are also being done of lipstick-size culture tubes, so women with recurrent UTIs can check their urine bacterial level if they feel symptoms coming on and take a dose of antibiotics.

▪ Urinary Tract Irritability ▪

Some women with symptoms of cystitis who have no bacteria in their urine may have *chronic cystoureteritis,* urinary tract irritability, or a *dysfunctional voiding reflex,* causing a sense of urgency even though only a small amount of urine is actually in the bladder.

"With a dysfunctional voiding reflex you have an intense urge to go to the bathroom. You have increased pelvic muscle tension because you feel that if you don't hold on, the urine is going to leak out. Because the bladder isn't full, you don't trigger the bladder contraction and bladder outlet relaxation necessary for relaxed urination," says Tamara G. Bavendam, M.D., associate professor of urology at the Allegheny University of the Health Sciences in Philadelphia. "The result is that you feel the need to strain to get the urine out, and there's a feeling of incomplete bladder emptying. These women are spending all their time in the bathroom feeling like they need to go and having trouble getting the urine out, because of an inappropriate sensation."

Associated with this voiding dysfunction is a loss of voluntary control over the pelvic muscles; the muscles stay tight when they should be relaxed, Dr. Bavendam notes. Causes include childhood urinary tract problems, past pelvic surgery, thyroid problems and neurological diseases. The same nerves that supply the colon supply the bladder, so irritable bowel syndrome may be linked to an irritable bladder through common nerve pathways. "No matter what the inciting factor, something about the sensory pathways of the bladder got turned on, and they never came back down to normal," Dr. Bavendam says.

Gynecological problems, such as fibroids pressing on the bladder or hormonal fluctuations during the menstrual cycle can also cause these symptoms, so a woman may need both a gynecological and urological workup, notes Dr. Bavendam. Some women may have especially sensitive urethras. In such women dysuria and frequency can result from exercise, vibrations during long car rides or even pressure from a bicycle seat.

Many women were routinely treated with antibiotics for this condition, even though there was no infection, and some patients do feel better temporarily. "One reason is that every bottle of antibiotics says, 'Drink with plenty of water.' And water makes things better. You start filling the bladder up, the urine dilutes and you start urinating more easily," Dr. Bavendam points out. "When women stop taking the antibiotics, they go back to poor drinking habits, and their symptoms return."

Drinking enough water, developing good voiding habits and avoiding acidic or spicy foods (see box below) can help. "That doesn't mean that women can't have these foods. Even limited intake of bladder irritants offset by drinking more water can dramatically decrease symptoms," notes Dr. Bavendam.

A dietary supplement called Prelief can help neutralize acidic foods. Pyridium, Uristat or similar bladder analgesics may help relieve symptoms in some women. Also effective is bladder "retraining" to increase bladder capacity and decrease the frequency of urination. Women are instructed to drink at least a quart of water over the course of the day and urinate every three to four hours, keeping a diary of both fluid intake and voiding.

∞ *Urinary Irritants* ∞

Sources: Tamara G. Bavendam, M.D., Allegheny University of the Health Sciences; U.S. Department of Agriculture; Vulvar Pain Foundation.

The following foods can be bladder irritants and should be avoided or consumed in small amounts by those with irritable bladder problems, interstitial cystitis or vulvodynia. Experts suggest women keep track of all foods that provoke symptoms.

- All alcoholic beverages
- Apples/apple juice
- Carbonated beverages
- Chilis/spicy foods
- Chocolate
- Citrus fruits/juices
- Cranberries/cranberry juice
- Coffee (including decaffeinated)
- Grapes, guava
- Nutrasweet
- Peaches
- Pineapple

- Plums

- Strawberries

- Teas/citrus herbal teas

- Tomatoes

- Vinegar

- Vitamin B complex

The following foods are among those high in oxalate, which can accumulate in urine and cause irritation of vulvar tissues:

- Parsley

- Chives

- Spinach

- Rhubarb

- Beets

- Beans

- Watercress

- Radishes

- Cocoa

- Caffeinated coffee

- Peanuts

Alternatives include noncitrus herbal teas; fruits with a low acid and high water content, such as watermelon, papaya, pears and apricots, and such low-oxalate foods as ginger ale, zucchini, water chestnuts, wild rice, alfalfa sprouts and butter lettuce. For vitamin C, substitute calcium ascorbate cobuffered with calcium carbonate.

─── ๑ *V i c k i ' s   S t o r y* ๑ ───

"I came down with interstitial cystitis when I was in my thirties and a second-year medical student. I'd had urinary tract infections occasionally

in the past, so I was put on antibiotics. But my urine culture was negative, and the antibiotics did not help. This was very debilitating pain.

"*My doctor was no help. He assured me that it was just stress. I saw ten urologists, two allergists, two specialists in infectious diseases as well as several gynecologists. Most of them didn't know what I was talking about and attributed it, again, to stress. Some said I should quit medical school; some said I should get married; some said I should change boyfriends.*

"*Finally I went to the medical library and came across an article on interstitial cystitis. As soon as I read the first paragraph, I was sure that's what I had. I copied the article and brought it to my urologist, who totally dismissed it and said, 'you couldn't possibly have this. This is a disease of elderly, postmenopausal women.'*

"*There was a test described in the article that could make the diagnosis of IC, a cystoscopic bladder distension and biopsy done under general anesthesia. I really had to beg this doctor to do it. But he eventually gave in, and the diagnosis was made. Knowing I had IC was an enormous relief.*

"*I was treated with DMSO,* dimethyl sulfoxide, *one of the standard medicines used in this disease. It did help. At least temporarily it relieved some of the symptoms for me.*

"*We started the Interstitial Cystitis Association, and after the first few newspaper articles and stories about it we got thousands and thousands of letters. But it was a big struggle in the beginning because no one had heard of interstitial cystitis. The problem is we look healthy, and people say, 'Nothing bad could be wrong with you.' They don't know what our lives are like. Some women can't travel, can't even go to the local supermarket. Many women are unable to have intercourse.*

"*But we have made progress. In 1982 everyone thought this disease was psychosomatic. Now there's general acknowledgment that this disease is real and that the pain is debilitating and women need help. So I think we've come a long way.*"

Vicki Ratner, M.D., is the founder and president of the Interstitial Cystitis Association. The above remarks are taken from a personal interview and printed with her permission.

▪ Interstitial Cystitis ▪

Interstitial cystitis (IC) is a chronic inflammatory condition of the bladder that causes nerve endings to be irritated by elements in urine, resulting in pain on filling, so the bladder holds less urine. Some experts call the disorder *painful bladder syndrome*. Whatever it's called, it may affect as many as 500,000 women, and costs almost $2 billion a year in lost wages and medical care.

The exact cause is not known. Women with IC do not usually have bacteria in their urine. However, new types of molecular testing, which can detect remnants of bacterial DNA in the urine, may reveal the presence of bacteria that don't usually test positive in a typical urine culture, says Philip Hanno, M.D., professor and chairman of the Department of Urology at Temple University School of Medicine in Philadelphia.

Another theory is that the cells lining the bladder are somehow "leaky" in IC patients and allow substances in urine to penetrate the bladder wall, inflaming the bladder muscle. "There may also be something abnormal in the urine of some IC patients. A significant proportion of people who have had their bladders removed and have *continent urinary diversions* made out of a section of bowel develop pain and irritation in the storage pouch. So it may well be a problem with urine," says Dr. Hanno.

Other research suggests IC may be an autoimmune problem, in which the immune system attacks healthy bladder cells, producing inflammation. *Mast cells*, which play a role in allergies and inflammation, have turned up in bladder biopsies of some women with IC, and 40 percent of IC patients have allergies as well.

There may also be a connection with other inflammatory disorders. A recent study by Drs. Ratner and Hanno and colleagues at Temple University, found that 25 percent of women with IC have also been diagnosed with irritable bowel syndrome, almost 20 percent have migraine headaches and 13 percent had endometriosis. In addition, the Temple University study found that other IC patients have been diagnosed with (or have occasional symptoms of) fibromyalgia, ulcerative colitis, chronic fatigue, lupus and asthma. There are probably multiple causes, which may be different in different women, suggests Dr. Hanno.

The most common IC symptom is an urgent need to urinate, sometimes upward of sixty times over twenty-four hours. There's also a burning or cramping pelvic pain before and after urinating. Sixty percent of patients experience pain during or after intercourse, possibly the result of pelvic muscle spasms caused by irritation. Symptoms can be mild to severe, constant or intermittent.

The Temple University study of women with IC found that as many as 10 percent also had symptoms of vulvodynia (page 111). "Interstitial cystitis is really a 'diagnosis of exclusion.' We have to rule out all other causes, including benign or cancerous tumors," says Dr. Hanno. According to diagnostic criteria set by the National Institute of Diabetes and Digestive and Kidney Diseases, IC can be diagnosed only if symptoms of pain and frequency are present with specific findings on *cystoscopy*.

In cystoscopy the patient is put under general anesthesia, the bladder is filled with water and drained (*hydrodistension*) and then a flexible lighted fiber-optic scope is inserted into the urethra so the distended lining of the bladder can be examined for tiny hemorrhages (*glomerulations*), ulcers (*Hunner's ulcers*) or cracks in the mucosa. Hydrodistension may even be therapeutic for half of patients. "It probably damages sensory fibers in the lining of the bladder, so it relieves pain and urgency temporarily," suggests Dr. Hanno.

The most effective treatment has been the drug dimethyl sulfoxide (DMSO), infused into the bladder by a catheter, weekly (or every other week) for four to six weeks.

A new drug, *pentosan polysulfate sodium* (Elmiron), was recently approved for treating IC. "When the drug is given orally, it's thought that some of it gets into the urine and coats the bladder and protects the lining of the bladder, much in the way Pepto-Bismol is said to coat the lining of the stomach," explains Dr. Hanno. A ninety-month clinical trial found Elmiron reduced pain and urgency in 38 percent of patients after three months and almost 60 percent of women who continued treatment after seven years.

A pilot study began in 1997 of *hyaluronic acid* (Cystisat), instilled into the bladder, where it's believed to provide a temporary replacement for defective mucus membrane. It's given once a week for four weeks, then monthly to prevent recurrence. An open-label study of the drug by its Canadian manufacturer found a 70 percent positive response.

Other treatments include the antidepressant amitriptyline (Elavil), which acts on nerve cells to reduce pain and tends to increase bladder capacity, and the antihistamine *hydroxyzine* (Vistaril, Atarax). Both drugs cause drowsiness, so they're usually taken before bed.

A solution of water and the blood thinner *heparin*, self-administered by catheter three times a week for two months, has helped severe symptoms, as does a solution of heparin with the anesthetic *marcaine, hydrocortisone* and *sodium bicarbonate.*

For IC patients who have bladder ulcers, use of a laser or electrocautery to destroy the lesion or surgical removal of the ulcer may relieve symptoms. But the laser may cause more harm than good, cautions Dr. Hanno.

However, none of these treatments cures IC. Various treatments can help the vast majority of patients for a period of time, with some going into remission. For 15 percent of women, no treatment works, and many suffer emotional isolation and depression in addition to pain. A 1987 study by the Urban Institute in Washington, D.C., found that half of women with IC are unable to work full-time; some are on disability. It also learned that patients with IC are four times more likely to consider suicide than the general population. Many rate their quality of life as worse than that of people undergoing kidney dialysis.

Stress can trigger symptoms of IC. "But women are very afraid to admit that because they may get sent off to the psychiatrist before anyone listens to them again," says Dr. Ratner. Stress reduction exercises or medication can help. Women with IC are also advised to avoid use of the diaphragm and to avoid or limit foods that can be bladder irritants (see page 127).

∞ *Bladder Cancer* ∞

The incidence of bladder cancer is four times higher among men than women, but women need to be informed about it since many of its symptoms can mimic urinary tract infection. More than 13,000 women are diagnosed with bladder cancer each year. Smoking, a major risk factor, contributes to a third of all cases and 37 percent of deaths from bladder cancer among women. People in certain occupations who may be at increased risk include hairdressers, painters, printers and workers in the dye, rubber, leather and chemical industries. Some animal studies have linked the artificial sweetener *saccharin* to bladder cancer. Studies also link heavy caffeine consumption and chlorinated water to bladder cancer, but the links are poorly understood.

Early symptoms include blood in the urine, usually associated with increased frequency of urination, pain with urination and a feeling of urgency. Often bladder tumors cause no symptoms and may be felt only during pelvic or rectal exams. Bladder cancer is typically diagnosed by cystoscopy to examine and biopsy the bladder under general anesthesia. In some cases cells are collected from urine samples and analyzed.

Treatment includes surgery, radiation therapy and, in later stages, chemotherapy. For patients with early cancers or those at risk for recurrence, a new therapy using a bacterium called *BCG* is instilled into the bladder to stimulate the immune system.

One method of surgery, *transurethral resection*, involves inserting a cystoscope through the urethra into the bladder to remove small tumors or destroy them with electric current. In late-stage cancer *radical cystectomy* may be performed, removing the bladder as well as the urethra, uterus, fallopian tubes and ovaries. Intestines can be used to create a continent diversion for urine, which is emptied via an abdominal port and a catheter, or a "neobladder" that can be emptied normally can be created, eliminating the need for a urine bag outside the body.

When bladder cancer is detected at its earliest stages, the five-year survival rate is 92 percent. Once it has spread regionally, however, survival drops to 48 percent, and to 8 percent when there's distant spread (*metastasis*).

෴ *Cheryle's Story* ෴

"*Incontinence is not an older woman's problem. I was in my late twenties when it happened to me. I was working and studying for my M.B.A. when I suddenly got a rash of urinary tract infections. I started to leak urine. My doctors treated the infections, but this was the Dark Ages where incontinence was concerned.*

"*The incontinence wasn't constant, but it was bad enough to make me feel it was unsafe to be caught anyplace where I couldn't find a washroom quickly. First I tried to deal with it by drinking as little as I could, but my bladder just became more irritated from the concentrated urine, and I would get these splitting headaches from dehydration. Gradually it began to change my life. Over time I virtually became a recluse.*

"*I switched to independent study so I wouldn't have to sit in a classroom and risk an 'accident.' Then it seemed easier just to leave my job. I started turning down invitations to go out with friends, but I never told anyone why.*

"I finally admitted the problem to a friend, who said, 'Do something about it.' When I started to research this problem. I saw how little information there was, so I began to write a book, and that led me in 1982 to start the Simon Foundation, which is dedicated to helping people with incontinence.

"I was in my early thirties when I finally got the correct diagnosis. I had a benign tumor deeply embedded in my spinal cord that was destroying the nerves of my bladder. They did laser surgery that lasted sixteen, seventeen hours and removed as much of the tumor as they could without further damaging the nerves. The incontinence improved somewhat, but there was enough damage that mine will never be a normal bladder.

"That is why I always tell people that incontinence is a symptom, and you need to find out what's causing the problem. Most people hate to talk about it. They feel it's shameful. But incontinence is a medical condition, no more shameful than needing eyeglasses, and it can be treated."

Cheryle B. Gartley is the founder and president of the Simon Foundation for Continence, a nonprofit organization based in Chicago and Toronto, and the author of *Managing Incontinence: A Guide to Living with Loss of Bladder Control* (Jameson Books). The above remarks came from an interview and are printed with permission.

▪ Urinary Incontinence ▪

More than one-fourth of American women between the ages of thirty and fifty-nine, and 40 percent of women over sixty, suffer from *urinary incontinence*, loss of bladder control and leaking of urine. It can be caused by damage from stroke or tumors to the nerves that supply the urinary system, abnormal bladder contractions, weakened pelvic floor muscles or pelvic tissue atrophy after menopause. Urine leakage can also be caused by constant straining from constipation, obesity and chronic smoker's cough (which causes pressure on the bladder).

Unfortunately most people do not seek help for incontinence. Women typically wait more than a year to even discuss the problem with a doctor. As Cheryle Gartley found, incontinence can severely constrict a woman's life. A recent survey by the Bladder Health Council found that almost half of women with urine leakage have cut back on physical and social activities. As many as 40 percent avoid sexual activity for fear of leaking during intercourse. A third of the women wore baggy garments to hide bulky incontinence pads or old clothing that could be easily washed. One quarter percent said they felt life was not worth living. But it doesn't have to be that way. In most cases all types of incontinence can be treated.

STRESS INCONTINENCE is the inability to hold urine when any abdominal pressure is placed on the bladder. Perhaps one in three women suffers some degree of stress incontinence.

The ligaments and muscles that make up the pelvic floor and support the base of the bladder are normally very strong, but they can be stretched or injured by pregnancy and childbirth. The muscles usually return to normal after a brief period of time, but in many women, having several children weakens pelvic floor support (or damages nerves controlling those muscles) to such a degree that the urethra and bladder neck move when they shouldn't. Sneezing, coughing and even laughing cause the abdominal muscles to press on the bladder, pushing urine out of the bladder.

Weakening of support tissues can be worsened by lack of estrogen after menopause. Estrogen receptors exist in the tissues around the base (*trigone*) of the bladder, and loss of estrogen can affect these tissues, causing a feeling of urgency and *urge incontinence*. Uterine prolapse, in which the uterus drops down into the vagina because of weakened muscles (see page 53), can also cause stress incontinence.

Some women experience only mild, occasional stress incontinence. If their bladders are full and they sneeze, they may leak small amounts of urine. Others may have a severe problem, emptying the entire bladder when they stand up.

"Most frequently patients seek attention when there is daily leaking of urine. They are already forced to wear some sort of protection, usually sanitary napkins, when they finally seek help," says Dr. Victor Nitti. (In fact, more women buy sanitary napkins for incontinence protection than for menstruation.)

URGE INCONTINENCE occurs when the volume of urine produced exceeds the capacity of the bladder. It's characterized by a sudden, uncontrollable urge to urinate so strong a person can't make it to the bathroom without leaking urine. This is frequently associated with abnormal, involuntary contractions of the bladder or involuntary relaxation of the urethra. Causes can range from simple urinary tract infections to strokes, brain tumors, multiple sclerosis, Parkinson's disease or Alzheimer's disease. As with Cheryle Gartley, tumors that involve nerves or muscles can also cause urge incontinence.

MIXED INCONTINENCE is a combination of stress and urge incontinence caused by a variety of factors.

OVERFLOW INCONTINENCE is a leakage of urine that occurs when the bladder is distended and does not empty completely.

REFLEX INCONTINENCE is often caused by spinal cord injury and stroke, which block nerve signals between the bladder and the brain, so a person does not sense when the bladder is full.

VESICAL SPHINCTER DYSSYNERGIA is a "discoordination" between the bladder muscle and the sphincter muscle. Although the bladder contracts normally, muscles below the bladder do not relax appropriately, so the bladder never empties fully. This occurs in diseases of the nervous system, and it can be difficult to treat, requiring medication, surgery and intermittent catheterization.

VESICAL-VAGINAL FISTULA is a tiny passage that develops in the urethra, where urine collects. It may develop during childbirth or as a result of pelvic surgery, radiation therapy or a tumor, or it may occur as a congenital malformation.

Diagnosing Incontinence

Telling the difference between a patient with a weakened pelvic floor and one with *urethral insufficiency* (a weakened sphincter muscle) or a problem sensing bladder fullness can be done with urodynamic testing. First a small catheter is placed in the bladder to fill it and measure bladder pressure. Another small catheter is placed in the rectum to measure abdominal pressure. Then the bladder is slowly filled, while pressures in the bladder and abdomen are recorded.

"The patient is asked to cough and strain during the test and also to tell us when she experiences bladder fullness and the urge to urinate. When the bladder is full, the patient empties her bladder," explains Dr. Nitti. "During the test we measure the urinary flow rate and take periodic X rays to get a picture of what is going on. We can see whether the sphincter muscle is tightening properly or whether there's leakage." Patients may be given antibiotics afterward to guard against infection.

Fistulas can be diagnosed by first filling the bladder, then emptying it using a harmless solution of blue dye. If the fistula is in the vaginal area, a tampon placed in the vagina will be stained at the site of the fistula. Another test, using saline solution in the vagina, can detect tiny air bubbles at the site of the fistula (kind of like air escaping from a punctured tire).

Do Kegels Really Work?

For years experts have advised women with mild stress incontinence, and women who have just given birth, to perform Kegel exercises to strengthen the pelvic floor muscle. Some clinical trials have found improvement rates of up to 77 percent for stress incontinence when women perform Kegels regularly. However, a 1996 study in *Obstetrics and Gynecology* warned that women need to keep on doing Kegels to maintain the effect. Those who continued to exercise three times a week or more five years after they had taken part in a six-month intensive Kegel regimen had less urine leakage and more pelvic floor strength. At the same time, a federally sponsored incontinence prevention project found that Kegels are an exercise in futility if women don't fully understand *which* muscle to contract and *how* to do it.

You can ask your gynecologist to help you isolate the proper muscle during a routine pelvic exam, or try this maneuver: In the bathroom consciously try to interrupt urination several times. If you do this properly, you should feel the contraction at the highest level of your pelvis, says Dr. Nitti. To do Kegels:

- Contract the pelvic floor muscle as hard as you can (without tightening the buttocks or bearing down), and hold for at least ten seconds.

- Exhale gently through the mouth with each contraction to keep from straining. Rest between contractions.

- Start by doing ten repetitions at least four times a day for at least six weeks; gradually increase the number and frequency.

- Do Kegels during a fixed part of your daily routine, such as in the shower, or incorporate Kegels into your exercise regimen.

"In addition to strengthening the supports of the bladder neck and urethra, Kegels can start a reflex that relaxes the bladder and may decrease the urge to urinate," notes Dr. Nitti. Not only can Kegels reduce trips to the bathroom, but some women say they also improve the intensity of their orgasms!

There are a number of techniques to help women learn Kegels. One is a variation of *biofeedback,* using tiny surface electrodes or a vaginal probe that is connected to a monitor to measure muscle activity. When the patient contracts the muscle correctly, the device lights up. Another teaching device is weighted vaginal cones, which a patient must hold on to by contracting the pelvic floor muscle. The cones come in progressively heavier weights, a sort of urinary weight training.

If women have nerve damage in the area, the muscles may not respond to conscious efforts to contract them. In this case the muscles can be electrically stimulated intravaginally to increase their tone. A 1995 clinical trial at six medical centers found that 62 percent of the women treated with electrical stimulation had at least a 50 percent reduction in stress incontinence, compared with 19 percent of women treated with a placebo device.

Medications for Incontinence

In addition to Kegel exercises and bladder retraining (page 127), a number of medications are used to treat urinary incontinence.

Tricyclic antidepressants and *anticholinergic* drugs can help block bladder spasms that cause urge incontinence. These drugs lower the levels of *acetyl-choline*, a neurotransmitter that sends chemical signals between nerve cells in the body. Anticholinergic drugs include *propantheline* (Pro-Banthine) and *oxybutynin* (Ditropan). Tricyclic antidepressants include amitriptyline (Elavil), *nortriptyline* (Aventyl) and *imipramine* (Tofranil).

New federal treatment guidelines say the antihistamine *pseudoephedrine* can be a first-line drug for women with urge incontinence. The guidelines say that estrogen replacement therapy (ERT) should also be considered as adjunct therapy for mixed or stress incontinence. ERT can help restore some tone to vaginal tissue and sphincter muscles lost due to lack of estrogen in women over age sixty; estrogen creams can also help. A recent review of twenty-three clinical trials of ERT found that it provided improvement rates between 19 and 89 percent in the management of incontinence in older women.

Some medications and even foods can aggravate incontinence. Alcohol and tranquilizers can dull nerve signals that tell the brain when the bladder is full. Diuretics can cause the bladder to fill more quickly and leak. Caffeine has the same effect.

Surgical Solutions

Not long ago hysterectomy and vaginal reconstruction were used to treat incontinence. However, studies show hysterectomy is not an effective treatment and may worsen incontinence.

For certain types of stress incontinence caused by urethral insufficiency, a common treatment today is a collagen implant, a nonsurgical procedure done on an outpatient basis. Under local anesthesia a thin needle injects a small amount of collagen into the top of the urethra around the bladder neck, adding bulk to the tissue and forming a tighter seal to hold in urine. "The urethra will function naturally afterward, opening and closing during urination," says Dr. Nitti.

However, only 25 percent of women will be totally dry after a collagen implant, 50 percent will have major improvement in their incontinence and 25 percent will not benefit. A 1996 study in a small group of women aged sixty-eight to eighty-five found collagen implants cured 83 percent, while the rest thought their incontinence was improved.

Newer types of implants that last longer than collagen are being tested.

If the implant treatment fails or a woman is not happy with the results, the muscles and *fascia* (fibrous tissues that cover the muscles) can be tightened surgically to support the bladder neck and urethra better. The surgery can be done laparoscopically, abdominally or, most commonly, transvaginally, with only a tiny incision just below the pubic bone.

Another procedure creates a "sling" from a strip of the patient's own fascia (or a synthetic substitute), wrapped around the urethra to restore support for the bladder neck. This surgery can be performed abdominally or through the vagina.

Side effects of these procedures can include reduced sensation in the vaginal area or the clitoris. But for many women, surgery is the only way to stay completely dry.

Among the techniques to treat stress incontinence is *videoscopic bladder neck suspension,* done laparoscopically, with no incision in the vagina. Sutures put between the outside of the bladder and the tissue just behind the pubic bone "lift" the bladder neck back to its proper position. There is only an overnight hospital stay, and most patients can return to work within two weeks.

Special pessaries, including the Incontinence Ring and the Introl bladder neck support prosthesis, can offer immediate relief of stress incontinence.

These flexible silicone devices fold like a diaphragm for insertion into the vagina. The ring has a small ball on one side that presses against the bladder neck; Introl has two support posts on the ring that rest on either side of the urethra to elevate the bladder neck to its normal position. Another new device, the Reliance Urinary Control Insert, is comprised of a tiny balloon inserted by a small catheterlike applicator that fits into the urethra. When inflated, the balloon prevents the flow of urine; when a woman wants to urinate, she removes the device. A multicenter study found that Reliance kept 80 percent of women completely dry.

c h a p t e r 8

Sexually Transmitted Diseases

Sexually transmitted diseases (STDs) have become a global epidemic. More than 55 million Americans currently have an STD, and around 13 million more, one quarter of them teenagers, will be diagnosed this year. *Every* sexually active person is at risk.

Just a few decades ago venereal diseases were discussed in whispers, and the stereotype of a VD victim was a man who had sex with a prostitute and was punished by getting "the clap." Public clinics were originally set up to treat men, so STDs in women weren't tracked. We now know sexually transmitted diseases affect *both* men and women in every social, racial and economic group.

Once there were only two known STDs, syphilis and gonorrhea, both treatable with antibiotics. Since the 1980s more than twenty sexually transmitted organisms have been identified, and some, like *human immunodeficiency virus (HIV)*, which causes *AIDS*, cannot be cured. While we've learned that women are much more vulnerable to STDs than men, the Alan Guttmacher Institute reports that women are still diagnosed and treated less often than men.

Because women have larger genital mucous membranes, they are more susceptible than men to invasion by bacteria or viruses during unprotected heterosexual sex. Viruses and bacteria are also deposited near a very vulnerable area on the cervix, and some experts believe that semen actually *neutralizes* the normally acidic vaginal environment and gives STDs a better chance to take hold. "With just one *single* act of unprotected sex with an infected partner, women are twice as likely to contract chlamydia or gonorrhea than men, and twenty times more likely to contract HIV," warns Machelle Allen, M.D., an assistant professor of OB/GYN who heads an STD clinic for high-risk women at the NYU-affiliated Bellevue Hospital Center.

Sexually transmitted microorganisms often produce little or no symptoms until serious infection sets in. If an STD goes undiagnosed or treatment is delayed, the infection may spread to the upper genital tract, causing permanent damage.

STDs have more serious consequences for women than for men, including cervical cancer, pelvic inflammatory disease (PID), ectopic pregnancy and infertility, according to Dr. Allen. Researchers now believe even mild chlamydial infections may set up a chronic low-grade inflammation in the uterus that may interfere with implantation of an embryo (see page 145). Women can also pass STDs along to newborns, including herpes, syphilis, *gonococcal conjunctivitis* (which can lead to blindness) and *chlamydial pneumonia*, which can become a chronic respiratory disease.

While the threat of AIDS has increased awareness about STDs, many women are in denial about the risk, according to a 1997 survey conducted by the Kaiser Family Foundation and *Glamour* magazine. The random survey of women aged eighteen to forty-four, revealed that *97 percent did not consider themselves at risk for STDs,* and only 15 percent even discussed the subject during their initial visit for gynecological care. Other surveys indicate many women feel "it won't happen to me" *even* if they are at high risk: those under twenty-five, with multiple sexual partners or whose current partners have had multiple sexual relationships.

"The person who looks like the boy next door, or the girl next door, can be infected just as easily as anyone," comments Dr. Allen. "Very often we see college girls or young professionals who have contracted human papilloma virus, who really can't fathom who could have infected them. They are totally shocked. What's most troubling is their lack of awareness of HIV and other infections that are transmitted sexually."

Indeed, another recent survey, by the American Medical Women's Association (AMWA), found that many women knew little about STDs other than HIV/AIDS; 63 percent said they had little knowledge of chlamydia, the most common STD. Only 11 percent knew that STDs were more harmful to women than to men. While almost half the women said they relied on monogamy for protection and 30 percent used condoms, 6 percent said they did *nothing* to prevent STDs.

Teenagers feel particularly invulnerable, despite statistics showing that young people from every walk of life between fifteen and nineteen are at the *highest* risk of contracting chlamydia, gonorrhea and pelvic inflammatory disease. Teens are becoming sexually active earlier, and girls are more likely to be on the pill (which provides *no* protection against STDs) than to use condoms. Adolescent girls also have a unique biological vulnerability to STDs (see page 148). Yet only about a third of sexually active teenage girls are screened each year for STDs.

It all adds up to an enormous risk, jeopardizing women's health, fertility and futures. Experts stress that women need to be concerned, informed, and take *preventive* measures.

∞ Chelsea's Story, Cont'd ∞

"Today people think about STDs and AIDS, but back in the 1970s it was not a major concern. I was very sexually active and I got gonorrhea in 1976 at college. They didn't know about chlamydia then, so it's possible I had that too. They gave me a shot of penicillin, and that was that. I don't recall ever having major symptoms, but looking back, I know I must have had PID.

"I don't recall anyone ever telling me gonorrhea could affect my future fertility or talking about PID. Of course now I know that gonorrhea can destroy the tubes. When I had my ectopic pregnancy twenty years later and they did a laparoscopy to check my tubes, they found adhesions around the tubes and ovaries and had to remove them. So I must have had PID but never even knew it. I certainly had no symptoms, that I recall."

▪ Chlamydia ▪

The number one STD threatening women is *chlamydia*, spread by the bacterium *Chlamydia trachomatis*. According to the American Social Health Association (ASHA), chlamydia is the most common STD in the United States, affecting as many as 4 million people a year!

Actually, the *true* number of cases is not known. Many chlamydia infections occur with other sexually transmitted diseases; half of women who have acute tubal inflammation have *both* chlamydia and gonorrhea. But unlike gonorrhea (or syphilis), cases of chlamydia are not required to be reported to health authorities. In some cases the damage is discovered years after an infection.

Chelsea's experience in college is not unique. A recent survey found that *half* of the women on *one* college campus had chlamydia! Between 20 and 30 percent of teenage girls have had it.

Chlamydia is particularly insidious because 85 percent of infections in women produce *little or no symptoms at all*. Recent research shows that up to 40 percent of untreated chlamydial infections travel to the upper genital tract, often spreading to the pelvic cavity before becoming evident, says Cheryl Walker, M.D., Director of Reproductive Infectious Diseases and Immunology at the University of California-Irvine.

When symptoms do appear, typically one to three weeks after infection, they may include an abnormal vaginal discharge (including an increase in the amount of discharge, a change in color or an unpleasant odor) and burning during urination, according to Dr. Walker. "If a woman has developed a pelvic infection, there may be moderate to severe lower abdominal pain, which will be distinct from cramping related to menstruation." (Men with chlamydia may have pain or swelling in the testicles.)

Fifteen known strains of *Chlamydia trachomatis* can cause genital infections. It has been implicated in pregnancy complications, including premature delivery, low birth weight, postpartum inflammation of the uterine lining (endometritis) as well as eye infections and pneumonia in the newborn.

There are now more accurate tests for chlamydia, which can be performed within ten to fifteen minutes in a doctor's office. One *immunoassay* detects whether the immune system has made *antibodies* in response to the presence of *C. trachomatis*. Another looks for antigens, proteins on the surface of the bacterium that trigger immune reactions. The most recently approved diagnostic tests make use of genetic technology to detect the DNA of *Chlamydia trachomatis* in small samples of urine. These tests can also use vaginal secretions, and results are generally available within twenty-four hours, according to Dr. Walker. One test, a DNA probe, looks for a specific *piece* of *C. trachomatis* DNA. Another new DNA probe in development searches for the DNA of *both* chlamydia and gonorrhea.

New treatment guidelines set in 1997 by the federal Centers for Disease Control and Prevention (CDC) call for taking the antibiotic *doxycycline*, 100 mg two times a day for seven days, or in a single dose of one gram of *azithromycin*. Other drugs used to treat chlamydia include *erythromycin, ofloxacin* (Floxin). Ofloxacin, a type of drug called a *quinolone*, is the only single agent approved for treating *both* chlamydia and gonorrhea. Any of these drugs may cause an initial serious reaction. Pregnant women are given different versions of erythromycin for seven to fourteen days.

As many as 20,000 women a year become infertile as a result of chlamydial infections. Swedish studies on pelvic inflammatory disease show that women who waited three or more days to seek treatment after noticing symptoms had a threefold higher rate of ectopic pregnancy and infertility than those who went for treatment within forty-eight hours. *None* of the women with chlamydial PID treated within two days had ectopic pregnancies or infertility, compared with 20 percent of those who delayed treatment.

In such cases a fragment of *C. trachomatis* may remain in reproductive tissues even after treatment to cause fertility problems later on. According to research by Joseph Hill, M.D., a director of reproductive medicine at Brigham and Women's Hospital in Boston, part of the protein of chlamydia may stay in the uterus even after full antibiotic treatment, causing a chronic low-grade inflammation. This may flood the area with immune cells and their products, which can be toxic to an embryo or prevent its implantation, resulting in infertility or early pregnancy loss.

Experts urge all sexually active women to be screened regularly for chlamydia, even if they have no apparent symptoms, so that "silent" infections do not go untreated. A 1996 study in the *New England Journal of Medicine* found that women screened and treated for asymptomatic chlamydia were 56 percent less likely to develop PID, compared with unscreened women.

▪ Gonorrhea ▪

Gonorrhea can have devastating effects on a woman's fertility. According to the ASHA, it afflicts more than one million people a year (about 40 percent women). Girls aged fifteen to nineteen have the highest rates of gonorrhea among females.

Infection by the bacterium *Neisseria gonorrhoeae* can cause inflammation of the cervix (*cervicitis*), urethra (*urethritis*), fallopian tubes, *salpingitis* and more widespread infections but may also be asymptomatic. The incubation period for gonorrhea averages three to five days but can be as long as fourteen days.

Women are up to 50 percent more likely than men to become infected with gonorrhea after a *single unprotected sexual exposure* to an infected partner, observes Jonathan Zenilman, M.D., associate professor of medicine and an STD researcher in the Division of Infectious Diseases at the Johns Hopkins University School of Medicine. "Gonorrhea is transmitted in semen or other secretions, and parts of the bacteria are very adept at adhering to cervical epithelium."

Many women with gonorrhea *do* have some symptoms, usually a cervical or vaginal discharge. There may also be painful and frequent urination, cervicitis and vaginal spotting. A puslike discharge can be seen from the cervix during an internal examination. (The most common symptom in men is a puslike discharge from the penis.) Ten to 20 percent of women have abdominal pain, indicating inflammation of the endometrium or fallopian tubes, or a tubo-ovarian abscess (a pus-filled cyst). *Gonococcal PID* usually develops a few days after a menstrual period begins, with fever and abdominal tenderness.

"There may also be infections of the pharynx in up to forty percent of women, which may look just like a strep or viral throat infection," Dr. Zenilman notes. Between 10 and 20 percent of women may have an anal-rectal infection, with a puslike discharge. A generalized infection may result in joint pains.

Gonorrhea can be transmitted to a fetus during pregnancy or at delivery. *Conjunctivitis*, the most common symptom of infection in newborns, is prevented in the U.S. by administering silver nitrate drops or erythromycin ointment to the eyes at birth. Gonorrhea is also associated with preterm labor and miscarriage.

The diagnosis is confirmed by culturing the bacteria from cervical or vaginal discharge. In nonpregnant women it is treated with ofloxacin or *broad-spectrum antibiotics* like *ceftriaxone* or *ciprofloxacin*, since strains of gonorrhea are now resistant to penicillin and *tetracycline*, according to Dr. Zenilman. Pregnant women receive ceftriaxone or erythromycin. Uncomplicated infections can be treated with a single injection of ceftriaxone or a single dose of oral *cefixime* or ciprofloxacin.

After treatment, patients need to have further cultures taken from the affected sites to make sure the infection is completely eradicated. The rectum is a common site for relapse in women. But being cured of one gonorrheal infection will not make you resistant to another since the bacterium mutates, notes Dr. Zenilman. Reinfection can also occur if either partner stops taking medication too soon, and the bacteria multiply again.

∞ Chelsea's Story, Cont'd ∞

"My having gonorrhea came home to roost eventually. When I finally got pregnant a year after we were married, we were thrilled. I was six weeks pregnant when I started having spotting. I went to my OB/GYN, who gave me a pregnancy hormone test. By then I was getting some cramping. When the test results came in, he told me the hormone levels were dropping and I was probably having a miscarriage or had an ectopic pregnancy.

"I was devastated. I had an ultrasound, and my doctor told me there was an ectopic pregnancy in the right tube and they had to operate immediately. The doctor was able to save my tube, but I never conceived again. I took fertility drugs, but when I turned forty, I sort of knew it was over for me.

"I went through a real grieving process. I cried the entire day of my fortieth birthday. There was almost no chance I could have a child, and I had probably done this to myself."

▪ Pelvic Inflammatory Disease (PID) ▪

Both chlamydia and gonorrhea can lead to PID, or *salpingo-oophoritis*, which afflicts more than one million women each year, many of them still teenagers. Between 10 and 40 percent of women with PID may become infertile because of damaged fallopian tubes. The rate of ectopic pregnancy in women who have had just *one* episode of PID rises six- to ten-fold, according to Dr. Cheryl Walker.

Pelvic pain is a hallmark of PID. "This can range from a mild low-grade continuous discomfort to a painful and severe disability. But only one in five women who have PID will have severe pain," says Dr. Walker. "Any new onset of pelvic pain, even if it's mild, even if it's not constant, should prompt a woman to see her health care provider immediately."

Other red flags: cervicitis, with a mucuslike discharge from the cervix that may easily go unnoticed, spotting between periods, a small amount of bleeding after intercourse and increased vaginal discharge with an unpleasant smell, a dark gray or green color and a gritty or bubbly quality, instead of the usual creamy or eggwhite consistency.

Mild symptoms may not be connected to a sexually transmitted disease.

"When tested, many of those women will have antibodies to chlamydia, but at least half will not recall having an infection," says Roberta B. Ness, M.D., director of the Epidemiology of Women's Health Program at the Graduate School of Public Health of the University of Pittsburgh, who has been conducting studies into pelvic inflammatory disease. "Studies have looked at women diagnosed with tubal infertility, and when they carefully question the women, it turns out they did have minor symptoms that were not construed as being pelvic inflammatory disease and consequently were not treated."

Teenagers may be more susceptible to PID because the cellular structure of the cervix is maturing. Most STDs invade the cervical canal or the thin outer layer of squamous cells around the cervical opening, rather than attack the thicker, more resistant lining of the vagina. Chlamydia and gonorrhea seem to target columnar epithelial cells, which in adolescence are more exposed to infection. Before puberty the single layer of columnar-shaped cells that normally line the cervical canal extends onto the outer part of the cervix, explains Dr. Walker. At puberty these cells begin to differentiate into the squamous cells normally found on the outer cervix and the vagina. But the change is slow, and the bull's-eye area of cell transition outside the cervix, called the *ectropion* or *cervical ectropy*, remains fairly large during adolescence.

"Because of hormonal differences, especially in young teenagers, cervical mucus tends to be a little more penetrable by chlamydia and gonorrhea, so we believe there's a higher rate of ascension for pelvic inflammatory disease," Dr. Walker says. Teenagers also have the highest rates of hospitalization for PID.

Sexual behavior plays a major role. While many teenagers describe themselves as monogamous, what they really mean is that they have only one sexual partner for a period of time, Dr. Walker notes. "Some were probably 'monogamous' with as many as five partners in a given year. Data from the CDC suggest serial monogamy is a huge problem for teens." Teenage girls are more likely to be on the pill than to use condoms, which protect against STDs. Moreover, the earlier a girl becomes sexually active, the more partners she's likely to have, increasing her risk of infection (and reinfection).

Overall, chlamydia causes half of the one million cases of PID diagnosed each year; gonorrhea is responsible for many of the others. Bacterial vaginosis, as well as the organisms associated with it, *Gardnerella vaginalis* and *Mycoplasma hominis*, and some strains of strep may also be associated with PID.

The initial infection may lower the amount of oxygen available in the vagina, allowing the overgrowth of other harmful bacteria (especially *anaer-*

obic bacteria, which do not need oxygen). If the infection remains untreated, the microorganisms invade and inflame the uterine lining, fallopian tubes and peritoneal cavity, explains the NYU infertility specialist Dr. John Quagliarello. The white blood cells fighting off the pathogens form pus, which can fill the tubes (*pyosalpinx*) and spill into the pelvis, causing more inflammation, pain, fever and a foul-smelling vaginal discharge. "Eventually adhesions form in the peritoneal cavity. There can also be tubo-ovarian abscesses filled with pus and widespread infection," says Dr. Quagliarello. Inflammation can also destroy the delicate, frondlike fimbriae at the ends of the fallopian tubes, preventing them from taking up an egg released from the ovary. "Gonorrhea and chlamydia can also damage the tiny hairs, or cilia, lining the fallopian tubes, preventing an egg from being propelled through the tubes to the uterus. If a fertilized egg becomes stuck in the tube, it results in an ectopic pregnancy."

Many women find out they've had PID only when tubal damage is discovered during an infertility workup or they have an ectopic pregnancy. When PID is suspected, women may undergo diagnostic laparoscopy to look for redness and swelling of the tubes and inflammation of the pelvic cavity, so treatment can begin before there's further damage.

Treatment of PID should begin as soon as there is a suspicion of disease, and it requires broad-spectrum antibiotic therapy because several microorganisms may be involved. Outpatient treatment can include an injection of cefoxitin, ceftriaxone or other cephalosporin drugs with one oral dose of *probenecid*, and/or fourteen days of doxycycline. Ofloxacin can be given twice a day with a second drug such as clindamycin, or metronidazole for fourteen days or 400 mg as monotherapy twice a day for two weeks.

Hospitalization may be required if there is fever, nausea and vomiting, if symptoms suggest ectopic pregnancy or pelvic abscesses, if the woman is pregnant, if compliance is an issue or if PID is so widespread that intravenous medication is required. Intravenous antibiotics, including cefoxitin, cefotetan, clindamycin or gentamicin are given every six, eight or twelve hours, depending on the dose.

The sexual partner is also treated, and women should abstain from sexual relations until therapy is completed. The CDC recommends repeat cultures seven to ten days after treatment is complete, and some experts recommend rescreening for chlamydia and gonorrhea four to six weeks after therapy.

But the challenge is to *prevent* PID in the first place, not only by primary prevention (such as abstaining from sex or using condoms) but also by secondary prevention, screening for chlamydia and gonorrhea. "Within the next few years we will have widespread use of either urine-based or vaginal swab-based DNA testing for both chlamydia and gonorrhea. And that may allow for a mass screening program that would detect many silent infections," says Dr. Ness.

Studies show that up to 40 percent of women being treated for lower genital tract STD infections may have endometritis, a sign of PID. Dr. Ness and colleagues are studying women who have had cervicitis (or whose partners have chlamydia or gonorrhea) and doing biopsies to see how many have endometritis, and what the risk factors may be, so high-risk women can be identified and treated appropriately, even if there are no symptoms of PID.

ꙮ *L o r i e ' s S t o r y* ꙮ

"I had been having these pains around the edge of my vulva, a pins-and-needles–like feeling. I was referred to a gynecologist/oncologist who did a colposcopy and found condyloma, papilloma virus. The condyloma was inside the inner lips and in the cervix. I had absolutely no idea! I had no warts like you hear about.

"The doctor did a biopsy of the vulva, which nearly sent me through the ceiling. He knew from the way I reacted that I would have to have the laser surgery under general anesthesia in the hospital. Which is what I did. After the laser surgery I had to keep a piece of cheesecloth between the vaginal lips to keep them from fusing together while they healed, and I had to douche with this orange stuff, Betadine and water, all the time to promote healing.

"Then, after it healed, the doctor gave me fluoracil cream. This stuff is basically like chemotherapy in a tube. What it does is slough away the skin cells and takes the condyloma with it. It didn't hurt going in, but on the second day of this, I was in agony, crying my eyes out. So the doctor said, 'Just do it once a week for three months.' But then it came back, and I had to do it again. So it was a total of six months, and my vagina and vulva were always burning. It makes you feel you never want to have sex again!

"My boyfriend was tested, and he had it too. But it's easier to treat a man. All he got was this little bottle of medication, and all he had to do was put a drop on every night until it went away while I had to go through that godawful laser surgery! Neither of us has had a recurrence since."

▪ Human Papilloma Virus (Condylomata Acuminata) ▪

According to the CDC, 24 million Americans are infected with the human papilloma virus (HPV), and 1 million *new* cases will be diagnosed this year alone! Among women under age twenty, one quarter will become infected during their first year of sexual activity, even if they have fewer than two partners.

There are more than seventy strains of HPV, which either cause genital warts (*condylomata*) or warts elsewhere on the body (contact with these warts does not seem to cause genital warts). Other strains are now known to cause cervical cancer. "More women will die between now and the year 2000 around the world of cervical cancer caused by human papilloma virus than will die of AIDS," warns Penelope J. Hitchcock, D.Vm., chief of the Sexually Transmitted Diseases Branch of the National Institute of Allergy and Infectious Diseases (NIAID). "Unfortunately too many women remain unaware that HPV causes cervical cancer as well as genital warts."

HPV types 6 and 11 are the most frequently associated with fleshy, cauliflower-shaped warts that grow in or around the vulva, anus and perineum and that spread to the skin of the thighs. They can also occur as flat condylomata within the vagina and on the cervix. Genital warts usually appear within four to six weeks after exposure, but because of HPV's long latency period, warts may not appear for months afterward. (In men, genital warts appear on the glans and urethral opening, on the shaft and the scrotum.) For unknown reasons condylomata can flare during pregnancy. Strains of HPV that produce warts are not generally associated with cervical cancer, although they have been found in tissues of vulvar cancer patients.

"Sometimes these warts will be obvious, but sometimes the lesions are subtle, even microscopic. The patient has some itching or burning, but you may not see anything," remarks Dr. Ilona Brandeis, an assistant professor of clinical obstetrics and gynecology at NYU Medical Center. "The examination is aided by the application of acetic acid, vinegar and water, which turn abnormal tissues white, so the lesions can be seen more easily. The diagnosis of HPV is then made by biopsy."

While a Pap smear can detect HPV, it will show only the viral presence in cervical cells. So flat condylomata in the vagina or on the vulva may be missed; the vinegar and water solution brings out the lesions during colposcopy.

Genital warts are removed by freezing with liquid nitrogen, with a laser, such chemical compounds as *podophyllin, podofilox* and *trichloracetic acid* or by electrocautery. It may take a few treatments to eradicate the warts and kills the virus in the affected cells. But HPV can remain elsewhere in the body, so genital warts can recur.

Cervical cancer is most often associated with HPV types 16 and 18, which usually produce flat condylomata. HPV is thought to insert its DNA into the DNA of cervical cells, setting the stage for *dysplasia*, precancerous cell changes and invasive cancer. Papilloma virus DNA is found in most cases of cervical dysplasia and in more than 90 percent of cervical cancers (see page 265).

Mild to moderate cervical dysplasia can be treated by freezing or electrocautery; if it has progressed to carcinoma in situ, a portion of the cervix is surgically removed. While this does not eradicate the virus, many experts believe the immune system eventually clears it from the body. Only about 1 percent of women with HPV infections develop cervical cancer. Several vaccines against HPV are now in clinical trials. (For more on cervical dysplasia and cervical cancer, see page 263).

▪ Hepatitis B and C ▪

Of the seven known hepatitis viruses, only *hepatitis B* and to a much lesser extent *hepatitis C* are transmitted sexually. They are spread through semen, vaginal secretions and saliva, among intravenous drug users sharing contaminated needles and by unsterilized instruments used for tattoos, body piercing and even manicures.

Hepatitis B and C do not affect the genital tract but cause chronic liver infection and damage, increasing the risk of liver cancer. The most common symptoms are fever, headaches, fatigue, muscle aches, loss of appetite, diarrhea and vomiting, but often there may be no symptoms. Severe cases of hepatitis C may result in jaundice, a yellowing of the skin and eyes.

Ninety percent of hepatitis B infections resolve on their own. Acute hepatitis C and chronic hepatitis are treated with immune modulators called *interferons*.

More than 400,000 Americans are infected with hepatitis B and C each year; more than 10 percent by sexually-transmitted hepatitis B. But hepatitis B can be prevented with a vaccine. Federal health officials recommend that all infants and adolescents receive three doses of the vaccine.

▪ Syphilis and Genital Ulcer Diseases ▪

Syphilis is among several STDs that produce genital ulcers and increase the risk of contracting AIDS. Around 120,000 new cases of syphilis are reported each year in the U.S., about 45 percent among women.

Syphilis is spread by a *spirochete*, a microorganism named *Treponema pallidum*, which lives in the genital tracts of infected people. Diagnostic tests detect the presence of this organism or the immune system antibodies produced in response to it.

The first symptom of syphilis, usually a painless ulcer on the vulva or vagina, typically appears ten days to three weeks after infection. The *secondary* stage produces flulike symptoms, swollen glands and a skin rash, with large red patches on the trunk and extremities, as well as mouth ulcers and hair loss. These symptoms may disappear, but the infection lingers in a *latent* stage, during which the disease is not contagious.

Untreated, about a third of people will reach the *tertiary* stage of syphilis and develop severe complications, including mental illness, blindness, heart disease and death. These can occur as long as ten years after infection. *Congenital syphilis*, in which infants contract the disease at birth from mothers in the early stages of infection, can cause severe and permanent damage.

In its primary, secondary and latent stages, syphilis is treated with injections of *benzathine penicillin*. The antibiotics tetracycline or doxycyline may also be used in nonpregnant patients. In pregnant women, penicillin or erythromycin is given. Sexual partners are treated whether or not they show infection. In the tertiary stage another form of penicillin is given. Monitoring is needed after treatment, with tests for the spirochete performed for up to two years.

A less common STD that produces genital ulcers is *chancroid*, caused by the bacterium *Hemophilus ducreyi*. After an incubation period of four to seven days, a painful, red, pimplelike lesion appears on the genitals. It fills with pus and ruptures to form an ulcer. Chancroid is treated with a single dose of ceftriaxone or seven days of erythromycin. Genital herpes—herpes simplex-2 or HSV-2—also produces genital ulcers.

People who have these diseases are three to five times more likely to get HIV if they have sex with infected individuals because genital ulcers create a portal for the AIDS virus.

∽ *K a t y ' s   S t o r y* ∽

"I have AIDS, and I am fighting to make the most of each day. I can't plead ignorance. I knew about HIV; I'd even helped raise money for a local AIDS organization, so I should have known better than to take the chance I did.

"I contracted the AIDS virus during a brief and foolish affair. I had been married for six years, but we were having problems, and I was introduced to a very attractive man by a mutual friend. I did ask about HIV, but he swore he was healthy. I later found out that he had tested positive for HIV several years earlier. Why didn't he wear a condom? Why didn't I insist? It's a mistake I'll regret as long as I have to live.

"About a month after our affair ended, I awoke dripping with perspiration, shaking with chills. I felt like I had the flu. I knew immediately I must have HIV, but when I got the results, I was just devastated.

"I had to tell my husband. He was horribly hurt and betrayed. And he was in shock that I had a fatal disease and that he might have it too. That I might have given it to him. He was tested several times, but the results came back negative.

"My husband filed to get sole custody of our son, and we divorced. We didn't tell my son at that time. But then I developed full-blown AIDS, and I had to tell my son about my illness, that I was going to die. It was the hardest thing I've ever had to do. All we could do was hold each other and cry."

• HIV/AIDS •

The human immunodeficiency virus (HIV) is a *retrovirus*, which inserts its genetic material (RNA) into the cells it attacks. HIV targets immune cells called *CD4 T-lymphocytes*, which normally help fight off infections. The virus splices its genes into CD4 cells, converting its RNA into new DNA. When the cell reproduces, it makes another HIV-altered cell, which sheds more virus. As fewer and fewer normal CD4 cells remain, the immune system becomes increasingly unable to fight disease. When CD4 levels fall below a certain point, a person has *acquired immune deficiency syndrome (AIDS)*, which is eventually fatal.

Being HIV-positive means that blood tests have detected immune system antibodies to the AIDS virus. While HIV replication can sometimes be slowed, until recently it could not be stopped, and half of all HIV-positive people developed AIDS within nine to ten years of infection, with 40 percent dying within that period. Combinations of new drugs have helped reduce deaths from AIDS.

When scientists first became aware of AIDS in the early 1980s, it was considered a disease of homosexual men. In 1985 women made up 5 percent of all AIDS cases, by 1995 women constituted 20 percent of AIDS cases and the numbers are rising more rapidly among women than any other group. Of heterosexually transmitted cases of HIV, 60 percent are now among women.

The World Health Organization estimates that by the year 2000, 13 million women around the globe will be HIV-positive and 4 million will die of AIDS. In the United States AIDS is now the third leading cause of death among women aged twenty-five to forty-four and is the leading cause of death among African-American women in that age-group. Almost 75 percent of American women with AIDS, and 84 percent of infected children, are black or Hispanic, most living in poverty.

"Today in many communities in the United States you do not have to have multiple sexual partners or engage in other risky behaviors to be exposed to the AIDS virus because HIV infection has become so common," observes Howard Minkoff, M.D., professor and director of Maternal-Fetal Medicine at the State University of New York (SUNY) Health Sciences Center at Brooklyn, a leading researcher into women and AIDS.

Adding to the urgency of the situation is women's greater susceptibility to HIV infection. Not only do women have a larger area of vulnerable epithelium, but they also receive a heavier dose of virus from semen than men get from vaginal secretions. Semen also neutralizes the normally protective acidic vaginal pH, "which may be why the transmission rate from men to women is higher than from women to men," says David Phillips, Ph.D, a virologist and senior scientist at the Population Council in New York. Phillips believes that HIV-infected CD4 cells in semen stick to vaginal epithelial cells and shed virus rather than directly infect cells, as chlamydia and gonorrhea do.

HIV infection does not produce irritation, discharge or other immediate symptoms. The earliest sign of HIV infection is night sweats, like those Katy experienced, perhaps a month after infection. There can also be flulike symptoms, low-grade fever, swollen glands, loss of appetite, weight loss and fatigue. A woman may also have bacterial pneumonia. But such symptoms might not raise concern if a woman isn't considered high-risk, delaying HIV testing and early treatment that can prolong life.

Recurring yeast infections despite topical or oral therapy are the most common gynecological symptoms in HIV-positive women; some women may have cervical dysplasia. Other gynecological symptoms can include amenorrhea, irregular periods and bleeding.

The onset of AIDS in about half of HIV-positive men and women can be characterized by a lung infection with *Pneumocystis carinii pneumonia (PCP)*. In 1993 the CDC broadened its definition of AIDS to include women with cervical cancer, recurrent bacterial pneumonias and tuberculosis, as well as CD4 counts below 200 per milliliter (ml) of blood. As part of the diagnostic criteria, women may also have candidal infections of the esophagus and more virulent genital herpes outbreaks. As a result, the number of women meeting the criteria for clinical AIDS has dramatically increased, notes Dr. Minkoff.

Federal health officials estimate that 6 percent of HIV-positive women become pregnant each year, and one quarter to one third of babies born to these women will be infected with HIV.

Reducing the HIV Threat to Babies

It's not known why some newborns stay free or eliminate HIV while others do not. "Mother to child transmission appears to occur around the time of birth. For example, we found that a longer duration of ruptured membranes just before birth correlates with a higher rate of transmission. The likelihood of transmission also seems to relate to the *viral load* of the mother," says Dr. Minkoff. (Viral load is the amount of RNA from the AIDS virus found in blood plasma; it also seems to predict how quickly HIV will progress to AIDS.)

The U.S. Food and Drug Administration approved prenatal use of the AIDS drug *zidovudine (AZT)* in HIV-positive pregnant women in 1994, based on a two-thirds reduction in maternal to fetal transmission seen in a major clinical trial of the drug. (Dr. Minkoff notes that transmission rates outside such studies may be somewhat higher.) A 1996 report in the *Journal of the American Medical Association* suggests that AZT's protective effect may be due to its ability to decrease viral load prior to delivery.

Other recent reports suggest that newborns may also be less apt to contract HIV if they are delivered by C-section. A randomized trial comparing vaginal delivery with cesarean section is under way in Europe. Clinical trials of two experimental AIDS vaccines to see if they can prevent maternal to fetal transmission of HIV are also under way in the United States. The trials, which began in 1993 at eight university research hospitals, involve HIV-positive pregnant women between sixteen and forty and will test the vaccines' safety as well as their ability to protect newborns.

New Treatments, New Hope

Although there's no cure for AIDS, new combination drug treatments are prolonging survival. It's hoped that AIDS will one day become a chronic, manageable illness rather than a death sentence.

More than a half dozen new AIDS drugs are now available, and more are on the way. None of these drugs kills HIV, but they interfere with its replication. Older AIDS drugs called *nucleoside reverse transcriptase inhibitors* (like AZT, *ddC* and *ddI*) interfere with the *reverse transcriptase* enzyme that allows HIV to invade CD4 cells; improved versions of these drugs have recently been approved, including *laminvudine* (Epivir). *Nevirapine* (Viramune) is a *nonnucleoside reverse transcriptase inhibitor*, which interferes with the enzyme in a different way. The newest drugs—*ritonavir* (Norvir), *saquinavir* (Invirase, Fortovase) and *indinavir* (Crixivan)—are *protease inhibitors*. They act later in HIV's reproductive cycle, disabling an enzyme that helps infected cells divide. Combined with other drugs, protease inhibitors can reduce HIV to virtually undetectable levels for long periods, and have helped cut deaths in the U.S. by about 20 percent (but only 7 percent among women). However, some people have developed resistance, and a reservoir of virus may remain.

At the same time, the goal of developing a vaccine to prevent HIV infection has remained elusive. "Because HIV mutates so often, it's hard to design a single vaccine to produce an immune response against it," concedes Dr. Minkoff.

Katy's Story, Cont'd

"I have had HIV for more than eight years, AIDS for nearly four years. I feel that the new drugs have given me a fighting chance, and I hope I will have many years left. I am not afraid to die. But I will keep fighting as long as I'm able.

"I am now doing volunteer work at an AIDS hospice, and I have been doing some public speaking in my community because I want people to

> know the epidemic is far from over and we can't afford to be silent or complacent. My message to women is a warning: If it can happen to me, it can happen to you. Protect yourself. Please."

▪ Prevention: The Best STD Treatment ▪

Because many women don't recognize that they are at risk for STDs and AIDS, they don't take adequate steps to protect themselves or get screened.

"As a nation, we are still very uncomfortable about our own sexuality. And even though information about STDs is readily available, too many people are not in the habit of protecting themselves," warns Dr. Penelope Hitchcock. "We have to make safe sex as automatic as seat belt use. It's not enough to carry a condom; you have to have some sense of how you're going to talk to a partner about using it. But the first step in changing behavior is to believe that you're at risk."

All women who are heterosexually active, especially those who have more than one sexual partner or who have engaged in unprotected sex, should ask to be tested for chlamydia and gonorrhea when they go for their regular GYN exam, advises Dr. Hitchcock. Women at high risk may need Pap smears every six months, rather than once a year, to check for cervical dysplasia, HPV and other infections. STD transmission among lesbians is typically very low, but it increases if women are bisexual.

"Women should also be alert for unusual vaginal discharge, lower abdominal pain, painful sexual intercourse. These all should be considered signs of an STD infection and brought to a physician's attention," counsels Dr. Ilona Brandeis. Too many women douche after finding unusual discharge, ridding their vagina of its natural protection and increasing the risk of spreading infection, she notes. Watch for warning signs in your partner, such as penile discharge or lesions. If either of you have any symptoms or have reason to suspect that you have been exposed, avoid sexual contact, get screened and get treated.

A woman who is taking oral contraceptives is still at risk for STDs, stresses Dr. Machelle Allen. "We have a long way to go to educate women that pregnancy is not the *only* consequence of sexual activity." All sexually active women who are not in strictly monogamous, long-term relationships, and who are on the pill, should also be using condoms.

Women of every age should practice safe sex; a recent survey by the Center for AIDS Prevention Studies at the University of California, San

Francisco found that 10 percent of people over fifty had risk factors for HIV/ AIDS, including multiple sex partners or partners at risk. But even among these high-risk older individuals, 85 percent had never used a condom. Federal health statistics show that new AIDS cases among people over fifty rose by 17 percent between 1990 and 1992. Older women are more vulnerable because of thin vaginal tissues and less robust immune systems.

Latex condoms used with the spermicide nonoxynol-9 (N-9) provide the most reliable currently known barrier against STDs and HIV. Lambskin condoms are more permeable by microbes. A 1997 study found that nonoxynol-9 alone appeared to be ineffective against transmission of HIV, chlamydia and gonorrhea. The large two-year study involving almost 1,300 African women found a long-lasting vaginal film containing N-9 offered no more STD protection than did a placebo. In lab tests N-9 killed HIV in the test tube, but "while spermicides kill sperm, they may not act on *other* cells present in semen, which could be infected with HIV," explains virologist David Phillips. Studies indicate that frequent use of nonoxynol-9 can also cause vaginal irritation, which may counteract any protective value.

The National Institute of Allergy and Infectious Diseases (NIAID), which conducted the N-9 study, is also funding research into microbicides, which may provide a broad spectrum of protection against STDs as well as prevent pregnancy (see box below).

Barrier methods such as the *diaphragm* and *cervical cap* alone are not effective. The female condom also shields the vagina and vulvar area from STDs which cause lesions, such as herpes (but many women find it awkward to use). "Dental dams" protect from infected semen during oral sex, but neither is widely used.

The possible role of oral contraceptives (OCs) against STDs is yet unclear. Studies in Sweden suggest that oral contraceptive users who contract PID may have milder cases and less infertility. OCs thicken cervical mucus, which some experts say may provide some protection against the spread of pathogens to the upper genital tract. But other studies report that OCs may have other effects that accelerate the progression of HIV once a woman is infected.

Microbicides: The Future of Prevention

The U.S. government has pledged $100 million to help create microbicides—vaginal gels, films, ointments or suppositories—to protect women against STDs. "Many women are unable or even afraid to ask their partners to use a condom, and some men refuse outright. An inexpensive, easy-to-use, undetectable microbicide would give *women* the power to protect themselves," remarks Sharon L. Hillier, Ph.D., director of Reproductive Infectious Disease Research at the Magee-Women's Hospital in Pittsburgh. "Microbicides might be formulated with or without spermicidal activity for women who wish to become pregnant."

Hillier has developed a suppository that would deliver extra lactobacillus to the vagina. "Lactobacillus produces lactic acid and hydrogen peroxide, both of which kill bacteria and viruses. A constant level of lactobacillus could make the vagina and cervix more resistant to infection."

Hillier and colleagues will test the experimental suppository among sexually active young women to see whether once-a-month use decreases the number of STD infections (as well as bacterial vaginosis). The girls will be given counseling to help them make better sexual choices, including abstinence, and given condoms for safe sex.

The research team will also be studying other potential microbicides, including the spermicide *benzalkonium chloride* (which is used in Europe and Japan), and the disinfectant *chlorhexidine* (contained in mouthwashes, hand soaps and a lubricant used for GYN exams in pregnant women) to see how they affect the vaginal environment and chlamydia, gonorrhea, HIV, genital herpes and trichomoniasis.

Other microbicide research funded by NIAID involves a vaginal gel containing *PMPA*, a compound with action similar to the AIDS drug AZT. Preliminary tests in female monkeys found that the PMPA gel stopped transmission of the simian AIDS virus.

Taking another tack, scientists at Johns Hopkins are testing a buffering gel that could potentially maintain the protectively low pH of the vagina in the presence of semen, while not disrupting its natural "flora" or causing irritation. Such a gel might be combined with other antimicrobial agents.

For now, most experts stress that the *best protection a woman has against STDs are latex condoms used with nonoxynol-9,* along with common sense, good judgment and, if need be, assertiveness in insisting that a man wear a condom.

Negotiating condom use can be difficult for women among certain ethnic and racial groups, concedes Dr. Machelle Allen. For example, in some Latino subcultures and other groups where male dominance is the cultural norm, discussing sex is taboo and prime importance is placed on having babies, there may be major resistance to talking about condoms, much less using them.

"When women try to make the point that condoms benefit both partners, some men may turn it back on her, saying, 'Who have you been with, what have you got, that I have to be protected?' Or they become enraged at the implication that they have been with other women," she remarks. "Some women may even be subject to violence from their partner if they insist the man wear a condom. So not only do we have to empower women, but we have to educate the men. And that cuts across all cultures."

Women need to be selective, limiting the number of sexual partners. Before you become intimate, you *must* talk about your sexual histories and find out if your prospective partner has (or has had) an STD and if he is cured, advises Dr. Allen. This can be hard at the start of a new relationship, when romance often overshadows reality. But it's vital to your health.

If you *do* become infected with an STD, seek out any previous sexual partner and notify him or her. This won't be easy either, but it can prevent illness and infertility in others and help stop the spread of STDs. (Of course, abstain until you're cured.)

One final point: "Sexual activity tends to be more irresponsible when it is related to any kind of drug use, and that includes alcohol," warns Dr. Allen. "We put a lot of emphasis on illicit drugs and STDs, but not enough on alcohol, which is a growing problem among college-age women as well as many professional women."

So take care that alcohol doesn't cloud your good judgment.

Your Reproductive Choices

American women have unprecedented freedom in their reproductive choices. But yearly the U.S. still has 3.6 million unplanned pregnancies, one of the highest rates among developed nations. *Half* of all unintended pregnancies occur when couples use contraception incorrectly or inconsistently; the other half occur when couples fail to use any contraception. If most women are sexually active, why aren't more using birth control?

A 1996 report from the Institute of Medicine (IOM) cites limited choices in contraceptive methods as one problem; more choices would allow people to find a method they'd be more likely to use. The IOM report also blamed regulatory, liability, political and social factors for hampering new contraceptive development.

"Contraception has also been linked with abortion by certain conservative groups, which lobby against funding for family planning clinics, whether they provide abortions or not, and limit access for women," remarks Luella Klein, M.D., director of Women's Health Issues for the American College of Obstetricians and Gynecologists and a professor of GYN/OB at the Emory University School of Medicine. In addition to fear of lawsuits, low profits have reduced the number of firms doing contraceptive research. Only three new birth control methods have been approved over the past decade: Norplant hormonal implants; Depo-Provera, an injectable contraceptive, and the female condom. But few women are using them. Some methods can be expensive, and private health insurance often doesn't pay for contraceptives.

Lingering fears about safety also inhibit contraceptive use. Surveys show that only one quarter to one fifth of women believe birth control pills, diaphragms and spermicides are safe; 10 percent deem intrauterine devices safe. "Except in very rare instances, contraceptives are safer, have fewer side effects than pregnancy and are a lot less expensive," says Dr. Klein.

Our attitudes toward sex, which stress romance over responsibility, are also to blame. "In this country we still think of sex as somehow sinful and do not teach responsible sexual behavior," Dr. Klein remarks. "Sex is portrayed in the media as having no consequences; people are 'swept away' by the moment. Some people may feel that you can't be 'swept away' using a condom. And some women, particularly teenagers, are often not in a position of power to refuse sex or negotiate condom use."

Although newer contraceptives are in the works, "what women need most *right now* is accurate information about existing choices so that they can choose a method that's right for them and use it properly," says Dr. Klein. This chapter provides up-to-date facts on reproductive choices, including emergency contraception and nonsurgical abortions.

◌ *Anna's Story* ◌

"I have been taking the pill on and off since I was fifteen. I hated the first one; it was a higher estrogen pill. It made me fat; I had headaches; my breasts hurt, I had longer and heavier periods. The second one had a much lower dose of estrogen. I stayed on that pill until I got married and decided to get pregnant.

"After I had my second child, my doctor recommended a new triphasic pill. At first I had some spotting, but it eventually stopped. I'm very happy with it. I have friends who say they're afraid to take birth control pills, but one of them has also gotten pregnant by accident twice. I told her that wouldn't have happened with the pill."

▪ Oral Contraceptives ▪

Oral contraceptives (OCs) are the most effective reversible birth control; less than 1 percent of women who use them correctly will become pregnant over a year. More than forty years after its introduction, the birth control pill is used by more than 10 million American women and 60 to 70 million women worldwide.

Birth control pills contain man-made estrogens and/or progesterone (progestins), in sequential doses. The continuous estrogen interferes with the normal hormonal feedback that triggers ovulation, blocking the rise in follicle-stimulating hormone (FSH), so ovarian follicles do not mature; progestins stop the mid-cycle surge in luteinizing hormone (LH), which prevents release of an egg. Progestins produce a thick cervical mucus that acts as a barrier to sperm, reduces contractions in the fallopian tubes, slows egg transport and makes the uterine lining less active and hospitable to a fertilized egg.

The original birth control pills, introduced in 1960, contained high doses (up to 150 micrograms) of *ethynyl estradiol,* which caused many adverse side effects, such as blood clots and strokes. Today there are more than 40 kinds of pills with much lower, far safer doses of estrogen and lesser levels of progestins.

There are two basic types of pills: combination pills containing both estrogen and progestin and all-progestin "minipills." Combination pills are taken for twenty-one days, then omitted to allow withdrawal bleeding (shedding of the endometrial lining). Minipills are taken all month. Combination pills are either *monophasic, biphasic or triphasic,* meaning they contain one, two or three different doses of hormones.

Most pills on the market are monophasics, containing fixed doses of estrogens (either ethynyl estradiol or *mestranol*) and progestins. Higher-dose monophasics (Ortho-Novum 1/50, Ovcon-50, Ovral) contain 50 micrograms (mcg) of estrogen and varied doses of progestin. So-called second-generation, low-dose pills (including Ortho-Novum 1/35, Lo/Ovral, Nordette, Loestrin 21) contain 20 to 35 mcg of estradiol and 0.15 to 1 mg of progestin. A new pill, Alesse, is the lowest-dose OC currently available, with 20 mcg of estradiol and 100 mcg of the progestin *levonorgestrel.* Biphasic pills (Nelova 10/11, Ortho-Novum 10/11) have a constant dose of estrogen but two doses of progestin.

"Third-generation" oral contraceptives contain *newer* progestins, *desogestrel* or *norgestimate,* which may have fewer side effects because they have fewer androgenic properties (see pages 168–169). The pills currently sold in the U.S. include a monophasic containing norgestimate (OrthoCyclen), a triphasic (OrthoTriCylen), and monophasics containing desogestrel (Ortho-Cept, Desogen).

Most triphasics (Ortho-Novum 7/7/7, Tri-Levlen, Tri-Norinyl) provide three doses of progestin over twenty-one days; *Triphasil* varies the dose of estrogen and progestin, while the new *Estrastep* gradually increases estrogen over the cycle with a constant 1 mg dose of progestin. Pill colors vary with the hormone dose; placebo "reminder" pills may be included for the off week.

Minipills (Micronor, Nor-QD, Ovrette) contain either 0.075 mg of nor-gestrel or 0.35 mg of norethindrone. While minipills do not contain enough progestin to affect ovulation, they produce a thick cervical mucus and make the uterine lining less active.

Which to Choose?

The different doses of hormones may provoke different and varying degrees of side effects, and a woman may need to try more than one type to find a pill that she's comfortable taking.

"Estrogen is probably responsible for headaches, nausea, increased vaginal discharge and weight gain, as well as some cardiovascular effects," explains Livia S. Wan, M.D., a professor of OB/GYN and director of the Family Planning Division at the NYU-affiliated Bellevue Hospital Center. "Progestins cause breast tenderness, acne, moodiness, sometimes facial hair growth, and they may affect cholesterol." Minor side effects usually resolve within the first one to three months of pill use. "If a symptom does not go away, we try another formulation."

Spotting or "breakthrough bleeding" affects one quarter of pill users during the first three months and is more common with all-progestin pills since there's no estrogen to maintain the endometrial lining, says Dr. Wan. With combination pills, spotting may result from low levels of either estrogen or progesterone at critical points in the cycle, and a short course of oral estrogen may help manage it. If spotting continues after three months, a medical evaluation is needed to rule out other causes. Conversely, periods may stop in long-term users. While it's not medically harmful, some women may be upset by it (or worry they're pregnant). Switching to another pill with a higher dose of estrogen can restore withdrawal bleeding.

Pill users who experience increased frequency or intensity of migraines may be candidates for minipills. If migraines occur only during menses, elimination of the pill-free period may help. Minipills may also be advisable for women who have endometriosis or those at greater risk for endometrial hyperplasia—e.g., women with polycystic ovarian syndrome (see page 74). Women can use the minipill as early as three weeks after childbirth.

Low-dose combination pills can be used to stabilize hormone levels in perimenopausal women. "Healthy perimenopausal women who are not smokers can take low-dose pills right up until menopause and then switch to hormone replacement," says Dr. Wan. "In fact, Loestrin and Alesse contain 20 mcg of ethynyl estradiol, which is close to the dose of 0.625 of conjugated estrogen in Premarin." However, abnormal bleeding needs to be monitored carefully (see page 26).

A woman wishing to take oral contraceptives needs to have a complete physical, including breast, pelvic and abdominal examinations, blood pressure check and a discussion of past medical problems (as well as family history). Since OCs have a slight risk of hypertension, blood pressure should be rechecked three months after starting the pill. However, starting on the first Sunday after your period (if it's more than five days after the onset of bleeding), you'll need a backup method of birth control, says Dr. Wan.

"If a woman forgets a pill, she should *not* stop taking her pills but should take the missed pill as soon as possible and use a backup method of birth control," says Dr. Wan. "If two pills are missed, take both as soon as possible, take two pills the next day, then finish the pack as usual. If three pills are missed, follow the packet instructions and use a backup contraceptive."

A 1996 industry-sponsored study of 1,800 pill users found that 25 to 50 percent stopped taking the pill within the first year of use, the most common reasons being bleeding and weight gain. Almost half of the women forgot to take one or more pills per cycle (increasing the risk of pregnancy), many because they didn't establish a pill-taking routine. The study found that women are *less likely to forget* if they take the pill in the morning *at breakfast* and *more likely* to forget to take the pill *at bedtime*. Women were also more likely to forget pills if they didn't read or understand the packet instructions.

Other things you should know about taking the pill:

• Missing pills increases your chances of spotting or breakthrough bleeding in between periods.

• Monthly bleeding will be different; it may last the seven off days and may be heavier at first. As the endometrium becomes less active, there may be less flow (or none at all).

- Premenstrual symptoms may be lessened on the pill but may not be eliminated. Even though you're not ovulating, there are still some natural hormonal shifts, and PMS may well be due to other factors besides estrogen and progesterone. PMS symptoms can also shift to the hormone-free days.

- Some women experience a drop in libido because low-dose combined pills suppress testosterone production. Switching to certain triphasics may help; a survey of 364 women aged eighteen to twenty-six by San Francisco State University suggests that triphasics that vary the progestin dose may increase sex drive and satisfaction.

- Progestins can cause depression, and you may need a different dose pill if it occurs.

- Certain antibiotics, such as penicillin or tetracycline, may interfere with OCs. Sulfa drugs may be used instead (or use backup contraception). Check on other possible drug interactions with your pharmacist.

- *Progestins also stimulate appetite.* If you're taking a high-progestin or an all-progestin minipill (or using Norplant or Depo-Provera), you may *unconsciously eat more.* To avoid weight gain, experts advise pill users to reduce calories and exercise.

- Avoid high-salt foods to minimize fluid retention; check package labels for sodium content. Taking diuretics (under the direction of a physician) may help.

- Taking extra vitamin B_6 (50 to 200 mg) may lessen side effects like breast tenderness; try slow-release formulas.

- However, taking one gram of vitamin C daily to prevent (or treat) colds is not recommended. It can *increase* blood levels of estrogen in low-dose pills by as much as 50 percent!

- *Pills do not protect against STDs; you must use condoms.*

The Facts About OC Risk

Even though the doses of hormones in today's pills are very small and the risks relatively slight, a recent survey by the Kaiser Family Foundation found that only one quarter of reproductive-age women consider birth control pills "very safe."

Studies since the 1960s have found the primary risks of OCs are cardiovascular: high blood pressure, blood clots and strokes. These are mostly associated with older, high-estrogen–dose pills.

Smokers fall in the highest-risk group, facing a 40 percent increased risk of heart attack and a 20 percent higher risk of stroke. Cigarette smoke makes blood platelets stickier, increasing the chances of clot formation. *All women over age thirty-five who smoke are advised* not *to take oral contraceptives.*

Experts say higher doses of estrogen can cause high blood pressure by triggering increases in blood *plasma* volume (plasma is the fluid that transports blood cells), which lead to resistance in smaller blood vessels, causing blood pressure to rise. Between 2 and 5 percent of otherwise healthy women taking birth control pills with estradiol doses *over 35 mcg* may develop high blood pressure; experts say that lower-dose pills carry little or no risk of high blood pressure for most women.

Higher doses of hormones can also increase frequency of blood clotting, leading to heart attacks and strokes. Higher-estrogen pills are also associated with a slightly increased risk of developing blood clots in deep veins (*deep vein thrombosis*), usually in the legs. Such clots can be dangerous if they break away and travel to blood vessels in the lungs or brain. Again, the problem is most severe among smokers.

For most women, the clotting effects of pills appear fairly modest. A case control study among more than one million women aged fifteen to forty-four in a large California HMO reported in the *New England Journal of Medicine* in 1996 that use of low-dose pills did not appear to increase the risk of stroke. Studies by the World Health Organization (WHO) also conclude that the pill does not increase the risk of stroke or heart attacks. However, studies by the WHO conducted in seventeen countries said third-generation pills containing either desogestrel or gestodene may double the risk of deep vein thrombosis compared with older oral contraceptives.

Nevertheless, according to Walter O. Spitzer, M.D., a professor of preventive medicine at McGill University in Montreal and the author of another study of third-generation pills, the actual risk of blood clots would only affect two to three users out of every 10,000 women who take these pills. Dr. Spitzer's 1996 report found the risk of blood clots was actually *lower* with third-generation pills than earlier versions of the pill.

High doses of older progestins have also been associated with adverse effects on cholesterol. Pills with higher *estrogenic* action normally raise "good" HDL (high-density lipoprotein) cholesterol and decrease "bad" LDL (low-density lipoprotein) cholesterol, whereas pills containing highly androgenic progestins (norgestrel, levonorgestrel and *norethindrone*) raise LDL. But when a *low dose* of these progestins is used, the effects are counterbalanced by estrogen. In fact, the American Heart Association says that OCs containing newer progestins (desogestrel, norgestimate or gestodene) may even have *positive* effects on cholesterol, reducing the risk of heart attack.

∞ *Who Should Not Take the Pill* ∞

Sources: American College of Obstetricians and Gynecologists; *Contraceptive Technology*, 16th ed., 1994, Irvington Publishers, Inc.

Women with the following conditions should not take oral contraceptives:

• A history of heart attack or stroke

• A history of blood clots in the legs, lungs or eyes

• A history of blood clots in deep veins of the legs

• Chest pain (angina pectoris)

• Unexplained vaginal bleeding (until there's a diagnosis)

• Liver tumors (benign or cancerous)

• Known or suspected breast, endometrial, cervical or vaginal cancer

• A history of inherited or acquired clotting abnormalities

• Women over 40 who smoke

Women with the following risk factors may take birth control pills, but only under careful supervision by their physician:

• Well-controlled high blood pressure

• Elevated cholesterol or triglycerides

• Diabetes

• Migraine headaches or epilepsy

• Breast nodules, benign breast disease, abnormal mammograms

• Gallbladder or kidney disease

• History of scant or irregular menstrual periods

Oral contraceptives decrease the risk of ovarian and uterine cancer, but may slightly increase the risk of breast cancer. Past studies have found that oral contraceptives may increase breast cancer risk by as much as 15 percent; more recent research shows birth control pills do not increase the risk of breast cancer in general, except among women who took the pill for more than ten years and started it in their teens.

The latest studies, published in 1996 in the journals *Contraception* and the *Lancet,* analyzed data from fifty-four studies among more than 153,000 women in twenty-five countries and found only a small increased relative risk of breast cancer among current users, with the greatest risk occurring with OC use before age twenty. After the pill was stopped, risk gradually declined to nonsignificance after ten years. Interestingly, cancers diagnosed in women taking OCs were less advanced than in women who had never taken the pill.

A 1995 study in the *Journal of the National Cancer Institute* found that women under thirty-five who took the pill within the past five years or those who took the pill for ten or more years were twice as likely to get breast cancer than nonusers. Starting the pill before age eighteen and staying on it for more than ten years tripled the risk for women under age thirty-five. Women between thirty-five and forty-four had an increased risk, but at a much lower level than the younger women and with less effect from the duration of pill use. Women with mothers or sisters with breast cancer had a slighter higher risk than those who did not, and after age forty-five there was *no* risk associated with oral contraceptive use.

Studies show the pill may also carry a slight risk of benign liver tumors and gallbladder disease. See your physician if you develop jaundice, a breast lump or depression while taking OCs.

The "Hidden" Health Benefits

"The health benefits of oral contraception are one of the best-kept secrets in America," says David Grimes, M.D., professor and vice chairman of the Department of OB/GYN and Reproductive Sciences at the University of California, San Francisco.

In fact, a recent Harris survey on women's reproductive health issues found that 20 percent of women were unable to name any benefits of taking oral contraceptives other than preventing pregnancy; 12 percent said there were none. Only 7 percent knew that OCs could lower their risk of gynecological cancers.

"After as little as three to six months on oral contraceptives, the risk of ovarian cancer starts to drop, and it continues to drop with increased duration of use, so that after a woman has been on birth control pills for ten years the risk of ovarian cancer is reduced by 80 percent," explains Dr. Grimes. In fact, OCs may prevent as many as 2,000 cases of ovarian cancer each year in the United States.

One way OCs may prevent ovarian cancer may be by blocking ovulation. A 1997 study suggests that half of all ovarian cancers may be related to the number of times a woman ovulates during her life; the more ovulatory cycles, the more cellular proliferation, and the greater the chance for a cancer-causing genetic mutation to arise.

Birth control pills also cause the uterine lining to become less active, reducing endometrial cancer risk by as much as 50 to 70 percent. "The protection is strongest in women who have not yet had children. The benefits for ovarian and endometrial cancer persist as long as fifteen years after stopping the pill," says Dr. Grimes.

Because of lighter monthly bleeding and less iron loss, the pill reduces iron-deficiency anemia by 50 percent. It also cuts the risk of pelvic inflammatory disease by 50 percent. Women on the pill have fewer benign breast tumors and a reduced risk of ectopic pregnancies as well.

Scientists are also investigating its effects on osteoporosis. "A growing number of studies following women forward in time have shown the longer a woman stays on combined birth control pills, the more minerals she has in her bones. So she would enter menopause with stronger bones," says Dr. Grimes. "Whether or not this will translate into protection against fractures down the road remains to be seen."

Sue's Story, Cont'd

"I had a tubal ligation done when I was forty-three. I didn't like oral contraceptives. I am divorced, and I knew that I did not want to have children. I was going in for an endometrial ablation, so I figured, I'm going to be under general anesthesia anyway, why not have it done then?

"You are still ovulating afterward, so you still have periods. I have no regrets. It really made sex very worry-free."

Fig. 16: TUBAL STERILIZATION

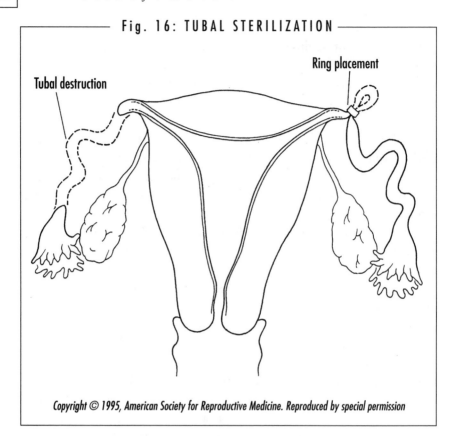

Ring placement

Tubal destruction

▪ Sterilization/Tubal Ligation ▪

More than 10 million American women have undergone tubal ligation, commonly called having the tubes "tied." The number of women relying on sterilization now tops 42 percent, making it currently more popular than the pill.

"The tubes may be tied and severed, or surgically blocked," explains Herbert B. Peterson, M.D., branch chief of Women's Health and Fertility at the federal Centers for Disease Control and Prevention and a clinical professor of OB/GYN at Emory University in Atlanta. If a woman is having tubal ligation right after she gives birth, a small abdominal incision is made. Otherwise it is usually done laparoscopically on an outpatient basis.

The latter most commonly involves electrocautery, "where you use electrical current to seal off the tube," Dr. Peterson explains. Other ligation techniques include applying a spring clip to the end of the tubes closest to the uterus, using a silicone (*Silastic*) band to close off a loop of each tube or (in postpartum tubal ligation) tying off the tube and removing a portion of the tube.

Tubal ligation is very effective, with a failure rate of only 0.2 to 0.5 percent. However, a long-term study of sterilization conducted by the CDC found that as many as 1 in 50 sterilized women in the study group became pregnant over a ten-year period. The study, which followed 10,685 women aged eighteen to forty-four for more than a decade, found that the risk of pregnancy was higher among those sterilized before age twenty-eight and those who had electrocauterization (suggesting that the electrical burn was not fail-safe). Women who underwent tubal ligation after childbirth had the fewest pregnancies.

Most Americans become sterilized around age thirty. More African-American women than whites choose sterilization, while more white males than blacks undergo vasectomy. Over four million men have had vasectomies, in which the tube carrying sperm from the testes is cut and sealed. Vasectomy, done under local anesthesia, actually carries *less* risk than tubal ligation, which requires general anesthesia, according to Dr. Peterson.

Surgical sterilizations can sometimes be reversed, but the success rate is better for vasectomies than for tubal ligations. Age, the amount of tube remaining and the length of time since the procedure are critical factors. However, anyone contemplating sterilization is advised to consider the operation permanent, stresses Dr. Peterson. Counseling prior to the procedure is important to emotional well-being afterward. "We found that six percent of the women in our study group had regrets and asked about having the ligation reversed. Young age at sterilization was by far the strongest predictor of later regret," he reports. "Younger women should strongly consider one of the reversible methods first."

✑ *Rachel's Story* ✑

"*I got my first diaphragm from planned parenthood when I was in college in the late 1960s. I was always afraid I'd forget to take birth control pills and bingo! I'd be pregnant.*

"*Using the diaphragm did take some forethought: I had to remember to take it with me if I spent the night and not 'forget' to put it in in the heat of the moment. In all the years I was single I met only one guy who used condoms. Most men assumed you were on the pill or left birth control up to you. I was not very much aware of STDs, but they were certainly out there.*

"My husband and I tried condoms for the first time after our son was born since I was told not to use the diaphragm for a while after giving birth. Frankly, I like them because they are a lot less messy than contraceptive gel, but my husband says he has less sensation with condoms. I have come to believe that the diaphragm enhances my orgasms. What's nice is we now have a choice of birth control, and we have incorporated both methods into our lovemaking."

▪ Barrier Methods ▪

Condoms, diaphragms, cervical caps and spermicides all work by preventing sperm from reaching an egg. The main side effects are allergies or sensitivity to latex or spermicides.

VAGINAL SPERMICIDES containing nonoxynol-9 are available in gels, creams, foams, suppositories and, most recently, longer-lasting films and gels. The gel *Advantage 24* adheres to the cervix and remains effective for twenty-four hours, unlike conventional spermicides, which must be applied two hours before intercourse. Spermicides are 79 to 87 percent effective when used alone, but when they are used with other barrier methods, the failure rate is much lower, and they protect against sexually transmitted diseases.

The DIAPHRAGM, used by 2 percent of American women, is a dome-shaped shield of latex attached to a flexible ring. Inserted behind the pubic bone and the cervix, it provides a large barrier to sperm. It must be used with contraceptive jelly or cream, and additional spermicide must be applied if a woman wants to have sex within six hours of her last intercourse. A diaphragm must be left in place for six to eight hours after making love, but it should be removed before twenty-four hours to avoid bacterial growth. It should be washed with mild soap and warm water and air-dried before it is returned to its case. Powder should not be used on a diaphragm because it damages the rubber, and talcum powder has also been associated with ovarian cancer.

A diaphragm will need to be refitted after a woman has a child or if she has gained or lost more than 10 to 15 pounds. "If a diaphragm is properly fitted, there should be no pressure or discomfort. If a woman is uncomfortable, she might need a different size or she may want to try the cervical cap. But she should try the diaphragm first," advises Dr. Wan.

The CERVICAL CAP is a small dome of rubber that fits snugly over the cervix. Used with spermicides, it may also help prevent STD transmission, but it still leaves most of the vaginal mucosa vulnerable to infections. Cervical caps are harder to insert than diaphragms and must be very carefully fitted. A cervical cap is squeezed and inserted into the vagina and fitted over the cervix to create a vacuum seal. It can be inserted up to forty-eight hours in advance but must be left in place for at least eight hours after lovemaking. However, additional spermicide is not needed for repeated intercourse during that period.

Cervical caps cannot be used by women who have ever had abnormal Pap smears, or who have chronic cervicitis or a history of toxic shock syndrome, according to Dr. Wan. A Pap test is repeated after the first three months of cap use. If it's normal, yearly testing is resumed. The cap cannot be used during the first six to twelve weeks postpartum, the first month after an abortion, during a period or when there's a vaginal infection.

The FEMALE CONDOM is basically an extended diaphragm that covers the vulvar area. Marketed under the name Reality, the device is comprised of two rings and a sheath of thin polyurethane closed at one end. The inner ring is placed over the cervix and secured behind the pubic bone, like a diaphragm. The outer ring covers the labia and part of the perineum.

"The female condom is a good choice for any woman who wants to protect herself from sexually transmitted diseases and does not want to leave the matter of condom use up to the man," says Dr. Wan. "It offers more protection than a diaphragm and is just as effective as a male condom in protecting against STDs."

The female condom is somewhat unwieldy and can take some getting used to. It has a tendency to ride up during intercourse if it is not sufficiently lubricated or to twist around if it is not inserted properly. The female condom should be as effective as a male condom, but if not used properly, about one in four women using it may become pregnant over the course of a year.

MALE CONDOMS are made of latex rubber, lambskin and new types of polyurethane. Latex and polyurethane provide the best protection against STDs. Lambskin is more permeable by microbes, but both are very effective in preventing pregnancy and transmission of STDs when used with a spermicide.

However, many men find condoms reduce sensation, while others believe it's not "macho" to wear one. About 18 percent of women rely on condoms. Usage is over 40 percent among teenagers and 20 percent among single women because of the STD protection. Newer male condoms made of polyurethane and other materials are stronger than latex and can be used with oil-based lubricants. They're a little baggier than traditional condoms, but they are also thinner and transmit heat better, so they may be more acceptable to men.

——————————— How Well They Work, How Much They Cost ———————————

Sources: The Alan Guttmacher Institute; Kaiser Family Foundation, 1993; Association of Reproductive Health Professionals

The following table shows the average cost and the percentage of women having unintended pregnancies for each method during the first year of use (in some cases cost estimates are based on average insurer payment to provider). Studies show that the effectiveness of short-term methods varies more by age and marital and poverty status than by method, suggesting that contraceptive failure may stem in part from improper and irregular use.

METHOD	PERFECT USE	AVERAGE USE	AVERAGE COST
No method	85.0	85.0	
Spermicides	3.0	30.0	$13/4 ounces
Withdrawal	4.0	24.0	
Periodic abstinence*	9.0	19.0	
Cervical cap	6.0	18.0	$69†
Diaphragm	6.0	18.0	$56†
Male condom	2.0	16.0	$1 each
Pill	0.1	3.0	$20–25/cycle
Copper-T IUD	0.8	1.0	$250–390**
Tubal ligation	0.2	0.2	$2,466.80****
Depo-Provera	0.3	0.4	$60–75/shot
Vasectomy	0.1	0.2	$755.70****
Norplant	0.04	0.05	$500–698***

       * *Rhythm method*
      † *Device and office visit for fitting (not including spermicide)*
    ** *Device and office visit for insertion—lasts 10 years*
  *** *Implants and office visit for insertion—lasts 5 years*
**** *Average payment to provider from insurer (ARHP)*

▪ Intrauterine Devices (IUDs) ▪

Intrauterine Devices (IUDs) prevent pregnancy by interfering with sperm transport and egg fertilization in several ways: Its presence in the uterus interferes with movement of sperm; copper contained in one type produces changes in uterine secretions that kill sperm. Both types of IUDs cause changes in the endometrium that prevent a fertilized egg from implanting.

IUDs are T-shaped. When the device is inserted into the uterus through a small hollow tube, the arms of the T are collapsed at its sides. Only two IUDs are currently available: the copper-T ParaGard, which can be used for eight to ten years, and the Progestasert, which must be replaced each year and is made of soft plastic material that slowly releases progesterone from the vertical portion of the T into the uterus. Recent studies show both cause a slight (or no) risk of infection and uterine perforation (usually self-healing) at the time of insertion.

The copper-T IUD is the most popular method of contraception world-wide; 25 to 30 percent of European women use it. "Studies by the World Health Organization show the failure rate after seven years is 1.5 percent, which is similar to female sterilization," reports Daniel R. Mishell, M.D., professor and chair of Obstetrics and Gynecology at the University of Southern California School of Medicine in Los Angeles and a noted researcher in contraception. "The IUD is also cost-effective. With a simple five-minute painless insertion, a woman can have very effective, reversible contraception lasting ten years, with minimal side effects."

However, less than 1 percent of American women are using IUDs, largely because of the fallout from safety problems with the Dalkon shield in the 1970s. After more than 10,000 lawsuits had been filed by women who claimed they contracted pelvic inflammatory disease because of the Dalkon shield, other manufacturers withdrew their products from the market, even though they did not pose the same high risk of infection. The Dalkon shield had a multifilament tail string made of material that allowed bacteria to ascend from the vagina into the uterine cavity. Today's IUDs have a mono-filament nylon tail like fishing line that does not pose that risk, according to Dr. Mishell.

"IUDS are recommended *only* for women who are in stable, monogamous relationships, who are at low risk for sexually transmitted diseases. For those women it can be a safe, effective method of contraception," says Dr. Livia Wan. IUDs can also be a good option for a woman who does not want any more children but doesn't wish to have her tubes tied, she adds.

Insertion can cause some cramping, and there may be spotting or bleeding between periods during the first few months of use. Fertility resumes immediately after the IUD is removed. IUDs should be inserted and removed only by a trained health provider. Women using them should check for the tail once a month to make sure the device has not been expelled during menses, which may happen in 5 to 6 percent of women, notes Dr. Wan.

A levonorgestrel-secreting IUD is available in Scandinavia and may also be marketed in the United States. Its advantages not only include use for five to seven years and less bleeding or pain but experts say it could be used in combination with estrogen for hormone replacement therapy.

∞ *What's on the Horizon?* ∞

A number of new contraceptives are in clinical trials or in development. They include hormone-secreting or medicated IUDs, vaginal rings containing progestins, short-term or biodegradable hormonal implants, transdermal patches that deliver ovulation-inhibiting hormones and, in the future, antifertility vaccines. Three new cervical caplike devices—the Oves Cap, a cervical cap with a small handle; Femcap, slightly larger and shaped like a sailor's cap; and Leah's Shield, which has an opening to let out cervical secretions while keeping out sperm—are being tested.

As mentioned in Chapter Eight, microbicides are being developed not only to protect against STDs but also to prevent pregnancy. New spermicides in the form of long-lasting vaginal films and new versions of the pill are also on the way.

Women often wonder why there aren't better contraceptives for *men*. The efforts being made in this direction include:

SPERM SUPPRESSANTS using high doses of testosterone to block or suppress FSH, which controls sperm production, are being tested in the U.S. and around the world. Studies in China, Australia and Europe found 97 percent of men produced little or no sperm, and fertility was greatly reduced. Other sperm suppressants using GnRH antagonists are also being tested.

CONTRACEPTIVE VACCINES for men are currently in safety trials. The vaccines use *LH-RF (luteinizing hormone–releasing factor)* to provoke immune system antibodies, which suppress androgen levels. To maintain their sex drive, men would be given testosterone.

Other possible vaccines may immunize men against FSH or produce antisperm antibodies to immobilize sperm.

SPERM DUCT PLUGS involve an injection of liquid plastic into the vas, or silicone plugs to obstruct the duct, so that no sperm get into the ejaculate. This would be a nonsurgical alternative to vasectomy and would have no effect on male hormones.

CHEMICAL STERILIZATION would use chemicals to scar the walls of the sperm ducts, blocking sperm from entering the ejaculate.

The *"MALE PILL"* is an extract of cottonseed oil, *gossypol,* taken daily as a pill to cause a drop in sperm production but not in androgens. It's currently under study in nine countries.

SPERM DISABLERS, another possible male pill, would be made of a compound that "blinds" sperm by blocking an enzyme that enables sperm to recognize eggs. The synthetic enzyme is being studied at North Carolina State University in animals but is several years away from human testing.

▪ Other Hormonal Methods ▪

DEPO-PROVERA is a long-acting, injectable progestin (*medroxyprogesterone acetate*) that has been used by more than 30 million women in 90 countries. Approved in 1992 by the FDA, it is used by 3 percent of American women. A single injection of 150 mg of Depo-Provera every three months blocks ovulation by suppressing mid-cycle surges of FSH and LH, thickening cervical mucus and making the uterine lining less active. The first shot is given within five days of menses to prevent unintended pregnancy. If a woman waits more than fourteen weeks between injections, she must have a pregnancy test. "After the second or third shot, a woman may not bleed, but Depo-Provera does not put a woman into menopause," says Dr. Wan. However, after stopping the injections, women may not regain fertility for six months.

Depo-Provera does not protect against STDs. Side effects are similar to other hormonal contraceptives: irregular bleeding or spotting initially, weight gain, headaches and fatigue. Studies by the World Health Organization suggest Depo-Provera may reduce the risk of endometrial cancer; there's no evidence yet about protection from ovarian cancer. Contraindications are similar to Norplant. Another injectable progestin, cyclo-provera, is under clinical investigation.

NORPLANT consists of six matchstick-size capsules made of a silicone material, Silastic, which releases the ovulation-blocking progestin levonorgestrel. Norplant was approved in 1990 after two decades of testing on more than 500,000 women worldwide. The implants are used by 1.3 percent of U.S. women. The capsules are implanted with a small surgical instrument called a *trocar* beneath the skin of a woman's upper arm, using local anesthesia. Levonorgestrel has the same general effects in preventing pregnancy as Depo-Provera, becoming effective in twenty-four hours, and remains active for up to five years. The implants are considered 99 percent effective. Fertility returns almost immediately after they are removed. Norplant provides no protection against STDs and must be used with condoms.

Of women on Norplant, 80 percent experience irregular menstrual bleeding, most commonly in the first six months after implantation. About a third suffer headaches or weight loss or gain, 20 percent develop mild acne and some women become depressed because of the progestin.

Contraindications to Norplant are similar to OCs. Women who should not use Norplant include those with histories of blood clots (phlebitis and thromboembolic disorders), women with liver disease and women with histories of abnormal bleeding. Women with high cholesterol need to be followed closely, since levonorgestrel is known to raise levels of "bad" LDL cholesterol. There is no indication the Silastic causes autoimmune disease. "Overall there were no major adverse affects seen in all the years of testing. In fact, Norplant is safer than the pill because it contains no estrogen," says Dr. Wan, who has been involved in clinical trials of Norplant and its two-capsule version, *Norplant II*. "After five and a half years of testing, we found that two implants are just as effective in preventing pregnancy as six." Norplant II has been approved by the FDA for up to three years of use. A single implant being tested was found to be less androgenic.

Norplant's major problems have been improper insertion, which can cause scarring and make the capsules difficult to remove, and "migration" of the capsules. Initially one million women had received the implants, but recently use has dropped dramatically with an avalanche of lawsuits by women claiming injury from botched implantation or removal.

▪ Emergency Contraception ▪

Another little-used form of birth control is emergency or postcoital contraception. These morning-after pills are regular birth control pills taken in two larger than usual doses within seventy-two hours of unprotected intercourse. This high dose disrupts the body's natural hormonal patterns, preventing fertilization or implantation and reducing the chances of pregnancy by about 75 or 80 percent, according to Allan Rosenfield, M.D., dean of the Columbia University School of Public Health and a professor of public health and obstetrics and gynecology. "However, this is *not* an abortifacient, since the medical definition of pregnancy begins at implantation of a fertilized ovum," he stressed.

While not officially approved by the FDA, the agency in 1997 declared that oral contraceptives used as morning-after pills are a safe and effective way to prevent pregnancy. The FDA says emergency contraception could prevent up to 2.3 million unintended pregnancies a year.

Eight brands of oral contraceptives can be used. The best-studied regimen calls for a total dose of at least 200 mcg ethnyl estradiol and 2.0 mg of norgestrel (1.0 mg of levonorgestrel) taken in two doses. With the high-dose pill Ovral, which contains 50 mcg estrogen, two white pills are taken within 72 hours of unprotected intercourse, and two more are taken 12 hours later. With lower-dose pills of 30 to 35 mcg, such as Nordette or Levlen, four light-orange pills are taken initially, and four more 12 hours later (with Lo/Ovral, each dose is four white pills). If the triphasics Triphasil or Tri-Levlen are used, four yellow pills (corresponding to cycle days 12-21) are taken in each of the two doses. The minipill Ovrette can be taken in two doses of twenty tablets, but is recommended only if women can't take estrogen.

Such high doses of hormones cause nausea and vomiting in about half the women who take them, sometimes severe enough to prevent the postcoital contraceptive from working. Some physicians give an antinausea drug at the same time. "This is not something women should use all the time. But we could have a significant impact on unintended pregnancy if this were an option of which more women were aware," says Dr. Rosenfield.

As with regular use of birth control pills and other hormonal contraceptives, morning-after pills are not advisable for women with severe liver disease, histories of blood clots or other circulatory problems.

The antiprogesterone drug mifepristone (RU-486), which prevents a fertilized egg from implanting in the uterine wall, can also be used as a morning-after contraceptive in a single, 600 mg dose taken within seventy-two hours of unprotected intercourse. A study in the *New England Journal of Medicine* found mifepristone effective with much milder side effects than high doses of birth control pills. (For more on RU-486, see page 183.)

Post-coital insertion of the copper-T IUD can be used as an alternative form of emergency contraception, for those women who want an IUD and have no contraindications to its use. It can be inserted up to five days after unprotected intercourse, preventing implantation, and is left in place for further contraceptive use.

∞ *N i c h o l e ' s   S t o r y* ∞

"Getting an abortion was the absolute worst experience of my life. I had too much guilt and regret afterward.

"With the birth control available in this day and age, I had no excuse for getting pregnant. I was seeing this really wonderful guy. I should have been on the pill since I am allergic to all the gels, foams and creams, but since I smoke, I was afraid to take the pill. We were using the rhythm method, but that didn't work at all. I happen to be very regular, and I knew immediately that I was pregnant.

"I went right away. I probably never would have done it if I hadn't had two small children. I'd known my boyfriend for only four months. I tried to think of every way not to do it, but I really had no choice. I do believe that life begins at conception. I was raised a Catholic, and they would say I killed my baby. I have to live with that knowledge every day. I had no other choice. But it took me a long, long time to get over it."

▪ Pregnancy Termination/Abortion ▪

According to the federal Centers for Disease Control and Prevention, 1.2 million abortions were performed among women aged fifteen to forty-four in 1994, the *lowest* number since 1976. Half the women who undergo abortions say either they or their partners were using contraception at the time they became pregnant. Most were white, single and younger than twenty-five. Around 43 percent had had at least one previous abortion; 49 percent had at least one child.

In January 1973 abortion was legalized in the United States in the landmark U.S. Supreme Court decision in the case of *Roe* v. *Wade*. The High Court reaffirmed the legality of abortion in 1983. Since then antiabortion groups have lobbied to have the ruling reversed and have pushed through passage of state laws restricting access to abortion, especially late-term abortions.

While abortion is legal, it is not always obtainable. The bitter ongoing political debate has made many practitioners shy away from providing abortion services, and picketing and violence have forced many clinics to close. According to the Alan Guttmacher Institute, there were 2,380 hospitals, clinics and physicians' offices providing abortions in 1992, down from almost 3,000 in 1982. The biggest decline has been an 18 percent drop among hospital providers between 1988 and 1992. The Guttmacher Institute says 84 percent of counties in the U.S. have *no* abortion provider; in nonmetropolitan areas, 94 percent of counties have no provider. One quarter of women must travel fifty miles from home for an abortion.

Surveys show that two thirds of the 40,000 OB/GYNs in this country do not perform abortions. Some doctors refuse on moral or religious grounds, some because of community pressure and others have *not even been taught how*. Only 12 percent of residency programs in obstetrics and gynecology currently offer abortion training. In an effort to rectify this situation, the Residency Review Committee has recommended that abortion training be offered by U.S. obstetrical residency training programs, but those with "moral or religious objections" may decline to take part.

Medical (Drug-Induced) Abortion

The situation is expected to change with the use of drug-induced abortions, which can be administered in the privacy of a physician's office away from abortion clinics, where the majority of surgical procedures are currently performed.

MIFEPRISTONE (RU-486) has been used with prostaglandins in Europe since 1981 to induce early abortions. Mifepristone blocks the action of progesterone, which helps prepare the lining of the uterus for implantation of a fertilized egg, so that the lining breaks down, menstruation occurs and the fertilized egg is expelled. Oral prostaglandins are used to induce uterine contractions, resulting in a process almost indistinguishable from an early miscarriage.

For more than a decade, women in three countries have used the mifepristone–prostaglandin combination for medical abortions; studies here and in a dozen other countries have shown it to be safe and effective. Mifepristone received FDA approvable status in this country in 1996 (it had been approved in 1988 in France and China and in 1991 in Great Britain). Because of the continuing controversy over abortion, the French manufacturer turned over U.S. rights for mifepristone to the nonprofit Population Council.

The administration of mifepristone requires at least three visits to a doctor or clinic, beginning with counseling, a physical examination and determination of the length of pregnancy. At the first visit the woman is given three tablets of mifepristone (200 mg each) and remains under observation for thirty minutes. During the second visit, thirty-six to forty-eight hours later, she is given two 200 mcg tablets of *misoprostol*, and remains under medical supervision at the clinic for four hours. French data indicate two thirds of women expel their fetus during this four-hour period; most women will abort within twenty-four hours after taking misopristol. The third visit twelve days later is to ensure that the abortion is complete; if not, vacuum curettage is done (this may be needed in 4 percent of women).

A large study in France involving 2,480 women found that the combination of drugs, taken within seven weeks of the last menstrual period, safely induces abortion in 95.5 percent of cases. The most common side effects were pain from uterine contractions in 82 percent of women and severe bleeding in 1.4 percent. Preliminary data from a similar safety and effectiveness study in the U.S. involving 2,121 women were nearly identical. Other trials indicate a lower dose of mifepristone (200 mg) is just as effective and will lower costs. The failure rate (requiring surgical intervention) was around 8 percent.

METHOTREXATE AND MISOPROSTOL, two widely available and inexpensive drugs approved by the FDA for treating cancer and ulcers respectively, have been shown to be just as effective as mifepristone in inducing early pregnancy termination. *Methotrexate* halts the rapid division of cells, in this case stopping early fetal and placental development (it has long been used to end ectopic pregnancies). Misoprostol is a prostaglandin, which induces contractions to empty the uterus.

The first study of the two-drug regimen was conducted by Richard U. Hausknecht, M.D., an associate clinical professor of OB/GYN at the Mt. Sinai School of Medicine in New York. The study involved 178 women (all less than sixty-three days pregnant), who received an injection of methotrexate and, five to seven days later, doses of misoprostol, as either tablets or vaginal suppositories. Dr. Hausknecht reported in 1995 in the *New England Journal of Medicine* that the combination of drugs was successful in terminating the pregnancies of 171 out of the 178 women, most of them within a day. The only side effects other than heavy bleeding were moderate cramping, nausea and diarrhea. A multicenter trial involving 300 women reported in 1996 in the journal *Contraception* had similar results. Like mifepristone, the dual-drug procedure requires three visits to the doctor.

The regimen would allow a woman to terminate a pregnancy almost "the minute she knows she's pregnant," says Dr. Hausknecht, instead of waiting the six weeks usually required for a surgical abortion. "In my initial study the vast majority of patients had had a surgical abortion and viewed the treatment as more private and less painful." (He has now tested the regimen on more than 1,350 patients, with a 3 percent failure rate.)

Drug-induced abortions require no anesthesia or surgery, and do not pose a risk of uterine perforation or injury to the cervix. They also offer a woman more privacy and control, away from the often turbulent atmosphere surrounding abortion clinics. However, while the drugs are simple to administer, they require absolute accuracy in the dating of each pregnancy by ultrasound which can be expensive and not always available, adds Dr. Hausknecht.

Side effects of mifepristone include nausea, weakness, fatigue, and, less commonly, headache. There may be light uterine bleeding in the two days before taking the prostaglandin. Side effects of prostaglandins include cramps and abdominal pain similar to a very heavy menstrual period, nausea, vomiting and diarrhea (sometimes requiring medication). A woman will also experience bleeding, either heavy bleeding lasting at least one week or moderate bleeding and spotting lasting one to three weeks.

A recent survey by the Population Council estimates that 60 to 70 percent of women would choose mifepristone over a surgical abortion. A third of obstetrician/gynecologists who don't currently perform abortions say they would be likely to prescribe mifepristone. Use of either of these drug regimens up to fifty-six days since a woman's last menstrual period would make over half of the women who currently undergo surgical procedures eligible for an earlier, drug-induced abortion, says Beverly Winikoff, M.D., Senior Medical Associate at the Population Council.

⎯⎯⎯⎯ ∾ *N i c h o l e ' s   S t o r y ,   C o n t ' d* ∾ ⎯⎯⎯⎯

"What I had was kind of like a D and C. I had it done at a clinic. I stayed in the recovery room for a couple of hours afterward and they gave me some antibiotics and sent me home.

> *"The people at the clinic were very nice, sympathetic and understanding—especially the doctor who performed the abortion. I had been in therapy since my husband and I separated, but nothing affected me like this. My therapist told me it was very important to grieve. I asked the clinic doctor, 'Will this feeling ever go away?' He said, 'No, you just learn to live with it.'*
>
> *"I believe abortion should be legal. It's not a good choice, but it's a choice some women need to have. We also need better birth control; maybe if I'd have had some alternatives, I would not have gotten pregnant and been faced with this awful thing."*

Surgical Abortion

Surgical procedures are quicker and require fewer office visits than drug-induced abortions. They are slightly more effective; a woman notices less blood loss and is unaware of the passing of the fetal tissue. Almost all abortions are performed during the first trimester, at or shortly before twelve weeks of gestation, when the risk of major complications is less than 1 percent. Several techniques are currently in use:

MENSTRUAL EXTRACTION can be performed up to the sixth week after the last menstrual period. It's a relatively simple outpatient procedure done under intravenous analgesia and/or injections of local anesthetic into the cervix (*paracervical block*). A hand suction device and a small flexible tube (*cannula*) are used to extract the contents of the uterus. The major disadvantages include a relatively high failure rate (failure to remove the embryo) and risk of cervical lacerations. Side effects include mild cramping, nausea, light-headedness and faintness.

SUCTION DILATION AND CURETTAGE is the most commonly performed abortion procedure in the United States, representing more than 90 percent of all abortions. The procedure may be performed until thirteen weeks' gestation and requires some cervical dilation. A disposable *curet* (a cigar-shaped scraping device) with attached vacuum suction is used to empty the uterine contents (which are sent for pathologic confirmation that the abortion was complete). It typically takes about fifteen minutes and may be done on an outpatient basis under local anesthesia at a clinic or in a hospital under general anesthesia. A woman can be sent home within one to two hours if local anesthesia is used.

Immediate complications may include uterine perforation and excessive bleeding caused by lacerations to the cervix or retained products of conception. Long-term complications include *cervical incompetence*, in which the cervix is unable to maintain future pregnancy without reinforcing, and infertility as a result of uterine scarring (usually the result of repeated D&C procedures).

Second-trimester abortions are more difficult since the cervix is not easily dilated and the fetus is larger.

DILATION AND EVACUATION is the most common method used in the early second trimester and is safe up to twenty weeks of gestation. It requires presurgical cervical dilation, using laminaria (dried seaweed, which absorbs secretions and slowly dilates the cervix overnight) or prostaglandin suppositories applied the day before surgery. The procedure takes approximately thirty minutes and can be performed on an outpatient basis using spinal *epidural* or general anesthesia in a hospital setting. Curettage aided by ultrasonography may be performed afterward to make sure the abortion was complete. *Oxytocin*, which causes uterine contractions, may be given intravenously during or immediately following the procedure, so contractions can be controlled and blood loss minimized. Side effects are similar to those experienced with a D&C. In general, dilation and evacuation has a low complication rate.

AMNIOINFUSION involves injecting solutions of saline or prostaglandins directly into the amniotic sac under local anesthesia, to induce abortion by bringing on labor. It is generally used after sixteen weeks of gestation and is usually performed as an inpatient procedure. Laminaria may be inserted the day before to dilate the cervix, and intravenous oxytocin may also be given to decrease the labor period. It's less costly and slightly more effective than dilation and evacuation. However, the procedure can be upsetting for the patient, who experiences labor and the expulsion of fetal tissue and placenta. Side effects include nausea, vomiting and diarrhea. Complications include cervical trauma, blood loss, fever, uterine inflammation and the possible need for a D&C afterward. The type of prostaglandin used cannot be employed in women with asthma, pulmonary hypertension, glaucoma, epilepsy or hypertension.

Third-trimester abortions are much less common, traumatic and mostly performed when the life of the mother is jeopardized by continuing the pregnancy or the fetus has died. Congress has tried to enact measures to outlaw the procedure; many states currently do not permit abortions after the twenty-fourth week of pregnancy.

After any abortion procedure, women are sent home with antibiotics to prevent infection and after-care instructions. These include abstaining from sexual intercourse and avoiding use of tampons, swimming and bathtub bathing for two to four weeks, as well as refraining from strenuous exercise of any kind and working long hours. Women are also cautioned to call a physician if they pass large clots or soak through two sanitary napkins in an hour. Women may take acetaminophen for pain, but not aspirin or ibuprofen since these may interfere with clotting. A checkup is required three weeks after the procedure.

Women who decide to terminate pregnancies by any means may suffer short-term emotional problems: conflict over their decision, mourning or guilt. However, studies do not find lasting negative psychological effects after abortions, even in highly religious women (although some admit to symptoms of depression only long afterward). Most abortion providers stress that patients need counseling before and afterward.

No matter which side one is on in the debate over abortion, experts agree there are entirely too many unplanned pregnancies. "It all comes back to people acting responsibly and how crucial it is for people not desiring pregnancy to use birth control or abstinence, depending on their religious views," concludes Dr. Charles J. Lockwood, chairman and Stanley H. Kaplan professor of OB/GYN at NYU Medical Center. "But thoughtful people on both sides of the abortion debate would agree the best way to prevent abortion is to prevent unwanted pregnancy in the first place."

Pregnancy and Postpartum

While the most visible reminders of pregnancy may be stretch marks, many unseen changes that take place in the reproductive tract can affect a woman long after she's given birth. This chapter focuses on changes and problems that arise before, during and after pregnancy. You'll also hear from women who "tell it like it is" about their childbirth experiences.

∞ *Anna's Story, Cont'd* ∞

"With both my children, I knew immediately when I was pregnant. I could just tell. It's hard to explain. It's this funny feeling you get. Your breasts feel tingly and extra tender; everything inside feels sort of full and I am always very regular. I have never been late a day unless I was pregnant."

▪ Expecting Changes ▪

Although a missed period is usually the first sign of pregnancy, some women, like Anna, seem to know right away that conception has taken place. You may not "miss" a period; spotting or bleeding may occur as the developing embryo implants itself in the womb, which may be mistaken for a lighter than normal period. You may feel a "tingling" sensation in the breasts or experience fatigue or frequent urination.

Most of the early signs of pregnancy are due to the effects of hormones, says Iffath Abbasi-Hoskins, M.D., director of Obstetrics at the NYU-affiliated Bellevue Hospital Center. "Massive amounts of hormones are produced by the placenta, and while they are intended to support the growth and development of the pregnancy, they have many effects on organs in the reproductive tract and elsewhere in the body."

The biggest initial surge is in progesterone, which is produced by the corpus luteum to promote placental blood vessel development to nourish the newly implanted embryo. The placenta eventually takes over progesterone production and also produces estrogen in much larger amounts than in non-pregnant women. (There's a rapid rise in estrogen in the months before delivery. Then both hormones take a nosedive. They return to prepregnancy levels around six weeks after the birth of the baby.)

Four days after fertilization the embryo begins to produce *human chorionic gonadotropin (hCG)*, the so-called pregnancy hormone. Blood or urine tests can pick up the earliest levels of hCG. Home pregnancy tests detect hCG in urine by changing the color of a specially treated stick. "Even if used correctly, home pregnancy tests may turn out negative because hCG levels were not high enough yet," remarks Dr. Hoskins. If you think you're pregnant but the test is negative, try another test in a week.

The placenta also produces *human placental lactogen (hPL)*, critical to the baby's growth and development, changing the mother's metabolism to make *glucose* (blood sugar) and proteins more available to the fetus. Along with other hormones, hPL stimulates milk glands in the breasts to grow and eventually to produce milk. Breasts may feel tender, heavier, fuller and, as early as two weeks after conception, become noticeably larger.

Some of the earliest signs of pregnancy are visible only to a physician's trained eye. The consistency and color of the vaginal area change, becoming a little more swollen and fleshy. The folds in the vaginal lining become more pronounced and change from pink to a bluish color. "This 'blueing' of the tissues is due to increased blood flow in the area. Other internal changes include softening of the cervix and a change in its position as pregnancy advances. The ovaries become somewhat smaller because they are less hormonally active," says Dr. Hoskins.

Women frequently have increased vaginal discharge, especially during early pregnancy, because of hormonal changes in the mucus-producing glands in the cervix, Dr. Hoskins explains. This discharge is thin and white and may have a mild odor. There's also an increased tendency for yeast infections because hormones can raise stored glucose in vaginal cells, decreasing friendly lactobacillus and allowing yeast to overgrow.

Up to 80 percent of women develop "morning sickness," the queasiness, nausea and vomiting that usually occur in the first trimester and can actually occur at any time of the day. Nausea is thought to be due to the effects of hCG, "which can act as a noxious trigger in an area of the brain, directly stimulating nausea and vomiting, or act with estrogen and progesterone to cause morning sickness," explains Dr. Lockwood. "The intensity of symptoms may correlate with higher levels of hCG, such as in women carrying twins."

One theory suggests that nausea and vomiting are a biological mechanism designed to prevent women from ingesting things that may have potentially toxic effects on a developing embryo, says Dr. Lockwood. While morning sickness usually goes away by the end of the first trimester, 3 percent of women develop *hyperemesis gravidarum*, severe nausea and vomiting that may require hospitalization (see page 195).

During pregnancy, digestion slows due to the increase in progesterone, and the enlarging uterus pushes on other organs in the abdomen and pelvis, resulting in constipation and heartburn. "The expanding uterus presses on the bladder, so the capacity of the bladder is decreased. There is also a lot more blood flow to the kidneys so the output of urine is increased, so you have to 'go' more often," says Dr. Hoskins. In the third trimester normal pelvic muscle relaxation and pressure from the growing fetus may cause some leaking of urine, especially with coughing or sneezing.

Up to 85 percent of women have minor abdominal cramps or pelvic pain during pregnancy, most often during the first and third trimesters as the uterus and surrounding ligaments stretch. "At first a woman may feel an achy, crampy, 'pulling' sensation in the pelvis," notes Dr. Hoskins. As the uterus enlarges more rapidly during the second trimester, tension on the muscles and ligaments may produce more discomfort. Late in pregnancy women may frequently feel stabbing pains inside the vagina, perhaps a loosening of the pelvic bones in preparation for labor, according to Dr. Lockwood. Warm baths or showers can soothe most aches and pains.

During pregnancy, blood volume increases by nearly 50 percent to supply mother and baby adequately with oxygen and vital nutrients. This rise in blood circulation causes small blood vessels in the skin over the breasts to become engorged, and many veins and arteries are more noticeable. Blood vessel distension causes varicose veins in the perineum, the anal area (better known as *hemorrhoids*, see page 208) and the legs. Pressure on the abdomen can result in *inguinal hernia*, a protrusion of intestines (or even fat) through a weak area of connective tissue in the groin area. Pregnancy can aggravate an existing hernia, and the labia may swell painfully. A woman may also have frequent backaches, worsening migraines, itching and darkening of skin pigment in the armpit, in the groin, around the nipples and in a line in the center of the lower abdomen, called the *linea nigra*.

Then of course there's weight gain. According to the latest guidelines from the American College of Obstetricians and Gynecologists (ACOG), a woman who is within her "ideal" weight range should expect to gain twenty-five to thirty-five pounds during pregnancy. Women should gain ten pounds in the first twenty weeks of pregnancy and about a pound per week thereafter, when the baby puts on most of its weight. Weight gain can be upsetting, but a large study suggests that fat stores may be *critical* to fetal health; failure to gain enough weight may lead to a low-birth-weight baby.

There is an unexpected bonus along with a bulging belly. While changing hormone levels may dampen sexual desire somewhat in the first trimester, during the second trimester increased blood flow to the genital area and the breasts can greatly increase their sensitivity, even to the point of feeling a heightened readiness for orgasm! Many partners feel more loving by sharing the experience of pregnancy.

∞ R a c h e l ' s   S t o r y ,   C o n t ' d ∞

"I never thought of myself as a high-risk pregnancy, but because of my age, I knew I would have to go for the amnio. I knew about the increased risks of Down syndrome and all that, but I was so happy to be pregnant I didn't dwell on it. My husband was more worried about it than I was at the time, so I only told him about the slight risk of miscarriage after it was over.

"*The amnio didn't hurt. I was more upset by the size of the needle. It is huge! And seeing it go into my belly on the ultrasound, so close to the baby, was unsettling. They numbed the area, but I could feel this uncomfortable pressure as the needle went in. My OB/GYN was great and talked me through it. Getting the normal amnio results was tremendously reassuring, as was seeing the baby on the ultrasound.*"

▪ What About Prenatal Testing? ▪

One of the first decisions that confront a pregnant woman is whether or not to undergo prenatal testing. Here's a summary of the tests and what they may be like.

ULTRASOUND is noninvasive, painless and can be done at any time during pregnancy to check on the growing fetus, to spot potential malformations and to help estimate the due date. A tiny embryo can clearly be seen as early as five weeks. During the first weeks a *transvaginal ultrasound* may be performed using a small vaginal probe. Later, *abdominal ultrasound* is done with a larger transducer and a special conduction jelly spread on the abdomen, providing a window on the growing fetus. In preparation you must drink several glasses of water, which can uncomfortably distend the bladder but makes the uterus more visible.

MATERNAL SERUM ALPHA-FETOPROTEIN (MSAFP) is a blood test done after the sixteenth week in most women to look for elevated or low levels of *alpha-fetoprotein (AFP)*, a protein produced by the fetus, present in amniotic fluid and in the mother's bloodstream. Elevated AFP is associated with an increased risk of neural tube defects, low levels with Down syndrome. But false positives are not uncommon. A more sensitive "triple test" for Down's may be done to measure AFP, human chorionic gonadotropin and estriol.

CHORIONIC VILLUS SAMPLING (CVS) involves removing a small amount of developing placenta to analyze for potential chromosomal abnormalities. *Chorionic villi* are fingerlike projections that attach the placenta to the wall of the uterus, explains Bruce K. Young, M.D., a specialist in high-risk pregnancies and the Herbert R. Silverman/Henry R. Silverman Professor of OB/GYN at NYU Medical Center. Because CVS does not sample amniotic fluid for levels of AFP, it cannot diagnose neural tube defects. The risk of miscarriage with CVS is 1 to 2 percent, and a number of studies have also linked it to a slightly increased incidence of limb malformations. "But the studies indicate that if performed between the tenth and thirteenth weeks, chorionic villus sampling is safe," says Dr. Young.

CVS is usually offered to women who are over age thirty-five, who have had a previous child with Down syndrome or who are at higher risk for chromosomal abnormalities or genetic diseases, such as sickle-cell anemia or Tay-Sachs disease. CVS is usually performed by inserting a small catheter through the cervix into the uterus under ultrasound guidance to take a small sample of chorionic villi cells (this may cause some cramping). It can also be done through the abdomen.

AMNIOCENTESIS is usually done after the fifteenth week to sample the amniotic fluid for AFP and to detect chromosomal abnormalities. It provides a little more genetic information than CVS and is usually offered to women over age thirty-five and those at higher risk for chromosomal abnormalities. Amnio (or CVS) can tell you the sex of the baby (if you want to know). The risk of miscarriage ranges from 1 in 200 to 1 in 400, according to Dr. Young. A recent study found the risk of miscarriage was eleven times higher in women who had early amniocentesis, between weeks eleven and fourteen.

Amniocentesis is a brief procedure that can be done in a physician's office or in an outpatient hospital setting. In preparation you must drink several glasses of water to fill the bladder so it can act as a conducting medium for the ultrasound guidance. First, the gestational age of the fetus, its position and the placement of the placenta are noted. Next, the abdomen is wiped with an antiseptic solution. A local anesthetic may be given to numb the area. A long, hollow needle is then gently inserted through the abdomen into the uterus and the amniotic sac. A small amount of fluid is withdrawn, as the doctor monitors the fetus on the ultrasound. The needle is withdrawn, and the tiny puncture may be bandaged. The insertion of the needle may be felt as pressure, or it may be more painful. Results from the amniocentesis usually take ten days to two weeks. Under development are new, more sensitive blood tests to assess fetal chromosomes, which scientists say may eliminate the need for CVS and amniocentesis or reduce the number of procedures.

GLUCOSE TOLERANCE testing for *gestational diabetes* is usually done between the twenty-fourth and twenty-eighth weeks of pregnancy. Gestational diabetes is caused by resistance to the hormone insulin, which regulates blood sugar; hormonal and metabolic changes during pregnancy make all women insulin-resistant, but only 1 to 5 percent will develop gestational diabetes.

Women over age thirty-five or who have family histories of diabetes may be most at risk, but one-hour blood glucose challenge tests are usually offered to all women. Glucose levels in urine are routinely measured during pregnancy, but more than 50 percent of pregnant women have excess glucose in their urine, so it's not a very accurate predictor of risk.

Rh STATUS TESTING is a blood test done early in pregnancy to determine if a woman has *Rh factor*, a genetically determined protein found on red blood cells. "If a woman is *Rh-negative* and the fetus is *Rh-positive*, the mother's immune system may begin to attack the fetal red blood cells," explains Dr. Young. However, an injection of *Rh immunoglobulin* will prevent this immune response. A woman who tests Rh-negative early in pregnancy will receive another blood test at around twenty-eight weeks to see if antibodies are forming. An amniocentesis and a sampling of blood in the umbilical cord may also be done to monitor the fetus.

Some women have underlying conditions that make them high risk and require not only prenatal testing but special care throughout pregnancy, according to Dr. Young. These include women whose mothers were exposed to the drug *diethylstilbestrol* (DES), used up until 1971 to prevent recurrent miscarriage and premature labor (see page 313). Women with lupus, rheumatoid arthritis, steroid-dependent asthma, histories of blood clots, cardiac, liver or kidney disease, hypertension, thyroid abnormalities, histories of preterm deliveries and twins or multiple pregnancies also require special monitoring during pregnancy.

▪ Warning Signs and What They May Mean ▪

With all the changes of pregnancy, a woman may be unsure of what's normal and what should prompt a call to the obstetrician.

SEVERE NAUSEA AND HYPEREMESIS affect one in every 300 pregnant women. If you are throwing up more than two or three times a day, can't keep anything down or have pain or fever, call your physician immediately, advises Dr. Lockwood. You should also notify your doctor if nausea and vomiting persist into the second trimester.

Hyperemesis is dangerous because if a woman can't keep food down, her baby won't get needed nutrients. "This has to be treated aggressively with antinausea medications," says Dr. Lockwood. "In rare cases it can be so severe that women may require hospitalization and *hyperalimentation*, an intravenous line to provide fluids and nutrients."

Severe nausea and vomiting can also be a sign of *molar pregnancy (hydatidiform mole)*, a rare condition in which an abnormal mass is formed in the uterus instead of an embryo. Caused by chromosomal problems in the sperm, the egg or both, a molar pregnancy must be removed surgically. Occasionally the "mole" persists and the rapidly dividing cells become malignant, so a woman must be given chemotherapy and monitored for recurrence.

BLEEDING AND SPOTTING occur in up to 25 percent of pregnancies and are not uncommon during the first trimester.

Bleeding during the first twenty weeks of pregnancy can signal potential miscarriage; bleeding between twenty and thirty-seven weeks may be a sign of imminent preterm labor. Painless vaginal bleeding during the third trimester can be a sign of placenta previa, blocking of the cervix by the placenta, posing a risk of hemorrhage before or during delivery. "If bleeding is bright red, heavy, lasts longer than a day and is accompanied by pain, cramping or fever, or if you seem to have passed clots or bits of tissue, it should prompt an immediate call to your doctor at *any* point during pregnancy," advises Dr. Lockwood.

SUDDEN WEIGHT GAIN AND FLUID RETENTION can signal the onset of preeclampsia (or toxemia), a condition causing high blood pressure. It's characterized by a *rapid* gain of more than two pounds in a given week and a sudden swelling of the hands, face, or feet as well as persistent headache, dizziness or blurred vision. Although women receive routine high blood pressure checks and tests for excess protein in the urine (*proteinuria*) to detect preeclampsia, they need to be aware of these physical symptoms.

Preeclampsia usually develops at about twenty weeks, when the mother's blood volume reaches its peak. It's most common in first-time pregnancies, in women over thirty-five, in patients with diabetes, lupus, chronic hypertension or kidney disease and in women who are overweight or carrying multiple fetuses, according to Dr. Young. Women with hypertension are at 25 percent greater risk for adverse outcomes.

Preeclampsia is linked to one quarter of premature deliveries in the U.S., and can increase the risk of having a low-birth-weight baby or stillbirth. When placental blood flow is hampered by hypertension, the fetus may become malnourished and oxygen-starved. In extreme cases, placental blood vessels may tear away from the uterine wall (*abruptio placentae*), leading to hemorrhage and premature labor. Left untreated, toxemia can progress to a more severe stage called *maternal eclampsia*, leading to convulsions, organ failure, coma and even death. "Fortunately this is rare. Preeclampsia is usually caught early and treated with bed rest and, if indicated, magnesium sulfate and antihypertensive medication," says Dr. Young.

A major randomized clinical trial reported in 1997 found no benefit to taking daily low-dose aspirin among 2,500 women who had diabetes, chronic hypertension, a history of preeclampsia, or who were carrying more than one fetus. This mirrors the results of several other large trials, and experts say women should not take aspirin unless prescribed. Results of the Calcium and Pre-Eclampsia in Pregnancy (CPEP) trial, also reported in 1997, found no difference in the incidence of preeclampsia among more than 4,500 women randomized to either calcium supplements or a placebo.

CRAMPING OR PELVIC PAIN that is moderate to severe, or *any* persistent pain, should be checked out by your doctor; it could signal miscarriage or preterm labor. Persistent pain could also be a sign of dehydration or upper urinary tract infections (which can also trigger preterm labor). Constant, severe abdominal pain can be a sign of abruptio placentae.

While occasional, slight contractions during the third trimester are not uncommon, some women do develop premature cervical dilation and uterine contractions, and measures are needed to stop or delay labor. Early uterine contractions may be felt as a "tightening" in the abdomen (sometimes with low back pain). If you feel more than five contractions in an hour, especially if they are accompanied by spotting or a watery discharge, contact your physician. A new test to detect preterm labor can now be used (see page 205).

OTHER RED FLAGS include any heavy or steady watery discharge from the vagina (a possible sign of premature membrane rupture), chills or fever (which can signal a serious bacterial infection) and painful urination (a symptom of urinary tract infection).

If you have any doubts about any symptom during pregnancy, no matter how minor it seems, don't hesitate to ask your doctor.

∞ Rachel's Story, Cont'd ∞

"*I knew I was not one of those women who could get by with breathing during labor, and I told my doctor well in advance that I wanted an epidural. Without it [the epidural] I would not have made it.*

"*To say labor pains are unique is an understatement. Labor pains are akin to having wild animals claw at your insides. But you can't go by me. I had a fourteen-hour labor, and my younger cousin almost dropped her baby on the hospital steps. But I'd do it all again in a minute!*"

▪ Labor Stages and Sensations ▪

As a woman gets closer to the birth of her child, she wants to know what will labor be like and how much will it hurt.

Labor has three stages. *STAGE ONE* consists of the early, active and transitional phases during which the cervix progressively thins and dilates, and uterine contractions become stronger in preparation for birth.

EARLY LABOR usually lasts from five to six hours (but some women go as long as twenty-four hours). During this phase the bands of muscle in the upper uterus contract, drawing up the cervix while special enzymes cause it to thin so it can begin to open; it dilates to four centimeters in diameter. Early labor contractions may be no more uncomfortable than menstrual cramps, lasting less than sixty seconds and occurring fifteen to twenty minutes apart. "It may feel like an intermittent pressure, fullness or aching. Some women have a backache or loose bowel movements," remarks Dr. Hoskins. The mucus plug that seals the cervix may become dislodged at this point, producing slight vaginal bleeding ("bloody show"). Some women, who are already several centimeters dilated, may not even notice early labor.

ACTIVE LABOR is reached when contractions get to be about three to five minutes apart. Now is certainly the time to head for the hospital or birthing center. Your "bag of waters" (*amniotic sac*) may have already broken. During active labor, contractions become much stronger, longer (about sixty seconds) and more frequent, as the cervix dilates from four to eight centimeters: about one centimeter per hour in a first pregnancy and more than two centimeters per hour if you've had a baby before, according to Dr. Lockwood. You may feel an uncomfortable tightening and tension in the abdomen, then a gradual lessening of pressure until the contraction is over.

"Each woman's threshold of pain varies, but most say breathing exercises are helpful during this phase," adds Dr. Hoskins. Some women opt for some form of pain relief or regional anesthesia. The length of active labor varies. A 1996 study at the University of New Mexico found that first-time mothers were in the first stage of labor an average of almost eight hours, compared with less than six hours for women who had children. The second stage of labor, during which the baby is born, was *considerably* shorter for women with children, seventeen minutes, compared with fifty-seven minutes for first-time moms.

TRANSITIONAL LABOR is the shortest, but most difficult, phase of active labor, during which the cervix fully dilates, from eight to ten centimeters. The pain is strongest because the uterus contracts frequently and with great intensity to stretch the last bit of cervix over the baby's head to begin the descent of the baby. Even with regional anesthesia, you'll feel the contractions becoming much stronger, longer and more frequent. Each contraction lasts about ninety seconds, with a minute or so in between. Some women may feel nauseated, and some vomit. An injection of local anesthetic may be given to numb the vaginal area for delivery or before an *episiotomy* (see page 200).

The *SECOND STAGE OF LABOR* is the period between full dilation and the birth of the baby. Along with contractions you'll feel a pressure in the pelvis and an uncontrollable desire to push. The combined force of your pushing and the uterine contractions will drive the baby down from the abdomen through the birth canal. How long you need to keep pushing varies. Some women need just a couple of good pushes; others push for two to three hours. (If you're not yet fully dilated, you may be told not to push, since it can cause bruising and swelling of the cervix.)

As the baby's head begins to crown, you'll feel a stretching and burning as the head stretches the skin around the vagina. Once the baby's head becomes visible, it is gently eased out of the vagina, followed by the shoulders and the rest of the body.

The *THIRD STAGE OF LABOR* involves the delivery of the placenta. For another five to thirty minutes contractions expel the placenta, and you shiver and shake. No one knows what causes the postbirth shakes. Some experts say it may be the shock to the mother's system (causing release of hormones called catecholamines), low blood sugar (since a woman usually hasn't eaten for many hours), the effects of anesthesia or release of prostaglandins into the blood after separation of the placenta.

The *POSTPARTUM PERIOD* may bring some afterbirth pains, resulting from uterine contractions, which control bleeding. Pains may be stronger if you breast-feed since it produces the hormone oxytocin, which stimulates uterine contractions. Pains can last up to five days and may be stronger after multiple births.

Urination may be difficult right after delivery because of a decrease in sensation resulting from pressure on the bladder as the baby's head moved through the birth canal; regional anesthetics can compound the problem. Reduced sensation can make it difficult to control urination fully, so there may be leakage. Normal urinary function usually returns in a few days, but some women may need a temporary catheter.

There is also a bloody vaginal discharge called *lochia*, which can last two to eight weeks, becoming progressively lighter in color and flow. Sanitary napkins are used during this period; since the cervix is still slightly dilated, women are advised to avoid intercourse and tampons for four weeks to avoid infections.

A woman who receives an episiotomy is usually given a squeeze bottle to rinse the incision after using the toilet. The stitches dissolve and the incision heals within two weeks postpartum. If the area becomes red, painful and swollen, it may be infected.

However, Dr. Lockwood and other experts say episiotomies may not always be needed and may increase the risk of urinary or rectal problems. A woman may be able to avoid an episiotomy by working closely with her obstetrician to control pushing in a way that has less potential for tearing. An episiotomy is needed in cases of fetal distress, to prevent tearing if the baby's head is large or if the baby's shoulders become caught during delivery.

∞ *A n n a's S t o r y , C o n t'd* ∞

"I had scheduled C-sections because I had broken my tailbone when I was a teenager in a skating accident. My doctor told me vaginal delivery was out.

"You're awake for the entire C-section, but they give you an epidural so you don't feel any pain. You feel a lot of uncomfortable pressure when they take the baby out. It's not so bad because you're so excited. It takes only ten or fifteen minutes.

"The worst part was when they sewed me up afterward. You can't see what they're doing. They are putting everything back where it belongs, but it felt like they were pulling me inside out. I was so scared I started to have a panic attack, hyperventilating and everything. They had to sedate me.

"My doctor had told me to leave the urinary catheter in, but I made them take it out right away because I didn't like it. Big mistake. I had to go real bad in the middle of the night. The painkillers had worn off, and I had to get out of bed and walk to the bathroom by myself. That hurt like hell. The next time I let them keep the catheter in.

"The second time around, with my daughter, the recovery was harder because I had a twenty-one-month-old child at home, I couldn't pick him up and I was doubly tired."

▪ When Medicine Must Intervene ▪

While most women go through labor and delivery with no problems, there are circumstances when intervention is needed.

INDUCED LABOR may be needed if the health of the mother or the baby is endangered late in pregnancy by such conditions as preeclampsia, diabetes or fetal growth retardation. A woman may also be induced if her bag of waters has broken and labor doesn't follow quickly (increasing chances of infection) or if pregnancy has gone beyond forty-two or forty-three weeks since the condition of the placenta may decline, the volume of amniotic fluid may decrease and the baby may not receive enough oxygen and nutrients.

Labor is sometimes induced or accelerated by breaking the bag of waters, to prompt production of more prostaglandins, triggering contractions. It's done by guiding a sterile tool into the cervix to pierce the membrane and should feel no more uncomfortable than a routine internal exam. Rupturing the membranes may shorten the first stage of labor by an hour or so.

Labor can also be induced using a synthetic form of the hormone oxytocin. These drugs (Pitocin, Syntocinon) are given gradually through an intravenous drip, producing contractions within thirty minutes. The contractions may be stronger and more frequent than natural labor, and labor may progress very quickly. Uterine contractions and fetal heart rate are carefully monitored during induction.

If the cervix has not already begun to soften, it will not immediately dilate in response to uterine contractions. In this case a suppository, gel or "ribbon" containing the drug *prostaglandin E2* may be inserted to soften the cervix.

REGIONAL ANESTHESIA can be administered during the most painful part of active labor and is usually given during a cesarean. Epidural anesthesia numbs you from your midsection on down, blocking pain messages from the nerves of the uterus and cervix. First, the anesthesiologist inserts a hollow needle that holds a catheter between the vertebrae of the lower back. The anesthetic will be pumped through the catheter into the *epidural space* outside the *dura*, the fluid-filled sac surrounding the spinal cord. A local anesthetic is injected to numb the area, but you'll feel pressure as the needle is inserted. Once the catheter is in place, it takes about twenty minutes for the anesthetic to become completely effective. Some epidurals allow you to walk around.

Some women may receive a *spinal block*, an injection of anesthetic into the fluid surrounding the spinal nerves, which takes effect quickly. A single dose of anesthesia is used, lasting two hours. Spinal blocks are used in about

40 percent of cesareans, epidurals in another 40 percent and general anesthesia for the rest. Medications are given in low doses and carefully monitored so effects on the baby, if any, are minimal. However, because these drugs are not without risk, you need to discuss regional anesthesia with your obstetrician before deciding.

FETAL MONITORING keeps track of the baby's heart rate and response to medications and may be used to watch for signs of fetal distress in women who do not choose analgesia.

External monitoring uses two belts, one placed low around the mother's abdomen, the other placed high on the uterus. The higher belt contains a gauge to record the frequency and strength of uterine contractions. The lower belt contains an ultrasound transducer to pick up fetal heart rate. They are connected to a monitor that simultaneously displays both readouts.

Internal fetal monitoring is more accurate, but more invasive, and can be done only if the membranes are ruptured. A tiny wire electrode is threaded through the birth canal and attached to the baby's scalp, where it directly monitors the baby's heart rate and cardiac electrical activity. A pressure-sensitive device may also be inserted between the baby and the wall of the uterus to monitor strength of contractions.

A new technology called *fetal pulse oximetry* measures the amount of oxygen in the fetus during labor; low oxygen indicates that the baby may be in trouble. The device measures oxygen by passing light through tissue, in this case inserting a probe that lies alongside the baby to measure the amount of light passed through the baby's cheek.

Fetal monitoring is somewhat controversial; some recent studies say the technology may be overused and inaccurate and may result in unnecessary cesareans. "But when used properly, monitoring should be a great help as a screening test for fetal distress. The obstetrician or midwife should be able to interpret the fetal monitoring readouts so as to minimize the risk of unnecessary cesareans," comments Dr. Bruce Young.

∞ C a r o n ' s   S t o r y ∞

"My C-section was an emergency, abruptio placenta. You start to hemorrhage inside. It was fairly close to my due date when I started to bleed, so I called my doctor. I was not in pain, I had no cramps and I was being calm. I had no idea what was going on, and no one at the hospital acted especially concerned. But meanwhile it seemed like I was bleeding quarts

> *of blood. By the time my doctor got there, I was practically in shock and the baby was minutes away from having no oxygen.*
>
> *"So they knocked me out and rushed me in for an emergency C-section. It was like two minutes to spare for my baby, which was starting to show signs of fetal distress. My doctor told me that they barely got my son out. But apparently because I wasn't in pain, no one thought anything was seriously wrong."*

A *CESAREAN SECTION* may be scheduled ahead of time if the baby's head is too large to pass through a woman's pelvis or if there are conditions that necessitate a quick delivery, such as placenta previa. A woman may also undergo a C-section if labor is not progressing (endangering the baby) or if the baby is in a breech (feet-first) position. During a scheduled cesarean a woman can be awake for her baby's birth; general anesthesia is often needed in an emergency C-section.

Most women will have either a *low-transverse incision* in the lower abdomen and uterus just above the pubic hairline or a *vertical incision* between the pubic hair and the navel; both are about six inches long. A transverse incision often heals better, and there's less chance of a rupture during subsequent labor. A vertical incision may be needed if the baby must be removed quickly, but it poses a greater risk for bleeding and subsequent uterine rupture, so it is used less often.

After a C-section the epidural catheter can be left in place for twenty-four hours to provide relief from pain. Full recovery takes four to six weeks. During those weeks pain from the incision may persist. Women are advised to avoid anything that puts strain on the abdomen, such as strenuous exercise and heavy lifting, for up to four weeks. You'll also experience afterbirth pains and heavier discharge than with a vaginal delivery.

▪ What About Next Time? ▪

Many women who have a cesarean wonder if they'll be able to undergo *vaginal birth after cesarean (VBAC)*. For most women, the answer is yes. Guidelines set by ACOG say vaginal delivery should be the treatment of choice in women who have had cesareans. Even having two cesareans doesn't mean a third child can't be delivered vaginally. However, women with high vertical uterine scars are generally not candidates for VBAC.

ACOG recommends that VBAC be performed only in a hospital, where there is continuous electronic fetal monitoring, and surgical and anesthesia teams are available if a repeat C-section is needed. Of the women who undergo VBAC, 70 percent have successful vaginal deliveries. But statistics show that only 20 percent of potential candidates are opting for VBAC. A woman's own fears are a factor, especially if her first labor was difficult. But experts say too many doctors perform C-sections simply because a woman had one with her last pregnancy, so the issue needs to be discussed with the obstetrician beforehand. There are special classes to prepare women for attempted VBAC.

While the numbers have started to decline in recent years, C-sections are still the most frequent surgical operation in the U.S., with cesareans performed in 20 percent of deliveries. Health advocates say many of those procedures were unnecessary. A recent report indicates women attended by midwives in the hospital may undergo fewer C-sections.

✸ *Miranda's Story* ✸

"I had three early miscarriages. I would just find out I was pregnant, then begin to bleed. I knew I was pregnant only because we were trying and I was following it so closely with home pregnancy tests.

"You're mourning a lot of things, not just the loss of the pregnancy. It's failure again. It's the loss of your hopes, the loss of your dreams. You wonder, Will this ever happen?"

▪ Miscarriage ▪

Between 14 and 18 percent of pregnancies end in miscarriage, usually during the first trimester. Up to 80 percent of early miscarriages are due to chromosomal abnormalities, according to Dr. Charles Lockwood. Luteal phase defects (low levels of the progesterone needed to sustain a pregnancy) may contribute to a number of the remaining losses, he says. Later miscarriages are mostly due to uterine abnormalities, to premature membrane rupture and labor or to an "incompetent cervix," one unable to remain closed during pregnancy. A procedure to close the cervix (*cerclage*) can prevent late miscarriage in selected women.

Pregnancy loss (and fetal growth problems) can also result from immunological problems, such as high levels of *anticardiolipin antibodies*, often found in lupus, which cause blood clotting in the placenta (see page 218). Women with these antibodies can take low-dose aspirin and heparin, which act as a blood thinner preventing miscarriage. "Success rates are about 70 percent with this treatment," says Dr. Lockwood.

Normal physical activity, most injuries and sex during pregnancy will not cause miscarriage. However, 1997 studies found that job stress, long periods of standing, heavy physical exertion, stress or working more than forty hours a week may increase the risk of preterm delivery. "But miscarriage is *never* the mother's fault," Dr. Lockwood emphasizes.

▪ Preterm Labor and Premature Birth ▪

Each year, over 400,000 babies in the United States are born too soon. While medical science has made great strides in saving the lives of "preemies," prematurity causes 74 percent of infant deaths. The greatest risk to the infant comes from labor that begins at or before thirty-three weeks. But only 25 percent of women who deliver prematurely are accurately diagnosed.

There's now a test, using a protein found in a vaginal smear, to help predict whether a woman is likely to deliver prematurely. "During labor the cells in the fetal membranes produce a large quantity of a protein called *fetal fibronectin* in cervical-vaginal secretions, starting about a month before a woman may develop contractions." says Dr. Lockwood, who headed the research team that developed the test. "The test can be used to find out which women are having contractions that may lead to premature labor and which are having Braxton Hicks contractions, or false labor, and will deliver at term." Dr. Lockwood's research found that 86 percent of the women with contractions who tested positive for fetal fibronectin prior to thirty-seven weeks delivered prematurely, while most who tested negative did not. (A later report found that *low* levels of fetal fibronectin at term could also predict which women would deliver late.)

"Most women who test negative can be sent home and checked again in two weeks. If a woman tests positive, she has a thirty to fifty percent risk of delivering preterm," Dr. Lockwood says. "If a woman is actively contracting, we can give drugs to stop contractions (*tocolytics*), treat potential infections with antibiotics, prescribe steroids to mature the fetal lungs to avoid fetal respiratory distress syndrome and order bed rest."

Tocolytic medications include *magnesium sulfate*, the most commonly prescribed medication given intravenously to stop contractions (studies suggest it may also help prevent cerebral palsy), and *terbutaline.*

If the contractions are successfully controlled or stopped, bed rest, or at least reduced activity, may be advised. Experts are divided over whether bed rest helps prevent preterm delivery. Dr. Lockwood says bed rest reduces both pressure on the cervix and stretching that may lead to premature contractions and increases blood flow to the uterus to reduce fetal stress.

Bed rest also helps increase blood flow to the placenta, so the baby receives more oxygen and nutrients, taking some of the strain off the mother's heart and kidneys. A woman with preeclampsia may be advised to rest on her left side several times a day, since blood exits the heart from the left side. If a woman appears in danger of preterm labor, she may be confined to the hospital, so contractions and cervical changes can be monitored.

Antibiotics are also given until infections (such as with *group B beta-streptococcus*) can be ruled out. "We have also become more aggressive in treating bacterial vaginosis. BV and urinary tract infections both may be triggers of preterm labor. Bacteria can produce toxins that break down the membranes around the bag of waters," Dr. Lockwood explains.

▪ Ectopic Pregnancy ▪

Ectopic, or tubal, pregnancy is a medical emergency because a ruptured fallopian tube could cause bleeding and infection of the peritoneum. Perhaps one out of every sixty pregnancies is ectopic, occurring most often in women twenty-five to thirty-four.

"A woman will miss her period and have all the signs of pregnancy. But on ultrasound you will not see a pregnancy in the uterus," says Dr. John Quagliarello, an associate professor of clinical obstetrics and gynecology at NYU Medical Center. "Eventually all women with ectopic pregnancies have irregular vaginal bleeding or pain, telling us something is wrong." Even if it is not visible on ultrasound, blood tests can confirm an ectopic pregnancy. Normally levels of hCG rise as pregnancy progresses; in ectopic pregnancy, hCG does not rise.

To prevent tubal rupture, an ectopic pregnancy is removed during abdominal surgery under general anesthesia, and the tube repaired with microsurgery. A tube may heal on its own after an ectopic pregnancy, but there's a risk it will recur. Even with in vitro fertilization, the embryo may still migrate and implant in a fallopian tube, according to Dr. Quagliarello. So a badly damaged tube may have to be removed. Early diagnosis and removal of ectopic pregnancy can prevent emergency surgery and infertility.

▪ Surprises After the Stork ▪

Pregnancy produces lasting changes in a woman's reproductive tract and genitals that can increase the chance of incontinence and other problems. Resumption of normal hormonal cycles helps get joints and ligaments back to their prepregnancy state, but a woman will have to work to get her body back in shape.

The ABDOMEN may still protrude after pregnancy, and its muscles remain lax even as the uterus returns to its normal size. If you didn't have a cesarean, you can begin a gradual exercise regimen right away to restore muscle tone in the abdomen and the rest of the body, says Dr. Iffath Hoskins. Kegel exercises should be part of any routine to help tone pelvic floor muscles (see below). However, if a woman has had a cesarean and muscle tissue has been cut, some of the repaired tissue is fibrous tissue, which may not respond as well to exercise, Dr. Hoskins cautions.

INCONTINENCE AND PELVIC FLOOR MUSCLE DYSFUNCTION may become problems when the normal pelvic muscle tone does not return after delivery. In some women the pelvic floor muscles may be damaged during delivery or prolonged labor. This can lead to urinary problems or to prolapse (page 53) later in life.

Reduced blood flow or nerve damage may weaken the pelvic support muscle and cause it to sag, observes Dr. Robert Porges. This can affect the bladder sphincter, causing urinary stress incontinence (see Chapter Seven). The damage may also affect the anal sphincter, causing some mild fecal incontinence, or the anal sphincter may be damaged by an episiotomy. "The episiotomy repair may achieve only a 70 or 80 percent continence," says Dr. Porges. "A woman may be able to control solid stools but may have some leakage with loose stools. This is a problem that is seldom discussed but that women need to be aware of."

A woman's pelvic floor muscle tone should be evaluated after childbirth (and as part of every GYN exam). The basic test is very simple: The physician will ask a woman to tighten the muscles around the vagina around his or her examining fingers. If a woman cannot contract her muscles or cannot contract them sufficiently, it indicates the need for some intervention. "This examination may not be appropriate at the normal six-week postpartum visit.

A woman may still have discomfort or weakness from an episiotomy; if she is nursing, there may vaginal dryness. We may need to have her come back at nine months or a year and at that point put her through some tests to see if she may be susceptible to pelvic floor dysfunction or prolapse later in life," comments Dr. Porges.

⸎ *Caron's Story, Cont'd* ⸎

"I developed hemorrhoids when I was pregnant with my first child, but they really got bad with my second pregnancy. It's an internal, knifelike, really severe pain. I didn't even know what was going on the first time it happened. It got to the point where any kind of abdominal pressure would bring it on. I would be laid up for days.

"The last time it happened I was in tears, the pain was so bad. My doctor sent me to the emergency room because she said there was always the possibility it could be something more severe, like an abscess. They found internal hemorrhoids, three of them, 'strangulated.' My first labor was long and hard and I've had two C-sections, but the recovery from the hemorrhoid surgery was worse than all of them together!

"No one really discusses hemorrhoids. Or they say they'll just go away. They don't. Maybe there was something that could have been done to avoid all this pain. Most women swap labor stories. Who swaps hemorrhoid stories?"

HEMORRHOIDS are distended, or varicose, veins in the lining of the anus that affect 20 to 50 percent of women in pregnancy. External hemorrhoids arise at the anal opening; internal hemorrhoids form in the rectum and anal canal. Minor hemorrhoids can go away, but most of the time they remain after pregnancy.

"Hemorrhoids develop due to pressure on the veins in the rectum from the growing uterus and can worsen during labor, when there is even more pressure, as a woman pushes the baby through the birth canal," says Kenneth Eng, M.D., a colorectal surgeon and professor of surgery at NYU Medical Center. "Constipation and chronic straining from hard stools also increase pressure on the veins and aggravate hemorrhoids."

The most common symptoms are intermittent bright red bleeding during the passage of stools, irritation, pain and swelling of tissues. Swelling occurs when continued pressure forces fluid from the small blood vessels into the surrounding tissue. A sensation of fullness and incomplete voiding causes more straining, which leads to prolapse of hemorrhoidal tissues. "Prolapsed hemorrhoids cause mucus discharge, which leads to itching, and you have difficulty maintaining hygiene, which causes irritation and rashes around the anus," says Dr. Eng.

Once hemorrhoids protrude, they are subject to ulceration and bleeding; internal hemorrhoids cause breaks in the tissue and bleeding as well as pain. In severe cases, prolapsed hemorrhoids can become strangulated—that is, pressure from swollen tissues cuts off blood supply to the area, leading to infection. As with Caron, this can cause extreme pain. Prolapsed hemorrhoids require a *hemorrhoidectomy.*

To avoid or minimize hemorrhoids after delivery, a woman should take stool softeners (such as Colace, Dialose, Surfak) to ease elimination and maintain regular bowel habits. Pain from hemorrhoids or an episiotomy may make a woman put off defecation, but this can lead to worse constipation and hemorrhoids. Drinking six to eight glasses of fluid a day and taking bulk-forming laxatives (like Metamucil) retain moisture and help avoid hard stools. Eating more vegetables and fruits (yes, prunes) can also help.

For minor hemorrhoids, Dr. Eng recommends warm sitz baths. Over-the-counter hemorrhoid ointments or suppositories (Anusol, Preparation H) can help relieve itching and swelling. Prescription ointments containing *hydrocortisone* (Anusol-HC) can help women with severe symptoms.

Surgery is usually a last resort. Some internal hemorrhoids can be treated as day surgery with local anesthesia by a proctologist or a colon and rectal specialist. The patient lies on her side while the *proctoscope* is gently inserted into the rectum and the hemorrhoid is grasped with tiny forceps. Tiny rubber bands are squeezed onto the neck of the hemorrhoid, which will then wither away and be expelled painlessly. *Cryosurgery* can be used to shrink distended veins, says Dr. Eng. Hemorrhoidectomy is done under general anesthesia, after a more extensive examination of the rectum. The hemorrhoid is clamped and removed with a surgical knife. Since rectal tissues are very delicate, recovery can be painful and can take two to three weeks.

However, don't assume rectal bleeding is due to hemorrhoids, warns Dr. Eng. Any episode of bright red rectal bleeding should be evaluated by a physician since it's a common symptom of *colorectal cancer,* the third most common cancer among women (see page 274).

---

๑ *A n n a ' s   S t o r y ,   C o n t ' d* ๑

"Two things no one warned me about: One was vaginal dryness while I was breast-feeding. I called my OB/GYN, and he told me when you're nursing, you have the vaginal lining of a sixty-five-year-old woman because your estrogen levels are so low.

"After I finished nursing my son, my breasts completely deflated! I went down a bra size to barely a B from a full C cup. And they are baggy and saggy and have stretch marks, and I just cried and cried. I was prepared to be fat for a while. I was not prepared for what happened to my breasts!"

The RETURN OF PERIODS is delayed while a woman breast-feeds; periods start up again in about four to six weeks in women who are not nursing. While some women do not ovulate until they stop nursing, this is not always the case, so birth control should always be used.

After childbirth some women may find their periods are more regular and menstrual cramps lessened. "The real reasons for this are unknown. It may be that the structure of the uterus is in some way changed, or production of prostaglandins is altered, or a hormonally related cycle of cramps is broken by pregnancy," comments Dr. Hoskins. Likewise, PMS may decrease (at least initially) because of lower hormone levels.

Your BREASTS may be enlarged after giving birth and while you breast-feed. They may also become engorged and painful with milk, sometimes developing an infection called *mastitis*. Many women like Anna do find their breasts are smaller and flaccid after breast-feeding ends. "You can't avoid most of this because there's very little muscle in breast tissue and there's more fatty tissue after pregnancy," says Dr. Hoskins. "Exercises that target pectoral muscles *beneath* the breasts may help. The more good support you give the breasts during pregnancy and lactation, the less likely you are to have pendulous breasts afterward."

---

๑ *P o s t p a r t u m   D e p r e s s i o n* ๑

More than half of all new mothers experience a brief bout with the "baby blues" shortly after delivery, and between 10 and 15 percent of women experience *postpartum major depression (PPMD)*, with symptoms lasting for weeks. Perhaps one or two out of every thousand new mothers suffer *postpartum psychosis*.

Some ways to distinguish between the "blues" and depression:

- The baby blues typically occur three to five days after delivery and lift after a week or so, while postpartum major depression may emerge weeks, months or even a year after giving birth.

- Women with the "baby blues" are usually euphoric, tired and weepy but don't feel the hopelessness typical of depression.

- Characteristics of PPMD include despondency, guilt, lack of appetite, sleep disturbances, feelings of inadequacy, problems with concentration or memory, extreme fatigue and irritability.

- Some women worry excessively about the baby's health or feeding habits and feel like "bad" or unloving mothers.

Thoughts about harming the baby may be a warning sign of *postpartum psychosis*, says Margaret Spinelli, M.D., director of the Maternal Mental Health Program at the New York State Psychiatric Institute. In this disorder a woman may seem fine for two to three days after delivery but soon becomes depressed and unpredictable, irritable and hyperactive, eating and sleeping very little. She may become paranoid, hear voices or have hallucinations "commanding" her to hurt or kill the baby. Postpartum psychosis requires immediate hospitalization.

PPMD is treated similarly to major depression, with medication and/or psychotherapy, according to Dr. Spinelli. Some antidepressants, secreted only in minute amounts in breast milk, may safely be given to nursing mothers. Recent research indicates that antidepressants started immediately *after* delivery and continued for three months may help avoid a recurrence of PPMD. Prophylactic medication can also help women with a prior episode of postpartum psychosis or *manic depression* (swings between euphoria and depression), which may worsen after pregnancy.

SEXUALITY can change during the postpartum period. Many women may feel unattractive, breast-feeding may change the sexual dynamics of a relationship and sex may even be painful, especially with temporary vaginal dryness during early lactation. Vaginal lubricants can help (see page 249). For some women, being on top helps control penetration and limits discomfort.

Some women report that having a C-section makes it harder to achieve orgasm. However, these changes may be due to pregnancy itself. "The incision used for a C-section rarely disturbs the pelvic nerves. Sexual changes may be due to nerve damage, tissue and muscle stretching in labor. Kegel exercises can help the vagina regain most of its prepregnancy tone," says Dr. Hoskins.

The main problem new moms have with sex is fatigue. Experts say parents need to make time for each other to reestablish intimacy. A woman needs to take time for herself, a key to coping with all the *other* changes having a child can bring.

When There's Infertility

The science of *assisted reproduction technology (ART)* can help many people fulfill their wishes for families. Thanks to ART, more than 40,000 "test-tube babies" have been born in the U.S. since 1981. But it's an expensive proposition, and the success rates are very dependent on age and the experience of the clinic. For women under forty, the take-home baby rate can be as high as 50 percent in good clinics, but the nationwide average is only 22 percent. However, rapid development of new high-tech procedures may help change that in the future.

▪ Getting Pregnant ▪

Six out of every ten women say they've tried to become pregnant at one time or another. But it isn't always easy. Ovulation usually occurs fourteen days before the start of the next menstrual period (day one being the first day of your period), when a surge in luteinizing hormone (LH) prompts the dominant ovarian follicle to expel a ripened egg. Most women ovulate within twenty-four to thirty-six hours of the LH surge.

Home test kits detect increased LH in urine and can reliably predict ovulation within forty-eight hours. Tracking ovulation by the rise in basal body temperature (oral temperatures from 98.6° to 99.3° around ovulation) is less precise. A recent study from Harvard Medical School reveals that a woman may be most likely to get pregnant if intercourse occurs *on the day of ovulation or the five days preceding it*, not right afterward, as previously believed.

It can take twenty-four to forty-eight hours for the sperm to travel to the tubes. If an egg isn't fertilized within six to twelve hours after it is ejected by the ovary, it dies off and is reabsorbed by the body. So timing is critical if a woman wants to become pregnant. The Harvard study tracked more than 600 women and found pregnancy occurred *only* during this six-day window of opportunity. Not surprisingly the chances of conceiving were related to the frequency of intercourse during this period.

A 1995 Harris survey found that it took an average of eight months for a woman to become pregnant, with younger women conceiving more quickly. "Many couples ask me what they can do to increase their chances of becoming pregnant. I tell them to have intercourse more often before and during ovulation. If intercourse is increased to more than four times a week, the rate of conception within six months increases from about fifty percent up to eighty-three percent," comments noted reproductive endocrinologist Anne Colston Wentz, M.D., former president of the Society for Assisted Reproductive Technology (SART).

Couples may experience sexual difficulties because of the anxiety and stress of trying to get pregnant. Stress hormones can disrupt ovulatory and menstrual cycles and lower testosterone in men, leading to lower sperm counts and less sperm activity.

For most couples, problems may be temporary. If a couple has tried to conceive unsuccessfully for a year or more, a formal diagnosis of infertility is usually made.

∾ *S a r a ' s   S t o r y* ∾

"*When we had our daughter eight years ago, I became pregnant almost immediately. I had an easy pregnancy, no problems. When Eileen was eighteen months old, we started to try again. I was only thirty, I figured in a couple of months I'd be pregnant. But months went by. Then it was a year.*

"*A fertility specialist found nothing wrong, so we consulted someone else. Again they found nothing. We did fertility drugs and had sex on a timetable, which I can tell you is not at all enjoyable. The specialist suggested we try insemination. So we did that, five times, and we had to plead with him to try again the last time.*

"The people at the clinic were sympathetic. Up to a point. They would say, 'At least you have one child.' I had always dreamed of a big family, but I guess it's not meant to be."

▪ The Causes of Infertility ▪

More than 2.3 million couples seek help for infertility every year. Most of the time the cause can be pinpointed after a thorough history and examination.

"Among our patients about 20 percent are not ovulating properly or are not ovulating at all. Another 20 percent have blocked or scarred fallopian tubes. About five percent have endometriosis. Another five percent may have a 'hostile' cervical mucus. About a third of cases are due to male problems, such as a low sperm count," says Alan S. Berkeley, M.D., professor of clinical OB/GYN and director of the In Vitro Fertilization Program at NYU Medical Center. "Only in about 5 to 15 percent of patients can we find no identifiable cause for infertility."

DELAYED CHILDBEARING has become a major reason for the inability to conceive these days, according to Dr. Berkeley. Many women put off starting families until their late thirties and into their forties, waiting to marry or establish careers. But every year a woman delays, the less likely she is to become pregnant and stay pregnant. "As a woman ages, her ability to ovulate healthy eggs and generate a hormonal environment that can adequately support a pregnancy becomes increasingly compromised," says Dr. Berkeley. Though men generate a new supply of sperm about every three months, sperm can develop chromosomal problems, and sperm production and motility also decline, inhibiting conception.

After thirty-five a woman not only has fewer eggs, but these may also have developed structural problems that lead to chromosomal abnormalities during early chromosome division. Up to 80 percent of early miscarriages are due to severe chromosomal abnormalities; the risk of miscarriage may be 50 percent for women after age forty-five. As a woman gets into her forties, her follicles also become increasingly resistant to follicle-stimulating hormone. "Rising FSH levels can be one indicator of fertility problems," Dr. Berkeley comments. Fewer of the remaining eggs are stimulated each month, further reducing the odds of conception.

Federal statistics show that about 40 percent of childless women thirty-five to forty-four years old have impaired fertility. Age is also a major contributor to *secondary infertility,* in which a woman has one or more children and is unable to become pregnant again. It's estimated that half the women who cannot conceive or carry babies to term already have one child.

However, "biologic age" and chronological age can be very different. "I have seen twenty-five-year old patients who are postmenopausal, and I have also seen forty-five-year-old patients who seem to get pregnant just like twenty-five-year-olds," comments Dr. Wentz. "Elevated FSH is not always incompatible with pregnancy. Levels can fluctuate from cycle to cycle."

SEXUALLY TRANSMITTED DISEASES (STDS) take a major toll on fertility at all ages. According to recent data from the Alan Guttmacher Institute and the Centers for Disease Control and Prevention, an estimated 100,000 to 150,000 women become infertile each year because of pelvic inflammatory disease (PID).

TUBAL FACTOR INFERTILITY (Fig. 17) is the cause of infertility in up to 25 percent of women. According to the American Society for Reproductive Medicine (ASRM), proximal blockage (near the uterus) is most often caused by previous pelvic infection, thickening and inflammation of the tubal wall, plugs of mucus or endometriosis. Distal blockages (near the fimbriae) are usually caused by pelvic inflammation, from infections or endometriosis. Also, previous tubal surgery (such as for ectopic pregnancy) can result in scar tissue or adhesions around the tube and ovary. Women whose mothers took the drug DES often have tubal abnormalities.

ENDOMETRIOSIS can cause tubal obstruction if scar tissue is on (or inside) the tubes. As many as 30 to 40 percent of women being treated for infertility have endometriosis. A 1997 study in the *New England Journal of Medicine* of more than 700 women found that even mild cases with no scarring or blockage can cause infertility, but if endometrial growths are removed or destroyed, a woman's chances of becoming pregnant are increased by 13 percent.

CHEMOTHERAPY can bring on premature menopause by destroying ovarian follicles. The risk increases with a woman's age and with the chemotherapy drugs used (*cyclophosphamide* most commonly causes ovarian failure) as well as with the dose, timing and duration of therapy. About 50 percent

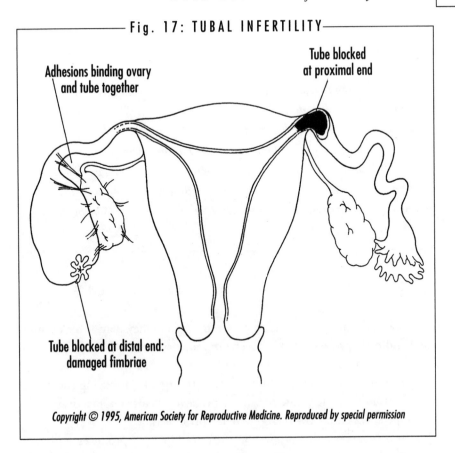

Fig. 17: TUBAL INFERTILITY

Adhesions binding ovary and tube together

Tube blocked at proximal end

Tube blocked at distal end: damaged fimbriae

Copyright © 1995, American Society for Reproductive Medicine. Reproduced by special permission

of women under thirty-five resume normal menstruation after chemotherapy and may be able to conceive.

OTHER CAUSES OF INFERTILITY include endocrine disorders, such as thyroid disease, diabetes and pituitary abnormalities, which can interfere with the hormones that regulate ovulation.

Alcohol, nicotine, marijuana, cocaine and other psychotropic drugs are capable of altering the genetic material of eggs and sperm. Some experts believe environmental pollutants may cause some cases of infertility. These include pesticides, which have "estrogenic" effects in the body and which some recent reports suggest may be lowering sperm counts worldwide.

∞ Miranda's Story, Cont'd ∞

"My problem was a combination of things. They discovered that I had a thyroid condition, Hashimoto's thyroiditis, which is hypothyroidism. So

even if I got pregnant, I wouldn't have been able to sustain the pregnancy. They put me on thyroid medication. Then there was my age. I was forty-four, and you don't know how many 'good' eggs you have left.

"*The first infertility clinic we went to totally overlooked my thyroid condition, and they didn't test sperm compatibility. We found another specialist who told us my husband was making antibodies to his own sperm. So then our doctor got my husband on steroids for a while.*

"*By this time we had made a conscious decision to go down two paths. We'd try infertility treatments, but we'd also start looking to adopt. We just said to ourselves, 'We want a child. It's getting later. Whichever way it turns out will be fine.'*"

▪ Infertility and the Immune System ▪

New research suggests that the immune system may play a role in infertility and early pregnancy failure. The immune system is able to distinguish between normal cells and proteins in the body (that which is "self") and foreign proteins and cells, such as bacteria (nonself), producing substances called antibodies in response to what is perceived as foreign, inactivating the interlopers, which is how the body fights off infection.

But in some people, for unknown reasons, the body produces antibodies against self. These *autoantibodies* attack and damage healthy tissue in the body. Autoimmune disease includes Hashimoto's thyroiditis (which targets the thyroid), *rheumatoid arthritis* (which destroys the lining of the joints) and *systemic lupus erythematosus* (which can damage any organ or part of the body, especially the joints, kidneys and blood cells).

In lupus, several types of antibody can interfere with the implantation and growth of an embryo. The *lupus anticoagulant antibody* and anticardiolpin antibodies cause clots to form in the early placental vascular system. This impedes embryo implantation and placental function, causing repeated miscarriage. Some researchers believe that autoantibodies produced in lupus and other autoimmune diseases may also contribute to repeated pregnancy failure and loss in women who carry these antibodies but do not have autoimmune diseases.

Studies suggest that the lupus anticoagulant and/or *antiphospholipid antibodies* (APL) may be found in as many as 25 to 33 percent of women who have unexplained early pregnancy loss. While some women with a history of repeated miscarriage who test positive may benefit from anticoagulants, the existence of immune-related infertility problems has *not* been well established, counters Dr. Berkeley, who says, "There are yet no large studies to show that these antibodies are a marker for infertility or for a lowered success rate with in vitro fertilization. At present this research is very speculative."

▪ The Infertility Workup ▪

An infertility workup includes a detailed medical history of both partners, a pelvic exam and a battery of blood tests.

The pelvic exam may reveal irregularities in the contour of the uterus or adjacent organs, which could indicate the presence of fibroids, ovarian cysts or swollen (and infected) fallopian tubes. Ultrasound or hysteroscopy may be done to check for any structural uterine defects (such as the T-shaped uterus found in DES daughters) or undetected fibroids. If endometriosis is suspected, laparoscopy may be performed to locate and treat it.

A hysterosalpingogram (page 80) is done to make sure the fallopian tubes are open. The procedure may even aid pregnancy by "flushing out" tiny, undetectable blockages in the tubes. "In fact, about twenty-five to thirty percent of patients will become pregnant within six months of a hysterosalpingogram," notes Dr. Wentz.

Blood tests include thyroid-stimulating hormone and prolactin levels. Hypothyroidism has been linked to luteal phase defects and anovulation. The hormone prolactin (which prepares the breasts for lactation) is believed to be needed to sustain early pregnancy; producing too much (hyperprolactinemia) inhibits the release of FSH and LH. This can be caused by hypothyroidism or a benign pituitary growth can lead to luteal phase defects, irregular periods and anovulation. Hyperprolactinemia can be corrected with replacement thyroid hormones or the medication *bromocriptine* (Parlodel). Tests for various antibodies are also done, including lupus antibodies, antinuclear antibodies (ANA) and APLs, especially if there's a history of recurrent miscarriage, blood clots in the legs or a low platelet count.

Levels of FSH and estrogen (in the early menstrual phase) are also measured to check for ovulatory dysfunction or perimenopause. A high FSH level may mean a woman is less likely to succeed with assisted reproduction (or any intervention).

"We do vaginal cultures for organisms that may be related to infertility and miscarriage, such as chlamydia or *mycoplasma*," says Dr. Berkeley. Another microorganism, Ureaplasma, produces no symptoms and can be found both in cervical secretions, where it may interfere with sperm transport, and in the uterine cavity, where it may interfere with embryo implantation. If any microorganisms are found, both partners are treated, then retested a few weeks later to make sure the infection has cleared. Cervical mucus may also be examined in a "postcoital test," by aspirating a sample of mucus two to twelve hours after intercourse right before ovulation. The activity of the sperm in the mucus (or lack of it) can indicate a "hostile" interaction, including the presence of antisperm antibodies.

Having had a cervical cone biopsy, laser or cryotherapy for dysplasia may lead to deficient or abnormal cervical mucus production, which can also be a factor in infertility.

The man's semen is also analyzed for low sperm count, low motility (low activity levels) and ability to penetrate an egg, as well as evidence of antisperm antibodies.

"Of the couples who come for basic infertility evaluation, a majority will become pregnant within a year," says Dr. Wentz.

■ Treating Infertility ■
Hormonal Treatments

Some hormone treatments are aimed at correcting imbalances in the feedback loop between the hypothalamus, the pituitary and the ovaries to regulate ovulation. Other hormonal treatments are designed to "hyperstimulate" the ovaries to produce more than one egg and to boost chances of conception.

CLOMIPHENE CITRATE (CLOMID, SEROPHENE) is most commonly used in women who don't ovulate or who ovulate irregularly because they don't produce enough FSH and LH at the right time during their cycles. Clomiphene stimulates the hypothalamus to release more GnRH, signaling the pituitary to pump out more LH and FSH. Clomiphene can also help women whose follicles do not mature normally because of low estrogen or who produce inadequate amounts of progesterone to sustain pregnancy (luteal phase defect).

Clomiphene is taken orally for five days each month, starting on the third or fifth day of the cycle, so that ovulation occurs around day fourteen. If a woman doesn't respond, the dose may be increased in the next cycle. Side effects can include hot flashes and ovarian cysts. Clomiphene can also cause a thick, dry cervical mucus that sperm cannot penetrate. If treatment to restore proper mucus production fails, a change in medication or insemination may be needed.

A majority of infertile women with hormonal problems will ovulate using clomiphene, and about 40 percent will become pregnant within six months, according to Dr. Berkeley.

HUMAN CHORIONIC GONADOTROPIN, hCG (PREGNYL, PROFASI), the pregnancy hormone produced by the placenta, may be added to the clomiphene regimen. Extracted from the urine of pregnant women, hCG is similar in structure and function to LH. It is given to a woman who produces a mature follicle but has no surge in LH by day fifteen of her cycle to stimulate its rupture. A physician may use ultrasound to determine the exact day on which to administer the hCG injection. It is also used in in vitro fertilization (IVF).

HUMAN MENOPAUSAL GONADATROPINS, hMGS (PERGONAL, HUMEGON), may be tried when a woman fails to respond to clomiphene and hCG. HMGs are made of equal parts of FSH and LH, both produced in high amounts after menopause, that have been extracted from the urine of menopausal women. These hormones directly stimulate the ovaries to produce several eggs in one cycle. Treatment involves one or two injections daily for a period of seven to twelve days, starting on days two to four of the menstrual cycle. If a woman has no other problem but anovulation, she can expect a pregnancy rate with hMGs close to that of normally ovulating women, says Dr. Berkeley. HMGs are also used in IVF and other assisted reproductive technologies.

FOLLICLE-STIMULATING HORMONE, FSH (METRODIN, FERTINEX) injections are used in a similar manner to hMGs to directly stimulate production of multiple ovarian follicles. Metrodin contains very little LH and may be useful in women who have normal or elevated LH levels but low FSH (a condition common in women with polycystic ovarian syndrome). It may be tried when a woman fails to respond to hMGs. New recombinant forms of FSH, Gonalf plus Follistene, are also being used.

GONADATROPIN-RELEASING HORMONE, GnRH (FACTREL, LUTREPULSE) and its analogs can be used in women who are not secreting the hormone naturally. GnRH is given via a special lightweight pump, which mimics the normal pulsatile release of GnRH by the body.

GnRH ANALOGS (LUPRON, SYNAREL) halt the production of ovarian hormones to enable women to respond better to hMG treatment and control ovulation more precisely. In in vitro fertilization, GnRH analogs are used to prevent the secretion of LH, which can cause follicles to release eggs before they can be harvested. They are taken as daily or monthly injections or as a nasal spray.

Women on these drugs are either followed by ultrasound and blood hormone assays (the most accurate way), with home ovulation kits or with basal body temperature charts, timing intercourse to increase their chances of becoming pregnant.

Superovulation plus Insemination

In cases of unexplained infertility, hormone treatments may be combined with insemination. This involves collecting the partner's (or donor) sperm, concentrating it and inseminating it into the cervical canal, the uterus or the fallopian tubes during a woman's fertile days. The greater the number of sperm and eggs, and the closer they are put together, the better the chance of pregnancy. Over 600,000 intrauterine inseminations (IUIs) are performed nationwide each year.

"All these therapies max out after about three cycles, no matter whether you are using clomiphene citrate or Pergonal with or without IUI. If you don't conceive within three or four cycles, you are less likely to be successful trying further," says Dr. Wentz. "It may be more cost-effective to move into early in vitro fertilization, which may get a couple pregnant sooner."

Women undergoing IVF are given injections of progesterone during the first twelve weeks of gestation to help the uterus maintain the pregnancy; a vaginal progesterone gel (Crinolone) was approved in 1997, enabling some women to avoid the injections.

Risks and Side Effects

It's estimated that more than two million American women have been exposed to fertility drugs over the past decade.

According to the American Society for Reproductive Medicine (ASRM), women taking Clomid can have up to a 10 percent risk of having twins, compared with 1 percent of women in the general population. There is a slight increased risk of miscarriage with clomiphene, as well as an increased risk of developing luteal phase defects and ovarian cysts. Side effects include hot flashes, mood swings, nausea, headaches, breast tenderness and depression.

Side effects of hMGs include rash at the injection site, breast tenderness, abdominal bloating, mood swings and extreme hyperstimulation of the ovaries. This *hyperstimulation syndrome* causes the ovaries to become painfully swollen, and in extreme cases, fluid accumulates in the abdominal cavity and chest, requiring hospitalization. One fourth of all pregnancies achieved with Pergonal are multiple births, with two thirds being twins and the other third triplets. With hMGs there is an increased risk of miscarriage and premature delivery, especially with multiple fetuses. Some patients pregnant with triplets or more choose to undergo *multifetal pregnancy reduction* to decrease such risks of prematurity as cerebral palsy, intracranial hemorrhage, respiratory distress and infant death. There's an average 10 percent risk of losing the pregnancy, but that drops to less than 5 percent in good hands.

The risks and complications of FSH are similar to hMGs, while those associated with GnRH are slight. Patients taking GnRH analogs often undergo a temporary menopause with all the associated symptoms, such as hot flashes and vaginal dryness.

"These drugs have been around for more than thirty years and are very safe when given for limited periods of time and monitored properly. There is no evidence they cause birth defects," Dr. Berkeley stresses.

A Question of Cancer

Recent reports suggest fertility drugs may cause increased risk of ovarian cancer. The theory is that just as oral contraceptives cut the risk of ovarian cancer by quieting the ovaries, so fertility drugs may have the opposite effect, increasing cellular proliferation, exposing cells to high estrogen levels.

A 1994 study by the University of Washington and the Fred Hutchinson Cancer Center among 4,000 women taking fertility drugs for six to eighteen years found a two and a half times greater than normal risk of ovarian cancer. However, use for less than a year did not appear to elevate risk. A 1993 report from Stanford University compiled data from three case-controlled studies and found that women who had taken unspecified fertility drugs (especially those who did not become pregnant) were nearly three times more likely to get ovarian cancer than women who conceived naturally. (It should be noted that never becoming pregnant raises ovarian cancer risk two to three times; pregnancy lowers risk by the same amount.)

At the same time, a 1997 case-controlled study from Denmark of over 2,000 women found no association between fertility drugs and ovarian cancer; other studies from Israel, Italy and China came to the same conclusion. Between 1980 and 1993 fifty-eight cases of ovarian cancer have been linked to fertility drugs worldwide, according to a 1995 overview in the *Journal of Women's Health*. "However, it is too early to predict the increase, if any, in the lifetime risk of ovarian cancer that may be caused by fertility drug exposure because so many of the exposed women have yet to enter the ages of highest risk," commented the authors.

Nevertheless, in 1994 the U.S. Food and Drug Administration ordered changes in the drugs' labeling to reflect recent information on risk. "It would be wrong for me to tell my patients that these drugs absolutely do not cause cancer. But the fact is there's no strong data yet to show that they do," comments Frederick L. Licciardi, M.D., an infertility specialist and assistant professor of OB/GYN at NYU Medical Center.

Answers may come in a few years from several studies funded by the National Cancer Institute and other institutions. However, until the data is in, experts say women with a strong family history of ovarian cancer should limit their exposure to fertility drugs. "These medications cause estrogen levels to rise to very high levels, but only for about one to two weeks. There are questions, all unresolved, about the role of estrogens in the development of breast cancer. Women with a family history of breast cancer, or who have had a previous breast cancer, and who are considering fertility treatment need to enter such treatments cautiously," says Dr. Licciardi.

DES daughters can take fertility drugs and may undergo IVF if needed, but because of problems with the uterus, they may have problems with implantation and preterm delivery. "Fertility drugs should be used for the fewest cycles possible, not only to reduce the body's exposure to the medications, but also because we know that the highest chance for pregnancy occurs in the first few cycles of therapy," stresses Dr. Licciardi.

Most patients start off with clomiphene citrate, and this should not be used for more than three or four cycles. The effectiveness of these cycles should be maximized by physician monitoring and the addition of insemination, he says. Likewise injectable fertility drugs should be limited to three to four cycles before going on to in vitro fertilization (which also requires fertility drugs). Older women should move quickly from step to step, because they don't have the biological time to waste on therapies that aren't working, adds Dr. Licciardi.

Miranda's Story, Cont'd

"What is IVF like? Disgusting and invasive for both the man and woman. My husband especially hated having to masturbate. It's painful *when they remove the eggs. You're sort of woozy from the sedative but awake. They go in vaginally, and they probe, and they tell you how many mature eggs you have. I had only two cycles out of four cycles that resulted in enough eggs. The first one didn't take.*

"They call you twenty-four, thirty-six hours later to tell you how many fertilized. Then you come back in for the transfer, which is kind of easy. They show you the eggs on a television screen, and you can see them being drawn into this pipette. You lie on your back with your knees against your chest. Then they put a speculum in and transfer the eggs through a catheter right into the womb. The transfer of the eggs is no more painful than an internal exam. Then you lie still on your back in the recovery room for three hours.

"Then there's the wait to find out whether or not you were pregnant. The big phone call. No matter how nice they tried to be about it, when they had bad news, it was always hard. I had tried insemination and had several miscarriages, and each time we had to start over again. It's an emotional roller coaster."

In Vitro Fertilization

In IVF, sperm and eggs are fertilized in a laboratory dish, and the resulting embryo is transferred to the woman's uterus where it is hoped it will implant and grow.

First a woman is put on Pergonal or Metrodin so that she produces multiple eggs. Ultrasound is used to monitor the development of the follicles to ensure that the eggs are fully mature, and blood samples are taken to measure estrogen, and sometimes progesterone and luteinizing hormone. When the follicles are mature, the patient is given an injection of hCG to trigger ovulation, so egg retrieval can be precisely timed.

Egg retrieval using *transvaginal ultrasound aspiration* is a minor surgical procedure that can be performed in the physician's office or an IVF facility with sedation or anesthesia. Guided by ultrasound, a needle is inserted through the upper vagina and into the ovarian follicles to remove eggs with gentle suction.

The sperm are "washed," separated from *seminal plasma*, to separate the most active (motile) sperm. (Donor sperm are also tested for infectious dis-

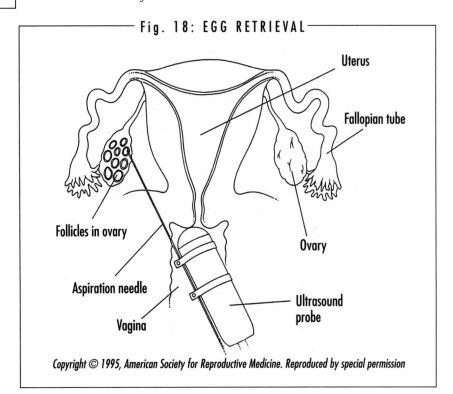

Fig. 18: EGG RETRIEVAL

Uterus

Fallopian tube

Follicles in ovary

Ovary

Aspiration needle

Ultrasound probe

Vagina

Copyright © 1995, American Society for Reproductive Medicine. Reproduced by special permission

eases, including HIV.) Each egg is placed in a separate laboratory dish prepared with IVF culture medium and mixed with sperm. The dishes are placed in an incubator, set at the same temperature as the woman's body, for two to three days. When the eggs have been fertilized and have begun to divide, they are transferred into the uterine cavity in an outpatient procedure that takes about ten to twenty minutes, rarely requiring only a mild sedative.

More than one embryo is usually transferred, increasing the chances of pregnancy (other fertilized embryos may be frozen for future IVF procedures). In some instances couples may have to make a difficult choice to "reduce" the number of fertilized embryos transferred to decrease the risk of multiple pregnancy and its complications. NYU and other IVF centers are also pioneering *embryo biopsy,* which removes a cell from an early multicell embryo to assess the risk of potentially serious genetic disorders.

While the delivery rate for a simple IVF procedure can be almost 50 percent for women under forty at the best centers, the success rate for basic IVF is about 22 percent nationwide.

Fig. 19: EMBRYO TRANSFER

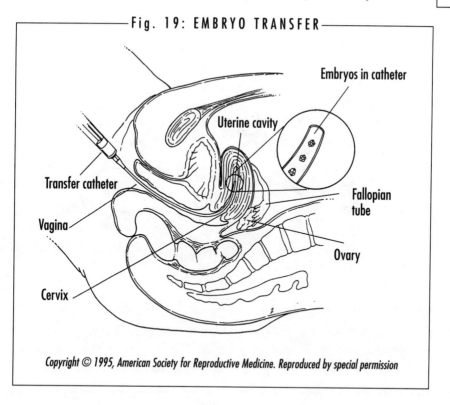

Embryos in catheter

Uterine cavity

Transfer catheter

Vagina

Cervix

Fallopian tube

Ovary

Copyright © 1995, American Society for Reproductive Medicine. Reproduced by special permission

---

Assisted Hatching

Assisted hatching is an IVF technique that helps the embryo implant in the wall of the uterus. After fertilization the egg begins to divide within its "shell," the *zona pellucida*. Normally about two days after the dividing embryo has reached the uterus the zona opens, and the embryo cells burst forth to burrow into the endometrium, a process known as *hatching*.

It's believed that in older women and women with other fertility problems the zona may become thickened, making hatching difficult. In assisted hatching, the zona's shell is treated prior to embryo transfer to weaken it and improve the likelihood of hatching. There are two hatching techniques:

> *ZONA DRILLING* involves making a small hole in the zona with an acidified solution to assist hatching. Also, an acid solution can be used to "digest" a small portion of the zona down to its innermost layer, so it's easier for cells to burst through.

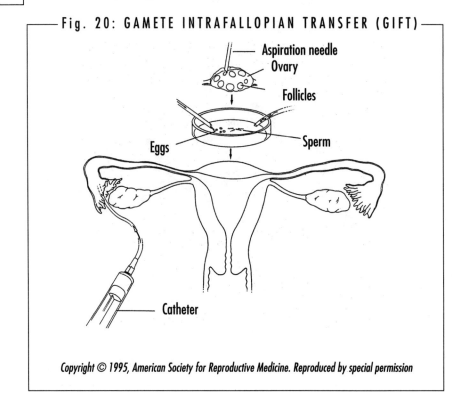

Fig. 20: GAMETE INTRAFALLOPIAN TRANSFER (GIFT)

Aspiration needle
Ovary
Follicles
Eggs
Sperm
Catheter

PROTEASE DIGESTION (PROD), a newer method, uses the natural enzyme protease to soften and thin the entire circumference of the zona, so cells can be expelled in a manner similar to natural hatching.

Candidates for assisted hatching are women in their forties and/or women who have failed previous IVF attempts.

Laparoscopic Procedures

Laparoscopic procedures to transfer the egg and sperm, or a fertilized embryo, directly into the fallopian tubes guided by laparoscopy are also done in many infertility centers.

GAMETE INTRAFALLOPIAN TRANSFER (GIFT) involves ovulation induction followed by egg retrieval using a laparoscope, under general anesthesia. One or two eggs are mixed with sperm, then injected with a catheter into one or both fallopian tubes using a laparoscope under general anesthesia. Fertilization can then occur in the fallopian tube with the embryo traveling to the uterus as in unassisted reproduction.

ZYGOTE INTRAFALLOPIAN TRANSFER (ZIFT) is a variation on GIFT in which the egg is fertilized in a laboratory dish but transferred before cell division begins. In this case the eggs are retrieved by transvaginal ultrasound aspiration and transferred to the fallopian tubes by laparoscopy the next day. The embryo will begin dividing in the tube and travel normally to the uterus for implantation.

TUBAL EMBRYO TRANSFER (TET) involves the transfer of a more developed embryo, a fertilized egg that has reached the stage of four- to eight-cell division, usually within twenty-four hours of fertilization. One reason for using ZIFT or TET rather than GIFT is to make sure the sperm are capable of fertilization.

These procedures can be used to treat women with unexplained infertility, mild endometriosis and cervical or immunological factors. However, women must have healthy, open fallopian tubes.

Although GIFT and its variations are effective, laparoscopy is still a surgical procedure requiring general anesthesia, according to Dr. Berkeley, who says, "In vitro fertilization is less surgically risky than laparoscopic methods, and IVF usually requires only intravenous sedation. When high-quality IVF is available, GIFT and similar techniques are not needed."

∞ *Miranda's Story, Cont'd* ∞

"The second IVF, I had multiple eggs implanted. When the pregnancy test came out positive and they took a sonogram, they saw only one embryo. A week later I was at a business meeting and I began to bleed. My doctor told me, 'Lie down; rest. If you're still bleeding tomorrow, we'll do another sonogram.' I came in, and there were two embryos! I now had twins! They said, 'We have no idea whether you'll lose one or two or none.' When I went back for another sonogram, I had lost the second embryo. But one was still there. My daughter was hanging on.

"By this time we had gotten far along in the adoption process. We went through a week asking ourselves, 'Do we still go through with it?' We knew we wanted two children. Friends of ours also have two children, one biological and one adopted ten months apart, and they said go for it. So we did. It was a very joyous time. Really, they were both miracle children."

What Are the Risks of IVF and GIFT?

When carried out by specially trained personnel in properly equipped settings, IVF and GIFT carry little risk. Laparoscopy carries the risk of any surgery requiring general anesthesia. With egg aspiration using an intravaginal needle there is a slight risk of bleeding, infection and damage to the bowel, bladder or a blood vessel in the area. When one or more eggs or embryos are transferred, there is always the risk of multiple pregnancy. With three or more fetuses complication rates increase, as does the risk of prematurity, low birth weight and congenital defects. Up to 30 percent of pregnancies achieved with IVF and fertility treatments result in multiple births.

There's a 2.6 percent chance of ectopic pregnancy with IVF and GIFT. As with all pregnancies (especially in older women) there is a 20 to 25 percent risk of miscarriage. There may also be first-trimester bleeding, which can signal possible miscarriage or ectopic pregnancy. However, early bleeding may be more common in women who undergo IVF and GIFT and may not indicate complications.

Using Donor Eggs

In recent years study after study has shown that while the ovaries shut down at menopause, the uterus is capable of maintaining a pregnancy if it is given the proper dose of estrogen and progesterone. Women in their mid- to late forties who have undergone premature menopause or chemotherapy or have had their ovaries removed for medical reasons can use donor eggs for IVF. "By far the largest group of women using donor eggs are those who are in their forties and have been trying to become pregnant for quite some time," says Dr. Licciardi, who directs the Donor Oocyte Program at NYU Medical Center.

Donor eggs come from women in their twenties or early thirties. "Generally they are people who really want to help other couples. They have a friend who couldn't get pregnant or they have a sister or they had read about it," says Dr. Licciardi. "They're screened psychologically, genetically and, of course, for all transmissible diseases." The donor and recipient are matched closely for physical characteristics. When a donor is accepted, she takes fertility drugs so that multiple eggs develop. She then undergoes egg retrieval, with around twenty eggs collected. IVF is performed in the same manner as women using their own eggs, except that the mother to be (the recipient) needs to take estrogen and progesterone to make sure that the lining of the uterus is prepared for pregnancy. The donor receives a fee for donating her eggs to compensate her for the time and physical requirements of the process. Every couple considering use of donor eggs (or donor sperm) must also see a counselor since there can be many psychological issues involved.

Surrogacy

Also fraught with psychological (and legal) consequences is the use of surrogates to carry a baby for another woman. A surrogate is implanted with an embryo, using eggs from either the legal mother or the surrogate, and with sperm from the legal father or a donor. In several highly publicized cases a surrogate mother decided she wanted to keep the child and sued for custody. At the same time some women have carried babies for their sisters or daughters and have forged unique family ties.

The Newest IVF Techniques

AUTOIMMUNE THERAPIES are being added to IVF in some women with suspected immune problems or autoimmune disease. Most commonly a baby aspirin a day is given to women with lupus to reduce the chances of miscarriage, hypertension, fetal growth retardation and preterm labor. Other therapies for women with lupus anticoagulants/antiphospholipid antibodies include low-dose aspirin along with injections of the anticoagulant heparin, with or without *intravenous gamma globulin.*

Aspirin-heparin therapy can increase the risk of bleeding during labor, so it is usually stopped at around 34 weeks. In some centers low-dose aspirin and the anticoagulant heparin are being given to otherwise healthy infertile women who test positive for APAs (or other autoimmune antibodies), in hopes of increasing the success rate of IVF. If a woman conceives, treatment may continue through part or even most of the pregnancy. However, there have also been no large-scale trials of aspirin or aspirin-heparin therapy, so the therapy remains unproved, cautions Dr. Berkeley.

Intracytoplasmic sperm injection (ICSI) has improved pregnancy rates dramatically. In ICSI a single sperm is injected directly into the egg's cytoplasm. Even in men who do not ejaculate any sperm at all (*azoospermia*), it is possible to retrieve sperm by doing a biopsy of the testicles. ICSI has a 60 percent fertilization rate and birthrates equal to or exceeding conventional IVF with no male infertility. ICSI embryos can also be frozen for later implantation.

"Given the high fertilization and pregnancy rates with ICSI, we believe it may eventually replace conventional IVF for many patients," says Dr. Berkeley. At present only large IVF centers with specially trained and equipped personnel are able to perform ICSI, but the technology is spreading.

The Future of IVF

On the horizon are several other promising techniques.

IMMATURE OOCYTE RETRIEVAL involves removing immature eggs (oocytes) from the ovary and bathing them in minute doses of hormones to mature them in the lab before IVF. The technique would avoid the need for powerful hormones to stimulate maturation of multiple eggs in the ovary, which not only have unpleasant side effects but add to the costs of IVF.

Jeffrey B. Russell, M.D., and colleagues at the Reproductive Endocrine and Fertility Center of Delaware reported in 1996 that they were able to produce embryos in seven out of the first eight patients who underwent immature oocyte retrieval; one woman became pregnant and gave birth to a baby girl. Although this represents only a 5 percent success rate, Dr. Russell thinks the pregnancy rate should improve as the technique is refined and physicians become more adept at it.

Researchers at the Jackson Laboratory in Bar Harbor, Maine, reported in 1996 that they have developed a way to "farm" multiple oocytes by growing them in culture. Egg maturation techniques are also being studied at NYU's IVF unit.

CRYOPRESERVATION is being done increasingly with IVF. Several eggs are fertilized, and the extra embryos are frozen and later thawed for transfer to the uterus. Almost seven thousand embryo transfers using cryopreservation are done a year. While freezing sperm for later use is a standard procedure, the freezing of eggs has been highly experimental. However, in 1997 the first births from frozen and thawed human eggs were reported. In the future, egg cryopreservation could provide an alternative for women at risk of losing ovarian function, either by surgery or chemotherapy, allowing the eggs to be matured later on in the lab and saved for the patient. It could also allow women to freeze eggs when they are young for use later in life.

OVARY CRYOPRESERVATION is another experimental procedure, which involves the freezing of parts of an ovary with liquid nitrogen for reimplanting after chemotherapy or radiation. In experiments at the University of Leeds in England with mice and sheep, scientists have shown that frozen parts of ovaries successfully survive freezing and produce eggs when reimplanted, allowing the animals to become pregnant.

Experts caution that only a handful of women undergoing cancer treatment have had parts of their ovaries removed, and it may take years to know whether the procedure even works, since the cancer would have to be fully in remission before ovarian function could be restored (and there could be potential danger for women with breast or ovarian cancers, which are driven by estrogen secreted by the ovaries).

CYTOPLASMIC TRANSFER is an investigational technique that takes a tiny amount of cytoplasm from a donor egg and injects it, along with a single sperm, into an egg from an older woman who has had trouble conceiving. The theory is that the transfer may somehow "normalize" the cytoplasm of the recipient egg, making fertilization and embryo transfer more successful. While a number of women have undergone cytoplasmic transfer at St. Barnabas Medical Center in Livingston, New Jersey, only two pregnancies have resulted, and there have been no clinical trials.

NUCLEAR TRANSFER would involve removing the nuclear material from the egg of an older woman and from the egg of a donor and inserting the older woman's genetic material into the enucleated donor egg, in an attempt to correct cytoplasmic and/or membrane problems that arise in "older" eggs. Right now such transfers are being tested in animals by David Keefe, M.D., director of the Infertility Service at Women's and Infants Hospital of Rhode Island, but if proved effective, it could be tried in human eggs in a few years.

☙ *S a r a ' s   S t o r y ,   C o n t ' d* ☙

"When you finally call it quits, you feel like a loser. You've failed at something you should have been able to do with no problem. But we just couldn't afford to continue when we knew the odds were against us.

"So you walk away, and it's a terrible feeling, like a door is closing on a part of your life. I keep wondering, I'm still young. Why did this happen to me?"

What Are Your Chances?

According to the yearly data gathered by Society for Assisted Reproductive Technology (SART) from 281 IVF programs in the U.S. and Canada, there were about 59,000 cycles of assisted reproduction technology in 1995, resulting in 11,631 deliveries (16,520 babies). The nationwide average take-home baby rate for IVF was about 22.3 percent; for women in their forties, the rate was less than half of that.

"The single most important variable is a woman's age in all success rates, whether it's drugs or whether it's IVF. The sad fact is that you are less likely to succeed with a woman who is in her mid- to late forties, using her own eggs," explains Dr. Berkeley. "Which is not to say that it can't be done, but the take-home pregnancy rates go down with every passing year."

According to SART data, a forty-plus woman using donor eggs has almost the same chance of delivering a baby as younger women (about 34 percent). While most studies say the age of the mother doesn't affect successful implantation with donor eggs, unpublished data have found an age-related decline in the implantation rate. And even after midlife women have become pregnant with donor eggs, they're still subject to age-related pregnancy and labor complications, such as hypertension, gestational diabetes, placenta previa and preterm labor, although most deliver without problems.

For ovarian stimulation and IVF in women over thirty-nine, 1995 SART data say there was a 10.6 percent delivery rate per egg retrieval without male factor infertility compared to a delivery rate of 27.5 percent for women under thirty-five. IVF using ICSI had an average of 23.5 percent success rate. For GIFT, the delivery rate among women over thirty-nine was 12 percent per retrieval (with no male factor infertility) versus 36.4 percent for women under thirty-five.

Mark V. Sauer, M.D., now director of Reproductive Endocrinology and Assisted Reproduction at Columbia-Presbyterian Medical Center in New York, first reported in 1993 that he and his colleagues at the University of Southern California at Los Angeles were able to initiate and maintain pregnancies in women through age sixty using donated eggs. In 1997 a sixty-three-year-old woman initially treated by Dr. Sauer had a baby girl using donor eggs. Since the first "menopause moms" made headlines, medical ethicists have questioned the wisdom of rewinding a woman's biological clock when she may not be around for her child's high school graduation. Some IVF programs have set age limits. At NYU the cutoff is age forty-six for IVF with a patient's own eggs and forty-nine for donor eggs. At one of the oldest programs in the U.S., the Genetics & IVF Institute in Fairfax, Virginia, the limit is fifty-five.

Choosing an Assisted Reproduction Facility

The American Society for Reproductive Medicine stresses that important considerations for choosing an IVF or GIFT program include the qualifications and experience of personnel, types of problems being treated, support services, cost, convenience and the rate of take-home pregnancies. The range of services offered by a program should also be considered. Some programs are equipped to offer combined IVF/GIFT, with more advanced techniques like ICSI.

A credible program will adhere to the guidelines from the ASRM and belong to its affiliate, SART. A majority of the 300-plus clinics in the U.S. and Canada are now members of SART. The IVF lab should have certification under the Clinical Laboratory Improvement Act (CLIA) of 1988 (having passed an independent, outside inspection) and be accredited by the College of American Pathologists (CAP). Office-based programs should be accredited by the Commission on Office Laboratory Accreditation (COLA).

"Be wary of programs that claim to have doubled or tripled their pregnancy rates. Although the registry rates are more than a year out-of-date because clinics must wait for delivery to list a successful pregnancy, rates do not change dramatically from year to year, unless a program changes drastically," says Dr. Berkeley. Centers may also inflate take-home pregnancy rates by selecting patients who have the *best* chances of success with IVF.

In recent years there have been a number of scandals involving IVF clinics, including one physician who impregnated women with his own sperm. Since 1991 the Federal Trade Commission (FTC) has won cease and desist agreements from a half dozen IVF clinics for deceptive advertising about success rates; another large clinic paid four million dollars to several hundred couples to settle a lawsuit over false success rate claims. So be wary.

Both CAP and SART require an IVF/GIFT program to have personnel on its staff who have been trained in reproductive endocrinology, laparoscopic surgery, sonography, hormone measurement, tissue culture and sperm and egg interaction. There should be a mental health professional available for counseling since infertility treatments can take a heavy emotional toll.

New York, California and Washington State now have state agencies to regulate embryology labs, but aside from voluntary membership in SART, there are no federal, state or medical regulations or standards governing the services or conduct of infertility clinics. The Fertility Clinic Success Rate and Certification Act, implemented in 1997, requires fertility clinics to report pregnancy rates to the Centers for Disease Control and Prevention; the data will be published yearly to help people choose a clinic. Britain (where the first test-tube baby was born in 1978) has regulated its programs since 1991, and Canada has taken steps toward regulating its clinics. ASRM is developing a series of guidelines for members that, among other things, will limit the number of embryos implanted to three or four to reduce high-risk multiple births.

Cost is also a factor. A *single* attempt at conventional in vitro fertilization can run up to $10,000; an ICSI cycle can cost upward of $12,500; IVF with donor eggs can cost up to $20,000 (including hormone treatments and fees to the egg donor). Multiply those numbers over two or three cycles, plus the costs of the infertility workup. Insurance coverage for IVF is not yet common; as of 1996, only ten states required coverage. Some 85 percent of the costs are borne by patients. (Listings for the ASRM, SART, CDC data, and other resources are in Appendix I.)

Choosing Adoption

Even with the availability of high-tech assisted reproduction, there are those people who will not want to put themselves through the rigors (or expense) of IVF. "Not every patient wants, or can afford, an in vitro fertilization attempt, even though for a particular couple it might be the most likely route to successful pregnancy," notes Dr. Wentz. "Physicians should discuss the full range of options, including adoption."

Even with the best technology, there are people for whom it will not work. "Anytime you do more than three IVF procedures without success, couples should seriously consider what they are doing and whether it's time to move on," advises Dr. Berkeley. The nationwide support group Resolve offers counseling that can help couples weigh their options (see Appendix I).

For infertile women struggling with the decision whether to undergo (or stop) assisted reproduction and try to adopt, we offer the following comments from Miranda:

"We all want a genetic connection to our children. We were in a support group with other couples who were infertile and were going to adopt. A lot of people were struggling with the lack of genetic connection, particularly that their parents would never accept it because lineage was important to them. It was an issue for me too because both my parents had died.

"But once I got through the mourning and understood what I really wanted, I realized that I can perpetuate my parents in other ways. I can pass along the family stories, the values. So we went through with the adoption and the pregnancy, and we now have two beautiful children, ten months apart.

"Pregnancy was nice, but I would have missed out on nothing that's wonderful about parenting had I ended up adopting two children. The quality of my feelings for these children is exactly the same, and the experience of getting to know a newborn is exactly the same.

"A lot of what my children become will be modified by the environment and way that we deal with them and the way we deal with life. But adopting has taught me that whatever is inherent in each child should be seen as theirs alone, not as an extension of someone else. It's a very special way to love anybody."

Midlife, Menopause and Beyond

Gynecological health cannot be viewed simply in terms of re-production and postmenopause. The dividing line isn't as clear-cut as that. Just as puberty gradually leads up to a girl's first period, the *climacteric*, or physiological process leading up to cessation of menses, takes place over many years. The average age of menopause is fifty-one, although in some women it can occur as early as age forty-four or as late as age fifty-eight.

No longer regarded as a hormone deficiency "disease," menopause is a normal biological stage in a woman's life, bringing special symptoms and health concerns. While hot flashes are the most well-known symptom of menopause, during these years more subtle symptoms occur that can be alarming if you don't know what to expect.

▪ Perimenopause: What's Happening to Me? ▪

Changes in ovarian function and reproductive hormones culminating in menopause actually begin ten years or more before periods stop. Ovarian function peaks in the twenties and early thirties; thereafter the ovaries are losing egg cells, follicles and the surrounding hormone-producing cells, leading to a gradual loss of estrogen and progesterone. The first signs of the climacteric may occur around age thirty-five, when fertility starts to decline.

As ovarian estrogen production lessens, the remaining follicles become more resistant to follicle-stimulating hormone (FSH), so a woman may not ovulate and menstruate every twenty-eight to thirty days. Among women in their forties, 70 percent have irregular periods—lighter or heavier bleeding, shorter or longer cycles, periods that stop and then start up again—or mid-cycle spotting. Only 10 percent of women abruptly stop menstruating.

"If a woman doesn't ovulate, there's no corpus luteum to produce progesterone. Estrogen may continue to build up the endometrial lining, but without progesterone, menstruation will not occur on schedule. This is why many women in their forties experience irregular periods," observes Nanette F. Santoro, M.D., director of reproductive endocrinology at the University of Medicine and Dentistry of New Jersey–Robert Wood Johnson Medical School. When menstruation does occur, the flow is heavy or there's spotting in mid-cycle. Overgrowth of the endometrium (or hyperplasia) can lead to cancer, so irregular bleeding must be checked out.

"Rather than a steady downward slide in estrogen, perimenopause is a hormonal roller coaster," says Dr. Santoro. This roller coaster effect disrupts the normal feedback loop among the ovaries, the hypothalamus and the pituitary. When the pituitary senses a dip in estrogen, it churns out extra FSH (and LH) to stimulate the ovaries, causing a spike in estrogen, which prompts the hypothalamus to pump out more gonadotropin-releasing hormone (GnRH) to stimulate the pituitary. Hormonal ups and downs usually trigger the varied symptoms of perimenopause because the hypothalamus also regulates blood pressure, body temperature, sleep and waking, appetite, sexual behavior and mood.

Only 10 to 20 percent of women in their forties experience hot flashes; many more experience hot flash equivalents, other symptoms affecting blood vessels and the nervous system (*vasomotor symptoms*), such as headaches, dizziness, palpitations, queasiness, pelvic discomfort, prickly sensations in the skin, insomnia or sleep disturbances (since hot flashes are more common at night). In perimenopausal women, hot flashes may feel more like brief sensations of heat, with or without the flushed skin and sudden sweating. Other symptoms can include irritability, fatigue, poor concentration and memory, mood swings and anxiety.

As estrogen declines, there's a gradual lessening of vaginal secretions, cervical mucus and lubrication during sexual arousal. While vaginal thinning and painful intercourse are more common after menopause, women in their forties may have some uncomfortable dryness (why some vaginal lubricants now contain spermicides). Lowered levels of estrogen may constrict blood vessels, reducing blood flow to the pelvis, so there's less engorgement during sex, changing sexual responsiveness. "Recent evidence also indicates testosterone may decrease in mid-cycle in women in their mid-forties who are still having regular periods, so it could lower libido," says Dr. Santoro.

Women with PMS may now see a worsening of their symptoms, with PMS symptoms such as bloating, breast discomfort and anxiety no longer being confined to the luteal phase of the cycle but sometimes felt all through the cycle.

But if a woman is still having periods, she may not connect any of these symptoms to approaching menopause. Experts say women who have had tubal ligations or hysterectomies but still have their ovaries may experience menopause somewhat earlier.

Oral contraceptives can help stabilize hormonal ups and downs and irregular bleeding during perimenopause. In fact, newer low-dose pills were actually formulated for the forty-something woman. With continuous levels of estrogen and progestin, the normal ovulatory process shuts down, providing a stable level of hormones. "There will be less buildup of the endometrial lining and only withdrawal bleeding, but that helps protect against endometrial hyperplasia. Most women will have considerable relief from pelvic discomfort and PMS-type symptoms," says NYU's Dr. Ilona Brandeis.

Low-dose pills will not delay menopause, but the end point may be less clear, Dr. Brandeis adds. Even with oral contraceptives, eventually estrogen will become low enough to push up levels of FSH. "We may have to monitor the FSH more closely than in a woman who is not on the pill, to determine at what point she can switch to replacement hormones, if that is what she chooses."

Physicians used to be reluctant to prescribe hormone replacement therapy (HRT) before a woman had stopped menstruating for at least six months. But there's growing recognition that the doses of oral estrogen and progesterone in HRT are much lower than those in oral contraceptives. Some reproductive endocrinologists are prescribing new cyclical or continuous regimens of HRT or the estrogen patch with a low-dose progestin to guard against endometrial hyperplasia (see page 276), but this is very controversial. Side effects may be less, but you'll need to rely on other forms of contraception.

"I never thought much about menopause. I knew you could start having irregular periods years before. But I have always been very regular. Since I had severe PMS, I was always much more concerned about that.

"One month my period came very early, and my PMS symptoms did not go away. I was really bloated, and the diuretic did not get rid of the bloating as it usually does. Then, a few days after my period ended, I started having mild menstrual-type cramps. I went right away to my gynecologist, but he said it was probably just a hormonal glitch and told me to keep track of my symptoms and call after my next period.

"I was early again, so I ended up having two periods in one month. I was sent for an ultrasound to see if there were any fibroids or uterine polyps causing the problem. But there were none. The lining of my uterus looked perfectly healthy. My ovaries also looked normal. The doctor explained that the irregular bleeding was probably due to my not ovulating every month anymore and that women in their forties commonly had that problem. He put me on low-dose birth control pills, which he said would help regulate my cycles.

"They made such a difference! No more PMS, very little bloating. No more weird cramps. And I feel very good knowing that the estrogen is going to sort of fill in the gaps hormonally until I do reach menopause."

▪ Checking Out Irregular Perimenopausal Bleeding ▪

Because irregular bleeding is so common in perimenopause, women are often sent for endometrial biopsies or dilation and curettage (D&C) to make sure there's no precancerous growth in the uterine lining. However, with newer, more sensitive transvaginal ultrasound, 75 percent of such diagnostic D&Cs could be avoided, says Dr. Steven Goldstein, head of the gynecological ultrasound unit at NYU Medical Center. "With *saline infusion sonohysterography* [*SIS*] we can easily distinguish between patients whose bleeding is anovulatory and is best treated hormonally and women with abnormalities in need of further intervention."

Saline infusion sonohysterography is a painless office procedure, usually done on days four to six of a woman's cycle, in which a thin catheter (the size of a thin strand of spaghetti) is inserted through the cervix to instill a teaspoon of sterile saline into the uterus. "Fluid enhances sound transmission, highlighting even small changes in the endometrium. We can see areas of endometrial thickening that will need sampling, instead of having to do a blind biopsy," explains Dr. Goldstein.

Studies show that endometrial biopsy, considered the gold standard for diagnosing bleeding problems, can actually miss 50 percent or more of uterine cancers because there is no way to sample the entire lining of the uterus. In contrast, studies have shown that SIS can help detect a majority of cancers in women with suspicious endometrial thickening, which shows up clearly on saline-enhanced ultrasound, so the exact area can be biopsied.

Two recent studies, one conducted by Dr. Goldstein at NYU and the other at the University of Texas, Health Science Center in Houston, showed that SIS not only was better than "blind" endometrial biopsies and D&Cs at finding problems (including cancers) but could also save considerable expense. Using ultrasound instead of endometrial sampling, 79 percent of the 433 patients in the NYU study were found to have no abnormalities and were able to be treated hormonally. "With SIS the only time women will go into the operating room for a D and C will be for treatment, not diagnosis," says Dr. Goldstein. The savings could be substantial: A biopsy followed by a D&C might run $4,000 in a big-city medical center, versus around $850 for SIS, including the office visit and initial sonogram. SIS can be used as well to follow postmenopausal women on hormones to monitor the thickness of the endometrium, also avoiding biopsies.

---

෨ *S u e ' s   S t o r y   C o n t ' d* ෨

"I was really not expecting to go into menopause. I was only forty-nine. My symptoms were really severe. I was not sleeping at night because of the hot flashes, and I could not remember things. There was anxiety; there was disordered thinking, inability to concentrate. It was scary. At first I blamed it on stress. My mother was ill; I had a new job. But I finally realized what was going on.

"When I look back, I realize it had started months before, when I had two periods very close together. When I finally saw my gynecologist, I told him I thought I was going into menopause. He laughed, but when he ran the tests, it turned out I was not starting menopause, I was well into it. My FSH was sky-high, and my estrogen was almost nil.

"I had an endometrial biopsy because my doctor wanted to check, since I was still bleeding. They dilate your cervix and take a pinch of tissue from the inside of the uterus. It hurts, like bad, bad cramps, but it's brief, thankfully. He said the tissue looked fine, so there's less for me to worry about."

▪ What to Expect in Menopause ▪

As menopause draws near, symptoms, especially hot flashes, may heighten. Between 50 and 75 percent of women may experience them to some degree within the two years before menstrual periods stop.

Hot flashes may be preceded by an aura, which includes dizziness, palpitations, headaches or a sense of unease. It begins with an intense sensation of heat, an increase in heart rate, flushing (as blood rushes to the skin) that seems to spread across the chest, neck and face, then an outpouring of sweat. As the sweat evaporates, skin temperature drops, and there may be chills. Hot flashes may last only one to five minutes, but it can take some women a half hour to recover. The frequency varies from woman to woman: Some have them once a week; others one or more times a day. Hot flashes are most common in the morning and evening, but they can also wake a woman up from a sound sleep. They can be triggered by stress, but anything that raises body temperature can bring one on: hot drinks, hot weather, hot rooms, hot or spicy foods, caffeine and even alcohol. (It's not a bad idea to keep a "hot flash diary," to see which triggers may be under your control.)

Even if hot flashes are not that frequent or severe, coupled with other symptoms, they may contribute to fatigue and a general sense of unwellness, especially if they disrupt a woman's sleep. While hot flashes and other menopausal symptoms are not "all in your head," a great deal of interaction between the mind and body is going on. A number of studies suggest that the severity of a woman's menopausal symptoms may have more to do with her feelings about getting older than to what's happening to her physiologically.

For example, a 1996 update from an ongoing study at the Center for Women's Health Research at the University of Washington, Seattle found that stressful life circumstances, coupled with a negative view of midlife, and health problems had a potent effect on the amount of vasomotor symptoms a woman experienced and the resulting emotional distress. On the other hand, the study of more than 500 women found those who viewed this stage in life in a positive way had less severe symptoms.

Menopausal symptoms can also can be culturally influenced. In the United States and other Western industrialized countries where aging is seen as a loss, women experience more severe symptoms. In contrast, studies show that women from cultures that view aging in a positive light experience few or no menopausal symptoms, even though they are undergoing the same biological process. For example, in Asian cultures age confers wisdom, and older people are highly valued and respected. Studies among Japanese women reveal that fewer than 20 percent have ever experienced hot flashes, compared with 75 percent of Americans. (However, this may also be due to the Japanese diet, which is high in soy products, which are plant estrogens.) In some cultures menopause is cause for celebration. A study of the Meo people of Thailand relates how menopausal women throw big parties to announce that they are no longer of childbearing age and thus deserve greater respect from everyone.

Although women may experience some mood disturbances, experts stress that menopause itself does not cause depression, which can occur at any stage of life and needs to be treated as a separate entity with antidepressants. "We see many women who have little or no menopausal symptoms, who feel terrific at this time of life," says Dr. Brandeis. However, she notes, some women who are extremely bothered by menopausal symptoms and have been put on antidepressants or tranquilizers can get complete relief with estrogen replacement.

When a woman has gone a full twelve months without bleeding, she is said to be in menopause, confirmed by blood tests for high levels of FSH. The ovaries don't shut down overnight, however, but continue to produce tiny amounts of estrogen for up to ten years. The adrenal glands produce the hormone androstenedione, which is converted to a less potent estrogen called estrone, and fatty tissues also produce small amounts of estrone. But it's not enough to prevent the effects of estrogen loss on bone and tissues. Testosterone production by the ovaries does not appear to drop as dramatically as estrogen (although some women report a loss of libido that could be related to low testosterone). However, the increased ratio of androgens to estrogens caused by the drop in ovarian estrogen can trigger acne and facial hair growth and can lower the levels of "good" cholesterol. Up to 50 percent of women experience hot flashes after periods have stopped.

Once a woman has entered menopause, she can consider taking replacement estrogen, which will relieve symptoms. The decision to take estrogen can depend on a woman's risk of heart disease, osteoporosis and breast cancer (see page 259).

Since fatty tissues produce estrone, studies show heavier women may have a buffer against major bone loss later on. While some experts believe heavier women may not need replacement hormones, this may not be true, according to Dr. Gloria Bachmann, chief of OB/GYN and director of the Women's Wellness Center at the University of Medicine and Dentistry of New Jersey–Robert Wood Johnson Medical School. "Overweight women may be just as symptomatic as a woman of normal weight. If a woman's mother and grandmother did not have particularly negative experiences with menopause, a woman may not be that symptomatic herself. But it's relative. Some women react more strongly to mild symptoms," Dr. Bachmann says.

---

൦ *S u r g i c a l M e n o p a u s e* ൦

Since removing the ovaries abruptly cuts off ovarian estrogen, women who undergo surgical menopause have more severe symptoms. "In natural menopause, forty-five percent of women will have severe symptoms, compared with ninety percent of women who undergo surgical menopause," says Lila E. Nachtigall, M.D., a professor of OB/GYN who heads the Women's Wellness section of the NYU Medical Center Women's Health Service. With natural menopause, the reduction in hormones is gradual, so a woman's body has time to adjust. Not only does the sudden absence of estrogen produce a jolt of hot flashes and other symptoms, but symptoms may take as long as eight years to go away, compared with two years with natural menopause, Dr. Nachtigall told a symposium at an annual meeting of the American College of Obstetricians and Gynecologists.

Dr. Bachmann told the same symposium that a woman who is about to undergo surgery to remove her uterus and ovaries should be fully informed of the likely symptoms, including a drop in sex drive since the ovaries are also a source of testosterone. Hysterectomy patients may need higher doses of estrogen than women with a natural menopause. When estrogen and androgens are measured before surgery, a more effective hormone replacement regimen may be designed. Testosterone levels vary from woman to woman, and some may only need small doses to restore energy and libido. Estrogen alone may boost sex drive 50 percent.

Drs. Bachmann and Nachtigall start the estrogen patch in the recovery room. "A woman has enough to deal with recovering from surgery without having to deal with hot flashes," Dr. Nachtigall observes.

▪ What You Can Do About Hot Flashes ▪

The most effective treatment for hot flashes and other menopausal symptoms is estrogen, but there are alternatives:

* *SOY PROTEIN*: Recent studies suggest that eating twenty to fifty grams of soy protein a day (in tofu, soy milk, soy flour or meat substitutes) may lessen the frequency and intensity of hot flashes. Soy contains plant estrogens, or *phytoestrogens*, called *isoflavones*, which have some of the same effects as synthetic estrogens but, because they are much less potent, may carry fewer risks. Studies are now under way at Tufts University and the Bowman Gray School of Medicine to look into the effects of soy on cholesterol, blood pressure and bone density.

* *VITAMINS*: Up to 75 percent of women may get relief from hot flashes with vitamin E, though it's not known exactly how it works. The recommended dose ranges from 400 to 600 international units (IU) twice a day. Dr. Santoro recommends vitamin B_6 for women with PMS-type symptoms, starting with a 50 mg dose and going up to 150 mg, if needed. A B_{50} complex tablet daily, or 500 mg of vitamin C, may help nervous system functioning. But remember, vitamins are powerful drugs and can be toxic in high doses, so don't overdo them, and consult your physician beforehand.

* *HERBS:* Women have turned to herbs for centuries for relief of premenstrual and menopausal symptoms. Many of these herbs, including licorice root, yams, fennel, unicorn root and black cohosh, are also phytoestrogens. Evening primrose oil, camp bark, sarsaparilla, chamomile tea and red raspberry leaves are said to relieve menopausal symptoms as well. Herbs are usually steeped as teas. While many women swear by herbs, doses are not standardized, and they can be toxic in

high doses. It may be wise to consult a naturopathic physician experienced with herbal preparations.

* *GINSENG:* The root of the ginseng plant is a potent phytoestrogen used in Eastern medicine in tea and other preparations to relieve aches and pains, including hot flashes. However, ginseng has estrogenic effects in the body, including overgrowth of the endometrial lining, and high doses can cause high blood pressure, gastrointestinal problems and insomnia.

* *HOMEOPATHIC REMEDIES:* Homeopathy is a two-hundred-year-old theory of treating medical conditions using small, very dilute doses of natural substances. *Estrex,* containing ingredients like yams, herbs and (supposedly) extract of animal testicles, is a homeopathic remedy for hot flashes and menopausal symptoms.

Other nondrug therapies include stress management, biofeedback, acupuncture, yoga and tai chi as well as Kegel exercises to strengthen the pelvic floor and reduce urinary incontinence.

There are a number of prescription medications that are used to treat hot flashes and other menopausal symptoms but they are not actually approved for this purpose, says endocrinologist Valerie Peck, M.D., a clinical associate professor of medicine and a metabolic consultant to the Bone Densitometry Unit at the NYU Women's Health Service. All the drugs listed below may interact or interfere with other medications and should be taken only under careful supervision.

* *BELLERGAL* is a combination of belladonna, ergotamine and phenobarbital that may help with hot flashes, sleep problems, irritability, mood swings, and headaches.

* *CLONIDINE (CATAPRES)* is a high blood pressure medication that relaxes blood vessels. Studies show it can reduce hot flashes by 20 to 45 percent. In higher doses, clonidine can cause dry mouth, insomnia and faintness.

* *METHYLDOPA (ALDOMET),* another antihypertensive, may cut down on hot flashes by as much as 30 percent. Side effects include nausea, dizziness and fatigue.

* *PROGESTINS,* such as medroxyyprogesterone acetate (Provera) and *megestrol acetate* (Megace), can also help reduce hot flashes. A 1994 study in the *New England Journal of Medicine* said Megace reduced the incidence of hot flashes by 85 percent after four weeks of low-dose therapy. Higher doses are used to treat selected cases of breast and endometrial cancer, so researchers think low doses may be safe for breast and uterine cancer survivors who cannot take estrogen.

▪ Moving Past Menopause ▪

Most of the gynecological problems women experience in the five to ten years after periods stop are due to the drying and thinning of estrogen-sensitive tissues in the urogenital tract.

Without estrogen to stimulate the growth of the vaginal epithelium and endometrium, these tissues thin and atrophy. The vagina becomes shorter and narrower, and there's a reduction in its folds (*rugae*), so the vaginal walls become less "elastic." Eventually the protective top layer of epithelial cells become nearly nonexistent. The vaginal lining becomes so thin and dry that it is easily inflamed and broken, little tears can form and the tissues can even bleed, according to Dr. Brandeis.

There is a drastic decline in secretions from the cervix and vagina as well as in vaginal lubrication during sex. Combined with shortening of the vagina, intercourse can become painful.

The pH of the vagina also becomes more alkaline, so there are fewer friendly lactobacilli and increasing vulnerability to infections. Chronic inflammation can develop in the vagina (*atrophic vaginitis*) or the uterus (*atrophic endometritis*), and it may cause spotting. Ultrasound may be helpful in distinguishing atrophic endometritis from endometrial hyperplasia.

As with skin elsewhere on the body, the vulva loses collagen and its fat cushion with estrogen depletion. These thinned, atrophic tissues are more vulnerable to injury and dermatologic problems. A woman may also begin to lose pubic hair.

Thinning and atrophy happen inside the urethra as well. With less vaginal tissue to cushion it, the urethra is more vulnerable to irritation and invading bacteria, which may cause burning on urination and more urinary tract infections.

There are also estrogen receptors in the bladder neck and bladder; estrogen depletion may lead to a diminished sense of urgency when the bladder is full. Postmenopausal women may experience urge incontinence (in which urine leaks before one can make it to the bathroom) or, as estrogen-sensitive muscles and supporting structures in the pelvis are also weakened, stress incontinence (leaking when pressure is put on the abdomen).

Rectal incontinence is also a problem in postmenopausal women. The most common cause is *obstipation*, straining to pass hard stools. Prolapse, obstetrical trauma, dysfunction of the rectal sphincter and nerve damage from disease or stroke can also cause rectal incontinence. This does not usually involve leaking large amounts of stool. The most common problem is difficulty keeping the rectal area clean; a woman may notice stained underwear. Behavior modification and muscle exercises can help; surgery is usually a last resort.

However, the major nongynecological health problems women face after menopause are a greatly increased risk of heart and blood vessel disease and osteoporosis, both resulting from estrogen loss.

Our bones are in a constant state of formation and breakdown; cells called *osteoclasts* break down bone minerals, while *osteoblasts* form new bone. Osteoporosis occurs when osteoclast activity exceeds osteoblast activity and so much mineral is lost that bones become brittle. "Recent research is investigating receptors for estrogen in osteoclasts and osteoblasts" explains Dr. Peck. "Lack of estrogen leads to increased breakdown and resorption of bone minerals."

As mentioned, the reduction in estrogen and increased influence of androgens cause adverse changes in blood cholesterol that lead to clogged arteries and increased risk of heart attack and stroke. Researchers believe estrogen loss also leads to decreased secretion of nitric oxide in blood vessels (the body's own vasodilator), contributing to high blood pressure.

▪ Weathering the Dry Spell ▪

Vaginal lubricants, estrogen cream and systemic estrogen all can combat vaginal dryness and atrophy of the genital tract.

Over-the-counter vaginal moisturizers are designed for daily use to reduce irritation and make intercourse more comfortable. Some are gels, like KY Jelly, Gyne-Moistrin and Lubrin; others are more liquid such as Vagisil Intimate Moisturizer and Astroglide. All are water-based formulations containing glycerine and other ingredients and have slightly acidic pHs to help avoid infections; they will not damage latex condoms. Replens and KY Long-Lasting are longer-acting and are applied two to three times a week. Replens artificially thickens the vaginal lining. KY Jelly also comes with spermicide.

Prescription estrogen cream (Dienestrol, Estrace, Ogen, Premarin) is a low dose of conjugated or other estrogen in an emollient base. Topical estrogen is absorbed by the vaginal tissues, restoring the normal cell structure. Studies show that within a week the vaginal epithelium will begin to thicken and there will be increased lubrication and relief from dryness and itching; within a month the normal cell structure of the vagina will be restored. By restoring moisture, estrogen cream helps makes sex comfortable again and reduces urinary tract infections. It should not be used as a lubricant for intercourse; a man can absorb some of the estrogen through his penis.

Estrogen cream comes with a plunger applicator you fill yourself or with a prefilled 1 gm applicator; the cream is inserted (usually at bedtime) every two to three days. A woman should work closely with her gynecologist to find the right product, dose and regimen (some women can develop allergic dermatitis). Estrogen cream must be used indefinitely to maintain the positive effects on the vaginal tissues. It may be used initially with systemic hormones to reduce genital symptoms quickly. After oral estrogens take effect, vaginal lubricants may be needed only occasionally.

Although estrogen cream is considered "local" therapy, some of the estrogen is absorbed into the bloodstream and has some of the same effects of systemic hormones. However, because only small amounts of estrogen get into the bloodstream, it will not have the same protective effects on cholesterol or bone as HRT. Women who use estrogen cream may also need to take progestins for ten to twelve days a month, to prevent the buildup of cells in the uterine lining.

Local estrogen therapy is now available as an estradiol-releasing vaginal ring, Estring. Made of a flexible plastic (estastomer) containing 2 mg of *beta-estradiol,* the ring is inserted into the upper vagina, where it releases a continuous local dose of estradiol for three months. Trials of the vaginal ring in almost 200 women at ten sites around the U.S. found it was as effective as estrogen cream in improving urogenital atrophy, including vaginal dryness, after fifteen weeks of treatment. Endometrial proliferation was more frequent in the cream users. Most women found the ring more acceptable than estrogen cream.

∞ *S u e ' s   S t o r y ,   C o n t ' d* ∞

"I'm very pleased with where I am right now physically, and physio-logically. I felt a complete difference in myself after I started taking estrogen. It was very dramatic. I am now taking estrogen with just a little bit of

progesterone. In the beginning it made me depressed, I gained weight and I was bleeding more heavily. So I stopped taking it. But my doctor wanted me to take it because it protects against endometrial cancer, so I started up again, but with a much smaller dose.

"It has not been bad. I haven't gained weight because I have been working hard and exercising. My mood has been pretty good. Overall, I feel like my body is functioning very well. I look well, and I have probably the best energy I've ever had, changing jobs and getting on hormones. It's definitely that postmenopausal zest!"

▪ Hormonal Therapies ▪

Hormone therapy after menopause is called *replacement therapy,* even though it does not really replace premenopausal estrogen levels. Use of estrogen alone is referred to as estrogen replacement therapy (ERT); estrogen in combination with progestin or other hormones is called hormone replacement therapy (HRT).

Postmenopausal estrogens have been prescribed for forty years, but the first formulations turned out to have serious drawbacks. A number of studies in the 1970s reported that women taking these high doses of estrogen were ten to fifteen times more likely to develop *endometrial cancer*. A number of studies since then have shown that unopposed estrogen causes an overgrowth of the uterine lining that, without progesterone to cause it to shed, continues to grow abnormally (endometrial hyperplasia) and can become malignant. Estrogen combined with synthetic progesterone, or progestin (HRT), eliminates that risk. Experts now agree that unless a woman has had her uterus removed, she should probably take HRT, if she chooses hormones.

Progestin does have side effects, including bleeding (which usually stops after a year or two) and PMS types of symptoms, which include bloating, tender breasts and depression. A woman may have to work with her physician to fine-tune HRT, balancing relief of menopausal symptoms with those caused by the hormones. For instance, since hot flashes tend to be bothersome at night, some women find taking estrogen late in the day provides more relief.

Oral estrogens include micronized estradiol (Estrace) and several modified plant-derived estrogens, including *estrone estropipate* (Ogen, Ortho-Est) and esterified estrogen made from soy (Estratab, Menest). The most commonly used is *conjugated estrogen* (Premarin), extracted from the urine of pregnant mares.

A number of synthetic low-dose progestins are used with estrogen in HRT: medroxyyprogesterone acetate, or MPA (Provera, Cycrin); *norethindrone acetate* (Aygestin) and "micronized" progesterone (Prometrium) made from finely ground soybeans.

There are currently three doses of conjugated estrogen available: 1.25 mg, 0.625 mg and 0.3 mg (the most commonly prescribed dose is 0.625 mg). Micronized estradiol comes in 1 mg and 2 mg doses; estropipate is available in a dose of 0.625 mg. Women are commonly given doses of estrogen ranging from 0.625 mg to 0.9 and 2.5 mg, if needed.

In pill form, estrogens can be given every day or in cycles of three weeks on and one week off (similar to oral contraceptives, but much lower doses). Estrogen can be supplemented by progestin in low or graduated doses, on a daily basis, or in a larger dose for ten to thirteen days a month, to allow for withdrawal bleeding. A 1997 study in the *Journal of the National Cancer Institute* said progestins must be taken at least ten days a month to be optimally effectively in preventing uterine cancer; most women are given low-dose progestins for seven to twelve days a month. Progestin doses range from 2.5 to 10 mg. New oral HRT formulations include Prempro, a single-pill continuous regimen combining 0.625 mg of conjugated estrogen and 2.5 mg of medroxyyprogesterone acetate, and Premphase, a cyclical two-pill regimen using a smaller dose (5 mg) of progestin, which some physicians are giving to selected perimenopausal women.

Studies suggest that oral micronized soy progesterone, taken twice a day, has fewer side effects than progestins and no adverse effects on cholesterol. However, there have been no studies of its effects on the endometrium. Progesterone creams made from yams or soy (Pro-Gest, PhytoGest, Yamcon) are also available, but these preparations are not standardized.

Oral estrogen is absorbed through the digestive tract and processed in the liver before entering the bloodstream. Studies show 0.625 mg of conjugated estrogen helps reduce the "bad" LDL cholesterol while increasing the "good" HDL cholesterol. However, oral estrogen may cause gallstones. Oral estrogen prevents osteoporosis by reducing bone breakdown and possibly increasing calcium absorption. New urine tests can monitor the amount of bone breakdown and determine if ERT or bisphosphonates are working. While the maximum benefits are derived from starting estrogen three to five years after periods stop, it can be taken after age sixty-five to prevent or slow bone loss, according to Dr. Peck.

Both oral estrogen and estrogen patches prevent drying and atrophy of tissues in the genital and urinary tracts and can reduce UTIs. A transdermal patch looks and feels like a thin, clear, round Band-Aid; it contains replacement hormones within a very thin membrane that allows a controlled amount to be absorbed through the skin. The patches are worn on the lower abdomen, upper thigh or buttocks and are changed once (Climara) or twice a week (Estraderm, Vivelle, Alora), although some doctors may prescribe them on a cyclic basis. The patch may cause skin irritation. Other patches containing a new progestin (Nestorone), a combination of estradiol and Nestorone, and a potent new synthetic androgen (MENT) are also being marketed, as well as a new very low-dose (.025 mg) estrogen patch, Fem Patch.

Since hormones from transdermal patches are absorbed through the skin, they enter the bloodstream directly and can be safely used by women with liver problems. Because transdermal estrogen initially bypasses the liver, it may have lesser effects on cholesterol, though some studies indicate it lowers LDL, and it may have similar benefits on bone and tissues to oral estrogen.

The tiny amounts of androgens normally produced by the ovaries, including testosterone, can also be supplemented. Small doses of synthetic testosterone *methyltestosterone* (1 to 1.5 mg) taken along with estrogen, or in tablets combining the two hormones (Estratest), may help a woman's sex drive as well as eliminate the breast tenderness experienced by some women taking estrogen. However, women taking these pills still need to take a progestin to protect the uterus. Testosterone can cause acne, growth of facial hair and a deepened voice, and it may also have negative effects on cholesterol and heart disease risk.

Of the more than 30 million postmenopausal women in the U.S., only 2 to 3 million are regular users of estrogen. And half the women who start hormone replacement stop after a year. One of the major concerns is the risk of cancer, but many women also complain about the menstrual-like bleeding. "Some women believe they will continue to have periods indefinitely if they take estrogen. But with combined, continuous estrogen-progestin, bleeding usually stops after a year or so," says Dr. Bachmann.

During the first year of therapy, when progestins are given for twelve days, bleeding should begin after day nine; earlier bleeding should be investigated. An endometrial biopsy may be recommended if bleeding is heavier or longer than usual. Saline infusion sonohysterography can also be done to make sure there is no abnormal growth or thickening of the endometrium.

▪ Hormone Replacement in the Future ▪

In years to come, there may be more choices in HRT. *Selective estrogen receptor modulators (SERMs)* are compounds that will selectively latch on to certain estrogen receptors and have estrogenic effects in some areas of the body (such as the heart and bones) but not in others (like the breast and uterus). Short-term studies reported in 1997 found the SERM *raloxifene* (Evista) increased bone density without causing endometrial hyperplasia or breast cancer. Raloxifene didn't dampen hot flashes, but is approved as an alternative to ERT in preventing osteoporosis.

Other new delivery routes under study include subdermal estradiol implants, a topical estrogen gel and a vaginal progesterone gel to protect the uterus without the side effects of progesterone. A six-month trial of the estrogen gel was conducted in 112 symptomatic postmenopausal women in Argentina. The gel was applied daily to a six-inch-square area on both arms and was found to be highly effective on menopausal symptoms; side effects included breast tenderness, fluid retention and bleeding. In the estrogen implant trial two tiny pellets were implanted in the groin area of 200 woman who were followed for ten years (half the women also received a small dose of testosterone). The implants relieved symptoms in 95 percent of women who had not been happy on oral estrogen. Prolonged use produced a rise in "good" HDL cholesterol and also prevented bone loss.

Also being tested is a progesterone ring, a plastic ring that secretes a continuous amount of progesterone to prevent endometrial hyperplasia without the effects of systemic hormone.

▪ The Risks and Benefits of Hormone Therapy ▪

A number of recent studies show that estrogen begun at the start of menopause substantially reduces a woman's risk of heart attacks and strokes, decreases deaths from all causes, prevents the bone thinning and fractures of osteoporosis and appears to protect against colon cancer and Alzheimer's disease.

However, many of these were "observational" studies (in which large groups of women were followed over many years, and their diet and health habits studied), rather than clinical trials comparing treatments, and the results may be skewed because women who elect to take part in such studies may be healthier and take better care of themselves than women chosen at random.

The largest observational study of heart risk and hormones is the Nurses' Health Study (which has followed different groups, or cohorts, among 121,000 nurses since 1976). Data published in the *New England Journal of Medicine* in 1997 said that women who took replacement hormones had a 37 percent lower chance of dying during the first decade of use and cut their heart disease risk by 53 percent. Women taking hormones for more than ten years had a 43 percent higher risk of dying of breast cancer, but those who stayed on hormones had a lower overall mortality rate sixteen years later. The mortality benefit dropped to 20 percent after ten years.

In addition, data from the longest observational study of estrogen users, published in 1996 in the journal *Obstetrics and Gynecology*, reported that women who took estrogen for at least five years after menopause had an overall death rate that was 46 percent less than those who did not take replacement hormones. Researchers found a 60 percent reduction in the number one killer of women, heart disease, and a 73 percent reduction in deaths from stroke. There was a slightly increased relative risk of breast cancer, but overall, the study concluded that women who take estrogen can "substantially reduce their overall risk of dying prematurely."

The benefits of HRT for some women may be considerable. The first major randomized clinical trial of estrogen and progesterone—the Post-Menopausal Estrogen and Progestin Intervention (PEPI) trial—showed significant benefits for ERT on certain heart disease risk factors, like cholesterol and clotting factors. Other studies suggest that ERT may reduce the number of fatty lesions in the arteries of postmenopausal women and keep blood vessels more supple, helping to prevent high blood pressure.

Two 1995 studies in the *Journal of the National Cancer Institute (JNCI)* say estrogen replacement may substantially lower the risk of colon cancer, cutting risk in half for women who used esyrogens for ten years or more.

Estrogen may also protect against Alzheimer's disease, which affects more women than men. Small, open clinical trials found that estrogen improved the cognitive functioning in one group of elderly women after six weeks of treatment; others had improved scores on a new test for dementia. Estrogen may boost blood flow to the brain via better cardiovascular health, increase energy uptake in the brain, prevent loss of key brain chemicals and protect brain cells. Larger prevention trials are under way.

Still to be determined is whether hormone replacement can prevent coronary artery disease, heart attacks and strokes over the long haul. Answers should come from the Women's Health Initiative (WHI). One arm of the WHI will evaluate the effects of HRT in a randomized trial among more than sixty thousand women over nine years; results may not be out until the year 2006 or later.

∽ *M i l d r e d ' s   S t o r y ,   C o n t ' d* ∽

"I went through menopause when I was fifty-three. My gynecologist thought I should be taking hormones to prevent osteoporosis since my mother had broken her hip when she was seventy. But I just didn't like how I felt. I gained weight, my breasts were very sore, I felt very irritable, I had headaches and I was bleeding again. So I stopped taking the pills after a year.

"Around the same time I developed some urinary incontinence. I would leak if I laughed too hard. My gynecologist prescribed some estrogen cream, but it did not seem to help much. I also developed what I was later told was prolapse, your uterus drops down into the vagina because your muscles are so weak.

"After I had a hysterectomy and surgery to repair the prolapse, the incontinence got better. My gynecologist said it wasn't too late to start estrogen to protect my bones. So I tried it again. I didn't bleed, of course, but I just didn't like it. A woman from our church gave me the name of a naturopath. But the herbs didn't do all that much for me, and they were very expensive. Instead I started walking, which the doctor says will help my bones, and I am back with my bowling league. So I am getting exercise. I am also taking calcium."

▪ The Estrogen Dilemma ▪

Many women either stop taking replacement hormones or avoid taking them because of reports that estrogen increases the risk of breast cancer. Dozens of studies of estrogen therapy and breast cancer have been conducted here and abroad, but the data are inconsistent and contradictory.

While the 1997 update from the Nurses' Health Study found an increased death rate from breast cancer after ten years of hormone use, a massive study by the American Cancer Society (ACS) suggests that estrogen replacement may actually *decrease* a woman's risk of fatal breast cancer. The ACS examined deaths among 422,373 postmenopausal women who had filled out lengthy health questionnaires in 1982 and found no increased risk of dying from breast cancer among those who had taken estrogen for eleven years or more. In fact, ERT users had a 16 percent lower risk of fatal breast cancer compared with nonusers. Those who started estrogen before age forty (for premature or surgical menopause) had a 40 percent decreased risk of dying of breast cancer.

Earlier data from the Nurses' Health Study found there was no increase in risk among women who took ERT (or estrogen and progesterone) for less than five years. And a case-controlled study comparing postmenopausal breast cancer patients with healthy women at the Fred Hutchinson Cancer Research Center in Seattle found no increase in cancer among hormone users compared with nonusers.

Experts concede the issue of estrogen and breast cancer risk may never be fully resolved since there are so many risk factors involved, including genes, early menarche, late menopause, never having children, obesity and alcohol use.

For many researchers, the question of risk centers on whether estrogen replacement may fuel the growth of existing, but undiagnosed, breast tumors. More than half of all breast cancers are *estrogen receptor–positive*—that is, tumor cells have receptors on their surface that pull in estrogen and use it as a growth factor. For this reason women who have had breast cancer (or have family histories of the disease) are not given hormone replacement. But even this is being questioned. Preliminary data do not show detrimental effects in the few short-term studies involving breast cancer survivors.

A 1997 review in the British medical journal *The Lancet* analyzed fifty-one epidemiological studies of hormone replacement and breast cancer over the past twenty-five years, involving 160,000 women from around the world. All of the studies found a slightly higher relative risk of breast cancer among women who had used HRT for more than five years, about comparable to the effects of delayed menopause among women who never used hormones. After five years of hormone use there was no significant excess of breast cancer cases. The increased risk was reduced after stopping hormones, and disappeared after about five years. The *Lancet* concluded that the risks of hormone replacement must be weighed against the benefits for HRT for individual women.

There *is* a clear association between endometrial cancer and ERT. Studies show that women who take unopposed estrogen have a two to eight times greater risk of developing cancer of the uterine lining than nonhormone users; the risk is nearly ten times greater after ten to fifteen years of estrogen use. A new study by researchers in the PEPI trial concludes that women are better off taking estrogen with progestin than estrogen alone. According to the 1996 report in *JAMA*, 74 of the 119 women in the PEPI trial who received ERT in the trial developed some type of endometrial hyperplasia, atypical cell changes or increased thickness and changes in the glandular structures of the endometrium, which have also been associated with later development of cancer. There were no differences in the number of abnormal endometrial biopsies among women who received placebos or those taking the three estrogen and progestin regimens.

The study concludes that if the yearly occurrence of such endometrial changes were to persist, a majority of the women taking unopposed estrogen would have more serious types of atypical hyperplasia within five years, raising "serious questions about the safety" of long-term ERT alone in women with uteri.

The researchers recommend that nonhysterectomized women who cannot tolerate progestin receive yearly endometrial assessment, and ERT should be stopped if endometrial hyperplasia is found. They note that most endometrial hyperplasia "will revert to normal with prolonged progestin administration."

P a t ' s   S t o r y ,   C o n t ' d

"I don't go to a gynecologist anymore. My internist does a pelvic exam and a Pap smear. I am nearly seventy, and it is just easier to see a general doctor for everything.

"I was never offered estrogen when I went through menopause. I don't know why it was never discussed. I was not all that bothered by the hot flashes; they didn't last that long. I had read all these stories about osteoporosis, and my daughter nagged me into going for a bone density scan. It turned out normal, so that's one thing I don't have to worry about. As long as I can get older without being a burden on anyone . . . My biggest fears are to be frail and immobile or to have Alzheimer's."

▪ Should You Take Replacement Hormones? ▪

The decision whether or not to take estrogen must be an individual one, based on each woman's health history and personal preferences and whether the benefits will outweigh the risks for *her*, stresses Sandra Kammerman, M.D., director of Ambulatory Care at the NYU Medical Center, who says, "There is no single, right answer for every woman on the question of estrogen. Any physician who unilaterally endorses estrogen is not doing patients a service. It ultimately comes down to what is comfortable and best for that woman."

Most experts agree that for most women the overall health benefits appear to outweigh the risks of long-term ERT. Those who gain the most benefits are women at higher risk of heart disease or osteoporosis. Women who should probably avoid postmenopausal estrogens include those who have family histories of breast cancer (although there are exceptions), past estrogen-dependent breast cancers or uterine cancers. Women with blood clotting disorders, *thrombophlebitis* (blood clots in the leg), high blood pressure or gallbladder disease should also avoid replacement estrogen. The American Heart Association (AHA) says estrogen replacement should be used cautiously in women with high triglycerides. However, *some* women in this group may be permitted to use estrogen cream on the advice of their physician.

Women at high risk of osteoporosis (such as small-boned, fair-skinned women of northern European descent) now have good alternatives to estrogen. A new class of drugs called *bisphosphonates,* including alendronate (Fosamax), not only prevents osteoporosis but also rebuilds bone lost after menopause.

"Many women don't think about their future health until they hit menopause because that's the time they will be making a decision about estrogen. But they should start taking preventive measures well before then to reduce their risk of osteoporosis and heart disease," says Dr. Kammerman. "It's deceptive to think that estrogen is the answer to everything."

If a woman does not have severe symptoms, such as hot flashes, or is not at risk for osteoporosis or heart disease, she may not need to consider hormone replacement. For many women, a diet low in fat, high in fiber, along with calcium supplements (and new osteoporosis drugs), and regular exercise may help keep the heart and bones strong, and lubricants can relieve uncomfortable dryness of the genital tract, according to Dr. Kammerman.

If a woman chooses to take estrogen, it should be part of a program of other preventive and healthy behaviors, including regular pelvic exams, Pap smears and mammograms. "Because reproduction is no longer an issue does *not* mean you no longer need to pay attention to the reproductive tract," Dr. Kammerman emphasizes. The risk of gynecological cancers rises sharply in the mature years, so neglecting GYN health in later life can be deadly.

Gynecological Cancers

It's estimated that more than 91,000 American women will be diagnosed with invasive cancers of the uterus, ovaries, cervix and vagina this year. But many women are unaware that bladder cancer, with some 15,000 cases a year, and colorectal cancer, which affects 64,800 women, can also invade the reproductive tract. In fact, colorectal cancer is now the *third* most common cancer (and cancer killer) among women, after lung and breast cancer.

Risk factors include genetics, family and reproductive history, exposure to hormones, sexually transmitted diseases or toxic chemicals and such life-style factors as diet, obesity, sexual behavior and smoking. Some of these cancers are easily diagnosed and treated in their earliest (even precancerous) stages, while others cause symptoms only after they are more advanced. Knowing the early warning signs, getting regular pelvic exams and Pap tests and making some simple lifestyle changes can help tip the odds in your favor. According to the American Cancer Society, 50 percent of people who develop fatal cancer could have been saved had they made use of available information on smoking, diet, exercise and early detection.

———— ∞ *Carol's Story* ∞ ————

"I guess no one is ever prepared for a diagnosis of cancer, but it took me completely by surprise. I had been constipated for a few weeks and feeling progressively more uncomfortable. I was not overly worried about it, but when I saw my gynecologist's face during the pelvic exam, it was clear something was wrong. He said he could feel a large mass between the bowel and the uterus. He tried to be reassuring, saying it was probably just a fibroid, but when he did the ultrasound, he scheduled me for exploratory surgery right away, and when they opened me up, they found cancer.

"It turned out to be a Stage III ovarian cancer, which meant it had spread through my abdomen. We were just in shock. Everything happened so quickly I didn't have time to go through the 'why me?' phase or even cry. All my husband and I could do was hold each other. He was trying to be strong, but at the same time he was terrified that I would die. And we had to face my daughter and sons. We were honest: I had cancer. It was bad, but I was going to get treated. They cried, we cried, we held hands, prayed and made this pact to fight it together."

▪ Cervical Cancer ▪

As many as 65,000 cases of noninvasive, cervical carcinoma in situ (CIS) will be detected in American women this year, and 14,500 cases of invasive cervical cancer will be found. While incidence rates have declined steadily over the past few decades, the mortality rate for African-American women is still more than two times greater than for white women.

Yet cervical cancer is a preventable disease. It can easily be detected in its precancerous stages with the simple, inexpensive Papanicolaou (Pap) smear, but not enough women are being screened: Half of all women newly diagnosed with cervical cancer have never had a Pap smear. A Consensus Development Conference convened in 1996 by the National Institutes of Health concluded that wider screening could prevent virtually *all* new cases of cervical cancer in this country.

How Cervical Cancers Begin

Unlike some tumors which grow hidden deep within the body, the abnormal cell changes, or dysplasia, which precede cervical cancer can usually be detected long before cancer ever develops. Physicians use several terms to refer to cervical dysplasia: *squamous intraepithelial lesion (SIL)*, (used on a Pap smear report) and *cervical intraepithelial neoplasia (CIN)* (used on a tissue biopsy report). *Intraepithelial* means abnormal cells are found only in the surface layer of cervical cells. Both SIL and CIN are considered precursors of cervical cancer. CIN is classified in numerical stages from mild to severe. As many as 2.5 million women will be diagnosed with mild cervical abnormalities this year, and virtually all of them will be cured.

Most cervical cancers and precancers arise in the area called the *transformation zone*, where there is a gradual transition between the multilayered squamous (scale-shaped) cells of the external part of the cervix to the single layer of mucus-secreting, columnar cells of the endocervical canal. Dysplasia can also occur on the portion of the cervix that protrudes into the vagina (ectocervix).

"The transformation zone is what we call an *area of unrest*. It is exposed to all the pathogens that are in the vagina. The cervix gets infected and sometimes ulcerated. So these reparative cells are the most likely to become damaged, grow abnormally or undergo a malignant transformation," says Rita I. Demopoulos, M.D., professor and director of Gynecologic Pathology at NYU Medical Center and a professor of surgical pathology.

A pap smear samples the topmost layer of squamous cells and columnar cells from the transition zone. Dysplasia is recognizable when these surface cells are stained, showing enlarged nuclei with an irregular outline. "This is actually a marker for changes taking place in the cell layers below since cervical cells grow from the bottom up," explains Dr. Demopoulos. "As more and more abnormal cells are produced, they progressively crowd out the normal cells and when the dysplasia fills all the layers, it becomes carcinoma in situ. When it breaks through the basement membrane into the connective tissue of the cervix, it is invasive cancer." This progression (Fig. 21) can take many years, providing a window of opportunity for early treatment.

Precancerous lesions in the upper layer of cervical cells are diagnosed in two basic categories. *Low-grade SIL* (or *CIN 1*) consists of early, abnormal cell changes most often found in women aged twenty-five to thirty-five, but it can arise at other ages. "A proportion of mild and moderate dysplasia will regress to normal over time," adds Dr. Demopoulos. But some early lesions

Fig. 21: HOW CERVICAL CANCERS DEVELOP

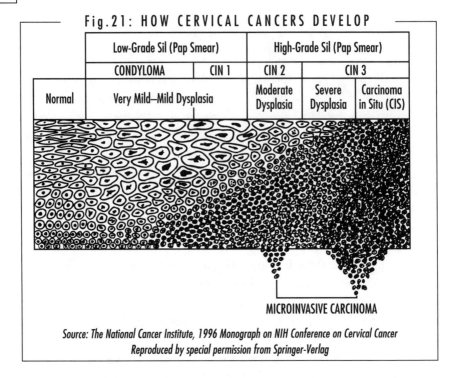

	Low-Grade Sil (Pap Smear)		High-Grade Sil (Pap Smear)	
	CONDYLOMA	CIN 1	CIN 2	CIN 3
Normal	Very Mild–Mild Dysplasia		Moderate Dysplasia	Severe Dysplasia / Carcinoma in Situ (CIS)

MICROINVASIVE CARCINOMA

Source: The National Cancer Institute, 1996 Monograph on NIH Conference on Cervical Cancer
Reproduced by special permission from Springer-Verlag

tend to grow larger, with the cells becoming more abnormal and more numerous. These worsening lesions are called *high-grade SIL* (on a Pap smear) and *CIN 2, CIN 3* (on a biopsy), encompassing moderate, severe dysplasia and/or *cervical carcinoma in situ (CIS)* and microinvasive carcinoma. High-grade SIL is most common in women ages thirty to forty. Only a small percentage of moderate to severe dysplasia go on to become CIS or invasive cancer but microinvasion can occur in some cases. Studies suggest that one quarter to one half of untreated CIS will progress to invasive cancer within five to ten years, but if the cancer is removed while it's in the in situ stage, it can be completely cured. Invasive cervical cancer is most often found in women over age forty.

Eighty percent of invasive cervical cancers are squamous cell carcinomas. The remaining tumors are mostly *adenocarcinomas*, cancers of glandular tissue that arise in the endocervical canal, or *adenosquamous tumors*, which contain both types of cells.

Most patients with cervical dysplasia or carcinoma in situ have no symptoms and the lesions are detected only with Pap smears or biopsies. Symptoms of invasive cervical cancer may include foul-smelling vaginal discharge and spotting after intercourse (indicating ulceration of the cervix). Even more advanced disease may produce sciatica (low back pain that radiates to the thigh) and swelling of the legs and feet.

∞ *New Knowledge About Risk Factors* ∞

Cervical cancer is the first major solid tumor shown to be caused by a virus. As many as forty million Americans may harbor human papilloma virus (HPV); one million active cases are diagnosed every year. Like any STD, transmission of HPV can be prevented by the use of condoms.

HPV is believed to insert its own genetic material into the DNA of cervical squamous cells, interfering with proteins that normally regulate cell growth, including tumor suppressor genes. HPV produces *koilocytic* (clear cell) changes that can be seen on a Pap smear or tissue biopsy. "There is an enlargement and wrinkling of the cell nucleus and a clearing of the cytoplasm around the nucleus. These are the first steps along the path to precancerous and then cancerous changes," says Dr. Demopoulos.

The two subtypes of HPV most strongly associated with cervical cancer are types 16 and 18. A 1996 gathering of international experts cosponsored by World Health Organization formally labeled HPV types 16 and 18 as "carcinogenic to humans" and types 31 and 33 as "probably carcinogenic." A 1995 study in the *Journal of the National Cancer Institute (JNCI)* reported finding genetic material of HPV in 93 percent of invasive cervical cancer specimens from twenty-two countries. HPV 16 was present in half of the tumor samples and many advanced cancers, while HPV 18 was found in 14 percent and in advanced cancers.

About 1 percent of women infected with HPV will go on to develop cervical cancer, according to Richard L. Sweet, M.D., professor and chair of the Department of Obstetrics and Gynecology at the University of Pittsburgh/Magee Women's Hospital. Adolescent girls who begin sexual activity before the age of eighteen are more likely to develop cervical cancer caused by HPV infection than women who delay having intercourse, Dr. Sweet told a National Institutes of Health Consensus Conference. The more sexual partners, the greater the chance of getting HPV. The panel strongly recommended that young people delay becoming sexually active as long as possible and limit the number of sexual partners.

The NIH panel also cited smoking as a risk factor, noting that women smokers are at four times greater risk of cervical cancer than nonsmokers. Recent reports have found clinical data linking smoking to cervical cancer. A 1997 report in *JNCI* said that tobacco-specific carcinogens called *nitrosamines* have been found in the cervical tissue of women smokers, where they may damage the DNA of cervical cells. In addition, smoking is thought to depress immune defenses against cancer.

However, a recent study in the British medical journal the *Lancet* found that 82 percent of women smokers diagnosed with mild dysplasia had a reduction in their lesions after quitting smoking (or cutting down) for six months, compared with less than 20 percent of those who kept on smoking.

There's also some suggestion that long-term use of oral contraceptives may slightly increase a woman's risk of cervical adenocarcinoma. A study from the University of Southern California comparing healthy women and women with cervical cancer found that those who used OCs for more than twelve years had more than a four times greater risk of cervical adenocarcinoma. So far there's no clinical evidence of cause and effect, but packages of birth control pills carry a warning of possible risk from prolonged use, and advise women on the pill to have yearly Pap smears.

Women whose mothers took the drug diethylstilbestrol (DES) during pregnancy are at increased risk of a rare type of cervical cancer. DES was prescribed between 1938 and 1971 to prevent recurrent miscarriage, and millions of women have been exposed in utero.

Recent reports indicate women with weakened immune systems, especially HIV-positive women, are also at greatly elevated risk for invasive cervical cancer. (However, AIDS and cervical cancer are found together in only a small percentage of women.)

The Pap Test

The Papanicolaou (Pap) smear, invented in 1945, has been credited with a 70 percent reduction in deaths from cervical cancer in the U.S. However, guidelines on how often women need Pap smears are the subject of some controversy. In general, annual Pap smears are recommended once women reach age eighteen or become sexually active. However, the American Cancer Society (ACS) and the National Cancer Institute (NCI) both say that after three consecutive normal tests doctors may allow selected *low-risk* women to have Pap tests as infrequently as every three years. Women who have had their uterus removed (including the cervix) may need Pap smears only once every ten years *if they have never had cervical abnormalities.*

A Pap smear is a simple, painless procedure performed during a routine GYN examination. After the walls of the vagina have been gently opened with a speculum (see page 307), a cell sample is taken from the exocervix, the external part of the cervix in the vagina, with a tiny spatula. Then a tiny disposable brush (cytobrush) is inserted into the cervical opening, or os, and turned clockwise several times. Both samples are then wiped gently across a glass microscope slide and fixed in place with a special spray. (A new method preserves the cell scrapings in liquid.) Slides are examined under a high-powered microscope by a cytotechnologist or cytopathologist, a person specially trained to look at cell samples. Among other things, the cytologist looks for the size of the cell nucleus and the degree of abnormality to determine either the grade of dysplasia or evidence of cancer, explains Dr. Demopoulos. The results are reported in standardized terminology known as the *Bethesda System*. If the cell sample was inadequate, a new Pap test will be ordered.

If Your Pap Test Is Abnormal

Your chances of having an atypical Pap test can range from 2 to 30 percent. But it doesn't mean you have cervical cancer. The test may reveal something as benign as a yeast or *Trichomonas* infection. In that case the doctor will treat the infection and order a repeat smear. If all's clear, nothing further is done.

In many cases a woman may receive a diagnosis of *atypical squamous cells of undetermined significance,* (ASCUS). ASCUS means that the squamous cells look abnormal but are *not* malignant, according to Dr. Demopoulos. Atypia can result from inflammation or the presence of the HPV (called *condylomatous atypia*).

"A woman with a finding of ASCUS may be brought back in three months' time for a repeat Pap smear. If the finding is the same, then she might proceed to colposcopy," says Dr. Demopoulos. If the repeat test is negative, Pap smears are done every four to six months for two years until there have been three consecutive negative reports.

If the finding is *low-grade squamous cell intraepithelial lesion (LSIL)*, it means the cell changes are either due to condyloma or CIN1. Although many cases of LSIL regress with no intervention, most physicians proceed to colposcopy and biopsy. Perhaps 20 to 30 percent of women will be diagnosed with CIN1 at some time.

However, uncertainty about the clinical significance of ASCUS and LSIL and the prospect of lawsuits have many practitioners opting for immediate colposcopy and biopsy, with no indication that it's beneficial. So the NCI is conducting a three-year randomized clinical trial to determine whether watchful waiting, immediate biopsy or DNA tests of cervical cells for HPV provide the best way to follow women with findings of ASCUS and LSIL.

Women with findings of *high-grade squamous cell intraepithelial lesion (HSIL)*—which encompasses CIN 2 and 3—go right to colposcopy and biopsy. A woman whose Pap test reveals atypical glandular cells may undergo further tests to determine the exact type of abnormality. If there's suspicion of adenocarcinoma, a cone biopsy will be done.

Colposcopy is a simple noninvasive examination using a special high-powered binocular microscope to examine the surface of the cervix, including the transformation zone. First, a solution of water and *acetic acid* (a component of plain vinegar) is applied to the cervix. Normal cells stay pink (the transformation zone has an almost transparent appearance), but dysplastic cells absorb the vinegar solution and become opaque, whitish patches. The degree of opacity, the color and the shape help indicate the nature of a lesion (genital warts are raised; dysplasia is flat).

The colposcope is then used to direct biopsies of the most suspicious-looking area. A local anesthetic may be applied, and a small amount of tissue is excised and sent to a pathologist for further examination. Colposcopy can be done in a gynecologist's office in around ten minutes, with only some mild cramping.

If invasive cancer cannot be ruled out either by colposcopy or by directed biopsies, the transformation zone may be removed for examination in one of two ways:

LOOP ELECTROEXCISION PROCEDURE (LEEP) uses a fine wire loop with low-voltage electric current run through it to remove the transformation zone for examination. The electric "hot wire" cuts and cauterizes (seals off blood vessels to prevent bleeding) the tissue as it passes through the cervical canal, explains Robert C. Wallach, M.D., director of Gynecologic Oncology at NYU Medical Center. "The edge of the tissue is singed by the hot wire, but the tissue is not appreciably damaged, so it can be examined by the pathologist." In most cases LEEP can be done under local anesthesia and sedation as an office procedure. The loops come in various sizes, depending on how much tissue needs to be removed. Loop excision can be used for CIN and cervical carcinoma in situ.

CONE BIOPSY (CONIZATION) gets its name from the cone-shaped tissue sample that results from wider and deeper removal of cells in the transformation zone. "Cone biopsy is done when it is necessary to have a microscopic view of the transformation zone, or if there is evidence of 'microinvasion' of abnormal cells beneath the surface of the cervix," explains Dr. Wallach. Conization can be done with a scalpel, a laser or a LEEP, and usually requires general anesthesia. In some cases conization is used as a treatment for CIN, and it has a cure rate of about 95 percent. In some women the cervix may be weakened after conization and may have to be stitched closed during pregnancy (cerclage).

Treating Cervical Intraepithelial Neoplasia

Treating premalignant lesions is controversial; some women are simply followed to see if the lesions regress. If treatment is undertaken, it is aimed at *destroying* abnormal tissue, says Dr. Wallach, by either laser vaporization or freezing.

CRYOSURGERY involves freezing and destroying abnormal cervical cells with a probe cooled by nitrous oxide, carbon dioxide or, less commonly, liquid nitrogen. Using colposcopy, the cryoprobe is inserted into the cervical canal, freezing the entire transformation zone to around minus sixty degrees centigrade, forming ice crystals. The resulting thermal shock kills the cells, which are subsequently sloughed off. Cryosurgery is usually done as two three-minute freezes in an outpatient setting requiring little or no anesthesia. Side effects include a foul-smelling watery vaginal discharge lasting about a month (as dead cells are sloughed off). The area heals in four to eight weeks, with little risk of infection. The cure rate for CIN 2 and 3 is over 90 percent.

LASER VAPORIZATION for CIN uses a carbon dioxide laser guided by colposcopy. The laser beam is directed into the cervix by a tiny hand-held wand called a *micromanipulator*. The light energy of the laser beam is converted to heat, which vaporizes the entire transformation zone. The procedure is painful and usually requires general anesthesia. Because there's very little dead tissue left, healing is faster than with cryosurgery, with epithelial cells regenerating in about a month. Laser vaporization is more expensive than cryosurgery.

While both treatments destroy abnormal cells infected with HPV, they cannot eradicate the virus. Freezing is somewhat less accurate for larger lesions than is laser vaporization, which can control the depth of tissue destruction. A 1995 study of almost 1,000 women found no indication that LEEP treatment, cryotherapy or laser vaporization adversely affected a woman's fertility or her ability to carry a pregnancy to term. However, especially in DES daughters there is a risk of cervical stenosis, or closure.

Experimental treatments for dysplasia include *transretinoic acid*, one of several derivatives of vitamin A, known to help abnormal cells "differentiate" back to a normal state. Results of a Phase III randomized clinical trial involving over 300 women with moderate to severe cervical dysplasia reported that 43 percent of those treated topically with transretinoic acid had regressions of moderate dysplasia (CIN 2), compared with 27 percent of women treated with placebos. There was no change in the severe dysplasia group. Researchers at the M.D. Anderson Cancer Center in Houston also reported in 1996 that tests of an orally administered drug called DFMO (*difluoromethylornithene*) may help halt the progression of neoplasia to cervical cancer.

Improving on the Pap Test

The cure rate for women treated for precancerous cervical lesions is well over 90 percent. But in some cases the diagnosis is delayed or never made. The false negative rate for Pap smears is estimated to be between 5 and 30 percent.

Cytotechnologists manually view thousands of slides under microscopes each day, and simple eye fatigue may cause an abnormal smear to be missed. Although cytology labs are required by the Clinical Laboratory Improvement Amendments (CLIA) of 1988 to select randomly 10 percent of all negative samples for a second analysis, abnormal smears may also be overlooked along the way. A 1990 federal law requires that cytology labs receiving Medicare or Medicaid reimbursements be certified every two years by the U.S. Department of Health and Human Services and that cytotechnologists be properly trained and be given enough time to study each slide adequately.

New computer technology may help in that process. Two new automated cervical cytology systems, AutoPap QC and Papnet, designed to replace random rescreening were approved in 1995 by the FDA. The systems will automatically rescreen all Pap smears designated as normal, then select at least 10 percent for a second, manual rescreening. Papnet can display abnormal cells in 128 computer-enlarged fields for closer viewing by the cytotechnician. However, the FDA cautioned that the system is not error-proof, and neither device is approved for the *primary* reading of Pap smears.

Sometimes a sample is tainted by blood or mucus, which smudges the slide made in the physician's office, so the test must be repeated. A smudge-free method of making Pap smear slides was approved in 1996. ThinPrep 2000 has the physician put the cell scrapings into a vial of liquid preservative to be machine-filtered at the lab, and the cells are spread cleanly on a slide so they can be better seen by the cytologist.

A new device that would add a "minicolposcopy" to the Pap smear has also been approved. Speculoscopy adds a tiny light bar to the device that holds the cervical os open during a Pap smear. After taking the smear, the doctor swabs vinegar solution on the cervix, and the "Speculite" shines a special wavelength of light that makes abnormal cells appear white and normal cells blue. One study found that the device almost tripled the amount of abnormalities found, compared with a Pap smear alone.

But none of these improvements will do any good unless women are screened regularly. A 1995 report by the Commonwealth Fund Commission on Women's Health and the UCLA Center for Health Policy Research found that four out of ten women had not had Pap tests within the past year. One third of women aged eighteen to thirty-nine had not been screened; more than *half* the women over age sixty had not had Pap smears. The lowest screening rate was found among Asian-American women, with 55 percent reporting they had not had Pap tests (compared with more than 40 percent of whites and Latinas and 37 percent of African-American women). Nearly three quarters of poor elderly women had not been screened. Lack of health insurance and the lack of access to a regular health care provider were key factors. Even though African-American women seem to have a good screening rate for cervical cancer, the report noted that they have a higher *mortality* rate, possibly reflecting diagnosis at a later stage of cancer or problems with access to treatment. According to the NCI, 54 percent of cervical cancers were diagnosed in white women while still in the localized stage, compared with 39 percent in black women. Forty percent of African-American women had regional disease, compared with 31 percent of white women, and almost twice as many blacks as whites were found to have distant disease.

∽ *C a r o l ' s   S t o r y ,   C o n t ' d* ∽

"*I was lucky that my oncologist was insistent on using the most powerful chemotherapy, Taxol and Cisplatin. I was given the chemo over twenty-four hours every three weeks, for six cycles of treatment. I don't remember much—except that I would stare up at the IV bag and dread what I knew was going to happen to me. After I got home I was so sick it was indescribable. I would lie in bed in complete darkness and wonder which was worse: the chemo or dying. I lost thirty pounds. I couldn't eat. I lost my hair. I tried to psych myself up by saying this was proof that the drugs were working. My oldest son shaved his head so I wouldn't feel so ugly.*"

Diagnosing and Treating Invasive Cervical Cancer

The staging of cervical cancer can involve diagnostic tests as well as exploratory abdominal surgery. CAT scans, magnetic resonance imaging (MRI) or ultrasound of pelvic organs may also be ordered as well as X rays to check the lungs. The inside of the bladder, rectum or lower part of the intestine may also be viewed with a fiber-optic scope.

Stage I cancers are confined to the cervix and can range from microscopic invasion to any size. Stage II cancers extend to the areas immediately adjacent to the cervix, the upper vagina or the pelvic area (parametrium), but not the sides of the pelvic wall. Stage III cancers extend to the pelvic wall or may have spread to the lower third of the vagina, or cause blockage of the kidney. Stage IV cancers have spread beyond the pelvis, involve the bladder or rectum or have metastasized to other organs. The five-year survival rate for Stage I cancers (with negative pelvic lymph nodes) is around 90 percent.

The 1996 NIH Consensus Conference on Cervical Cancer said that if the cancer is Stage 0 (carcinoma in situ), it may be destroyed with methods similar to those used for treating CIN, including a cone biopsy. For more advanced cancers that have *not* spread beyond the cervix, surgery or radiation are equally as effective, curing 70 to 90 percent of cases.

SURGICAL TREATMENT may be chosen as therapy for women with Stage I disease that has not spread beyond the cervix. Microinvasive lesions can be treated with a cone biopsy or simple hysterectomy. If the cancer has invaded deeper layers of the cervix, but not beyond it, the uterus can be removed, leaving the ovaries intact (since cervical cancer is not estrogen-sensitive). Nearby lymph nodes will be removed to check for cancer spread.

RADIATION THERAPY consists of external beam radiation, together with *intracavitary radiation*, or *brachytherapy*. "The choice of surgery or radiation therapy can depend on the size of the tumor, the patient's age and other medical conditions she may have. For example, we may recommend radiation therapy for a Stage I tumor that is large and may be difficult to completely resect, or for a patient with health problems who cannot have surgery," remarks Randy E. Stevens, M.D., an assistant professor and co-director of Gynecologic Radiation Oncology at NYU Medical Center. "For women with Stage I disease undergoing radiation therapy, the cure rate is equivalent to that of surgery. For Stage II tumors involving the pelvic area, Stage III and some Stage IV tumors, radiation therapy is the treatment of choice as the disease is too extensive to be completely removed."

The five-year survival rates for Stage I, Stage II, Stage III and Stage IV disease treated by radiation therapy are 85, 65, 35 and 10 percent, respectively.

External beam radiation treatments to the pelvis and/or *periaortic* area just above the pelvis (a likely area of cancer spread) are usually given five days a week for five to six weeks in a clinic or hospital setting. Treatments may be followed by brachytherapy (intracavitary radiation), in which one or more small hollow cylinders are inserted into the vagina, and a hollow tube inserted through the cervix into the uterus, then filled with radioactive material. Brachytherapy allows the radioactive pellets to be placed at or near the tumor site, and is essential to maximize chances for a cure. Brachytherapy can be delivered while the patient is in the hospital for two to four days (one or two sessions) or, more recently, once a week outpatient sessions for three to eight weeks.

Temporary side effects of external radiation therapy usually begin after the second week of treatment and include loss or thinning of pubic hair, mildly darkened skin, diarrhea, frequent urination and fatigue. The temporary effects of implants and intracavitary radiation can include frequent urination, diarrhea, vaginal discharge and fatigue.

The most common long-term effects include a narrowing of the vagina and occasionally loose stools. After treatment, use of a vaginal dilator markedly reduces vaginal narrowing, says Dr. Stevens. Women can resume sexual relations within a few weeks after treatment ends.

Women are followed by their gynecologist and a radiation oncologist, and have physical exams three to four times a year, with Pap smears and occasionally CAT scans of the abdomen and pelvis, for the first several years after radiation treatment.

CHEMOTHERAPY is indicated when there is spread of the disease to other parts of the body. The NIH consensus statement concluded that most active agent against squamous cell cervical carcinoma is *cisplatin* (Cisplatinum, Platinol). This drug is derived from the metal platinum and binds to the DNA of cells, preventing them from reproducing. The short-term response rate to cisplatin is about 30 percent. Side effects include nausea, hair loss, kidney and nerve damage, and increased risk of infections. Other drugs such as paclitaxel (Taxol) and isofosfamide have shown anti-tumor effects, and are being used with cisplatin. The NCI is sponsoring trials of concurrent radiation therapy and chemotherapy for some locally advanced cervical cancers.

BIOLOGICAL THERAPY, using a substance called alpha interferon, which helps the immune system fight disease, has been given for metastatic cervical cancer, but its benefits have not been confirmed. It may cause temporary flulike symptoms (fever, chills, muscle aches, weakness), loss of appetite, nausea, vomiting and diarrhea. Patients may develop a rash, bruise or bleed easily. Antiangiogenesis compounds to block blood vessel growth that feeds tumors are also under investigation. Systemic therapies for advanced cervical cancer are *not* curative, but can buy a woman extra time, emphasizes Dr. Wallach.

VACCINE THERAPY may prove more successful. Researchers are testing a genetically engineered vaccine to arm the immune system to destroy cervical cancer cells. Researchers at Johns Hopkins reported in 1996 that they had eliminated biologically similar tumors in mice with no side effects. Human clinical trials will be conducted in women with advanced cervical cancer who have failed standard therapy.

∞ *The Overlooked Female Cancer* ∞

Colorectal cancer is the third leading cause of cancer deaths among American women, yet most women know little about it and are not being regularly screened, according to Vicki L. Seltzer, M.D., chair of

Obstetrics and Gynecology at the Long Island Jewish Medical Center. There are several screening tools for colon cancer. *Flexible sigmoidoscopy*, an office procedure in which a lighted fiber-optic scope is inserted into the colon, and *colonoscopy*, a more extensive examination of the entire colon under intravenous analgesia or general anesthesia, can detect colon polyps, precancerous lesions that can be removed. Tests to detect blood in the stool (in which a patient places a small sample of stool on a specially treated card that is sent to a lab for analysis) and digital rectal examinations (which should be performed as part of a GYN exam) also play an important role in detecting colon cancer.

"The recommendations are that a rectal exam should be performed every year from age forty on, screening for blood in the stool annually from age fifty on and sigmoidoscopy after age fifty, every five years," says Dr. Seltzer. "If a woman has a parent with colorectal cancer, her risk increases considerably. So her screening may need to start at age forty, and may include colonoscopy."

Women tend to have rectal bleeding for some time before seeing a doctor, according to Dr. Seltzer, who observes, "They tend to blame bleeding on hemorrhoids and dismiss it. Women need to know that if they have *any* rectal bleeding, they *must* see their doctor right away."

There's a great deal of evidence that the risk of colon cancer can be greatly reduced by increasing the fiber and decreasing the fat in the diet and by exercising. A 1997 update from the Nurses' Health Study said that walking for just an hour a day could cut in half a woman's risk of colon cancer. Recent studies also indicate estrogen replacement may have some protective effects, as can aspirin. A 1995 study by the American Cancer Society of more than one million people found that those who took aspirin sixteen or more times a month had half the risk of fatal colon cancer than did nonusers.

Colon cancer is treated by surgery, sometimes combined with radiation. New surgical techniques can create a new rectum or new internal storage sac for feces, so many women today do not need a colostomy, an abdominal opening for stool to empty into a bag.

If colon cancer is found and treated in its early, localized stages, the five-year survival rate is over 90 percent. After the cancer has spread to nearby organs, the rate drops to 63 percent, and if there is distant metastasis, survival is less than 7 percent. So early detection of colorectal cancer is vital.

▪ Uterine Cancer ▪

Cancer arises most commonly in the uterine lining (endometrial cancer) and, in rare cases, in the wall of the uterus (uterine sarcoma). Of the estimated 34,900 cases of uterine cancer diagnosed this year, most will be found in women over fifty. The five-year survival rates for uterine cancer diagnosed in an early stage are 95 percent and 66 percent if the cancer has spread regionally. Because it is often caught early, the death rate is fairly low: about 6,000 deaths a year.

Endometrial cancer is estrogen-sensitive. Risk factors include prolonged exposure to the body's own estrogens (early age at menarche, late menopause), a history of infertility and failure to ovulate (for example, from polycystic ovarian syndrome). A major risk factor is having endometrial hyperplasisa, the abnormal growth of the cells lining the uterus that is a precursor to endometrial cancer. It is more common in women using estrogen replacement therapy (ERT) without progestin; women using unopposed ERT have a two to eight times greater risk of developing endometrial cancer than those who have not used estrogen. So unless there are special circumstances, women are advised to take progestin (either cyclically or continuously) along with estrogen to eliminate the risk of endometrial hyperplasia.

Conversely, women who have taken oral contraceptives containing estrogen and progestin have only about *half* the risk of endometrial cancer compared with those who have never used them. (But their risk of breast cancer may be slightly increased.)

Fatty tissue produces a form of estrogen called estrone; this may be why obese women are twice as likely to develop endometrial cancer as are women of normal weight. Women with histories of breast, colon or rectal cancer also have a slightly higher risk of developing endometrial cancer.

Detection and Diagnosis

The most common symptom of endometrial hyperplasia and endometrial cancer is vaginal bleeding after menopause or irregular bleeding during perimenopause. The bleeding may start as a watery, blood-streaked discharge;

later the discharge may contain more blood. Saline infusion sonohysterography (SIS) can measure thickening of the endometrium that signals endometrial hyperplasia or areas of cancer in the uterus; an endometrial biopsy is needed to make the diagnosis.

Endometrial hyperplasia is classified as mild, moderate or severe, depending on the amount of overgrowth in the endometrial cells and *stromal cells* (which support the endometrial tissue). There are two types of endometrial hyperplasia, and each is treated differently, explains Dr. Robert Wallach. " 'Simple' endometrial hyperplasia can be treated with D&C and possibly progestin. 'Complex' hyperplasia, where there is more glandular tissue and less connective tissue in between, is considered precancerous, and the treatment is surgery."

The majority of endometrial cancers are adenocarcinomas of glandular tissue. Other types include *adenosquamous carcinoma* (containing both squamous and glandular cells) and, less commonly, papillary serous or clear cell carcinoma.

If a biopsy finds endometrial cancer, additional tests are needed to determine the extent of the disease. The initial workup may include CAT scans, magnetic resonance imaging (MRI) and bone scans.

The staging of invasive uterine cancer is done during surgery. Before removing the uterus, the surgeon will use saline solution to take "washings" (*lavage*) from the abdomen and pelvis in an attempt to find any cancer cells present. If no cancer cells are detected, the washing is referred to as "clean." During surgery, the pelvic cavity, liver and intestines are also examined for evidence of metastatic disease.

Stage 0 is endometrial hyperplasia or carcinoma in situ. Stage I cancer is confined to the body of the uterus. Stage II cancer involves the cervix but does not extend outside the uterus. Stage III cancers have spread beyond the uterus but not beyond the pelvis; stage IV cancers have spread to other organs.

A pathologist also grades the tumor cells according to their degree of differentiation, or how closely they resemble normal cells. The more abnormally shaped, or poorly differentiated, the cell, the more aggressive the cancer. Tumor cells will also be tested for progesterone receptors. If the tests are positive, it means the cancer will respond to therapy with progestins.

∞ *Monitoring Women on Tamoxifen* ∞

Tamoxifen (Nolvadex) is a powerful synthetic hormone that blocks the proliferative effects of estrogen on breast tumors. It has been used since the early 1970s to treat advanced breast cancer and since 1985 as a routine hormonal therapy for breast cancer. Tamoxifen can prevent recurrences by up to 50 percent and may also prevent cancer in the opposite breast.

Although it interferes with estrogen in breast cells, tamoxifen paradoxically causes estrogenlike activity elsewhere in the genital tract. "Instead of a postmenopasual woman maintaining a thin, atrophic uterine lining, tamoxifen can cause the lining to become proliferative," says Dr. Steven Goldstein. "There can also be hyperplasia and in some cases polyps. Most of the time the hyperplasia is benign. But in some women it can be precancerous and, if left untreated, progress to endometrial cancer."

A number of studies show that the risk of endometrial cancer may be two to three times greater in women taking tamoxifen for five years or more. NCI now says there's no benefit to using tamoxifen beyond five years, but more studies are ongoing. The FDA advises women taking tamoxifen to have regular gynecologic exams, report any abnormal vaginal bleeding or discharge. Women taking tamoxifen need surveillance for endometrial changes, such as SIS (see page 241), or regular endometrial biopsies.

Treating Endometrial Cancer

For carcinoma in situ, women who wish to have children can be treated with D&C, followed by high doses of progestins to prevent recurrence. However, if fertility is not an issue, hysterectomy is recommended, says Dr. Wallach. Patients whose cancer has not spread beyond the endometrium can usually be cured with hysterectomy; lymph nodes are removed to check for spread. Early stage disease has a very low recurrence rate.

"For patients with Stage I carcinoma, the grade of the cancer and how deeply it extends into the muscle layer of the uterus are used to determine whether a woman will need postoperative radiation therapy," comments Dr. Randy Stevens. If there is no muscle (myometrial) involvement, radiation therapy may not be recommended, but the woman will be closely watched.

Treatment for Stages II and III uterine cancer combines total abdominal hysterectomy (with removal of the ovaries and tubes) with radiation therapy. Radiation treatments may be given pre- or postoperatively, and are most commonly delivered to the pelvis, says Dr. Stevens. Occasionally, if cancer cells have spread to the abdomen, radiation therapy may be delivered to the abdomen and pelvis; if there is cancer spread to the cervix or vagina, radioactive material can be placed in the vagina (see page 273).

Stage IV disease may be treated palliatively with radiation and hormonal therapy and, in some cases, chemotherapy.

Combining optimal surgery and radiation treatments, five year survival rates for Stages I, II and III are approximately 90, 75, and 50 percent, respectively, according to Dr. Stevens.

If a patient cannot undergo hysterectomy, radiation therapy will be used, combining intracavitary and external beam radiation, explains Dr. Stevens. With intracavitary radiation therapy for inoperable endometrial cancer, radioactive materials are put into hollow applicators and placed in the vagina and uterus. This can be done on an in-patient or outpatient basis.

Paclitaxel (Taxol) or *doxorubicin* (Adriamycin), either alone or in combination with other anticancer drugs, are the agents most often used against advanced endometrial cancer. Recurrent disease may be treated with radiation, progestin therapy, or chemotherapy. However, these treatments are not considered curative.

∞ *Carol's Story, Cont'd* ∞

"When we did the second-look surgery after my first chemo, there were more tumors. So I went through another round. My doctors believe that I am now in remission. I don't feel so much scared as guilty and sad for what my illness has done to my family. The kids have had to grow up a bit faster.

"But on the positive side, we are all much, much closer because we know each day is precious. They say there's maybe a twenty percent cure rate for cancer like mine. That's twenty women out of a hundred. Why shouldn't that one be me? We intend to keep fighting and trying to believe in miracles."

▪ Ovarian Cancer ▪

It's estimated that 26,800 women will be diagnosed with ovarian cancer this year. It's an especially deadly cancer, killing 14,200 women a year. While most ovarian cancers will be found in women over age sixty, according to the NCI, more than 14 percent are found in women forty-five to fifty-four, almost 10 percent among women aged thirty-five to forty-four, 6 percent in women aged twenty to thirty-four, and a very small number in those under twenty. Women under forty have a higher prevalence of localized disease, which has a higher survival rate.

A woman's average lifetime risk of ovarian cancer is only about 1.5 percent. The risk increases if a woman has never had children, has a family history of ovarian cancer or carries a mutation in two genes related to breast cancer, BRCA1 and BRCA2 (page 284). Women with a gene linked to family clusters of ovarian, endometrial and colon cancer are also at high risk.

A 1997 study from Duke University Medical Center suggests that half of all ovarian cancers may be related to the number of times a woman ovulates over her lifetime since ovulation requires cellular proliferation. The more ovulatory cycles, the greater the chance of a mutation in a tumor suppressor gene called *p53* that allows cells to grow out of control, causing cancer.

Conversely, oral contraceptives (which block ovulation) reduce risk. Each year of pill use lowers the risk of ovarian cancer by 5 to 10 percent, and after ten years the risk is reduced by 80 percent. Each full-term pregnancy a woman has lowers risk by about 20 percent. Breast-feeding also reduces risk (since it suppresses ovulation), as does having a tubal ligation.

New studies suggest that eating less saturated fat and more fiber may lessen the risk of ovarian cancer as well. A 1994 study of almost 1,000 women compared the dietary habits of women newly diagnosed with ovarian cancer with healthy controls. For every ten grams of saturated fat a woman ate each day, her risk of ovarian cancer rose by 20 percent. But every ten grams of vegetable fiber added to a woman's daily menu *lowered* her risk by 37 percent.

Making the Diagnosis

Unfortunately there is no effective means of early detection for ovarian cancer. Only a quarter of ovarian cancers are diagnosed in an early, highly treatable stage (and about 25 percent of those women still succumb within five years).

"Ovarian cancer is so deadly because it is usually not detected until it is in an advanced stage, with spread throughout the abdomen," observes Carolyn D. Runowicz, M.D., professor and director of Gynecologic Oncology at Montefiore Medical Center and Albert Einstein College of Medicine in New York.

The most common tumors, including serous cyst and mucinous cyst adenocarcinomas, which arise from epithelial cells on the surface of the ovary, can grow for some time before causing symptoms like abdominal pressure, indigestion and bloating. Germ cell tumors, which arise from the egg-producing cells in the ovary, are usually malignant; teratomas are a benign subset of germ cell tumors. Stromal tumors arise from the hormone-secreting tissues and may cause bleeding (due to high levels of estrogen) or "masculin-ization" like facial hair from high levels of androgens.

Most of the time, however, symptoms may be so vague that they are overlooked, says Dr. Runowicz. "The most common symptoms are swelling, bloating or discomfort in the lower abdomen. There may also be some loss of appetite and a feeling of fullness after eating very little." These symptoms frequently result from fluid build-up in the abdomen (ascites). Other symptoms include gas, indigestion, nausea and weight loss. As a tumor grows, it may press on such nearby organs as the bowel and bladder, causing constipation or frequent urination. Such symptoms and fluid buildup can also be caused by benign cysts, but only a careful workup and surgery can tell for sure.

That evaluation may include ultrasound to see if an enlarged ovary is due to a functional cyst or if there are suspicious areas. A woman may also undergo CAT scans, MRI, X rays of the lower bowel (lower GI series or barium enema).

Some women may be tested for elevations of the protein called CA-125, which is useful in detecting recurrences of ovarian cancer. "However, CA-125 can be elevated in other conditions, like endometriosis. And most women with abnormal levels of CA-125 do not have cancer," notes Giuseppe Del Priore, M.D., M.P.H., assistant director of Gynecologic Oncology in the Department of OB/GYN at NYU Medical Center.

A 1994 NIH Consensus Conference on Ovarian Cancer recommended that a woman suspected of having ovarian cancer be referred to a gynecologic oncologist and undergo meticulous surgical cancer staging. Consensus Conference guidelines say this should include careful examination and biopsies of pelvic and abdominal organs for evidence of spread. The surgeon should also biopsy pelvic lymph nodes and the *omentum*, a belt of fat inside the abdomen (a frequent site of spread), and take "washings" (samples of ascites) from the abdomen to see if cancer cells are present. However, some general surgeons or gynecologists untrained in cancer surgery may only biopsy the affected ovary. A 1996 NIH study examining the medical care of almost 800 women with ovarian cancer found that in 90 percent of early-stage cases, surgeons neglected to biopsy lymph nodes or other tissues to see if the cancer had spread. If only the affected ovary has been biopsied, the report said a *second surgery* should be done to take additional tissue samples to stage the cancer properly and "debulk" the tumor.

Stage I cancer is confined to one or both ovaries. Stage II disease is found on one or both ovaries and has spread to the uterus and/or the fallopian tubes and/or other areas in the pelvis. Stage III ovarian cancer has spread to lymph nodes or other areas inside the abdomen (such as the surface of the liver or intestine). Stage IV disease has spread to the inside of the liver or outside the abdomen.

Treatment always begins with surgery and usually includes chemotherapy. If the cancer is a "borderline" malignancy without evidence of spread or well-differentiated disease confined to one ovary, just the affected ovary can be removed with an excellent survival rate. "If there's any evidence of spread, chemotherapy will be needed," says Dr. Del Priore. "Malignant germ cell tumors are in general more responsive to chemotherapy, with survival close to 90 percent. In some of these tumors the unaffected ovary and uterus can be spared. Epithelial tumors have a much lower response rate, around 80 percent, and that is improving."

In more than half the cases women under age forty have a diagnosis of Stage I disease, and just the affected ovary and its tube can be removed to preserve fertility. In older women a total hysterectomy with removal of both ovaries and tubes is usually done. Removal of part of the tissue that stretches from the stomach to nearby abdominal organs (omentectomy) may also be recommended. Women with Stages I to III cancers will be given systemic chemotherapy and, in rare cases, external beam radiation to the abdomen and pelvis. Intraperitoneal radiation can be given using a radioactive phosphorus called *P32*, a one-time treatment that has been used instead of chemotherapy for some early-stage patients. In Stage IV cancers as much of the cancer as possible will be removed, followed by chemotherapy.

Chemotherapy Advances

Newer chemotherapy agents and new ways of administering older drugs are prolonging survival considerably.

PACLITAXEL (TAXOL) has become part of the first-line chemotherapy agent against ovarian cancer. Taxol was the first of a group of drugs called *taxoids*, extracted from the bark or needles of the Pacific yew tree, which fight tumors by gumming up components of the cell's "skeleton." Recent clinical trials show Taxol, approved for use against advanced ovarian cancer since 1992, to be even *more* effective when combined with older platinum drugs. Most recently a randomized clinical trial of 410 women, reported in 1996 in the *New England Journal of Medicine,* found that adding Taxol to first-line chemotherapy regimens improved overall survival in women with Stages III and IV ovarian cancers.

TOPOISOMERASE INHIBITORS are a new class of agents that attack ovarian cancer from a different angle: blocking enzymes cancer cells use to repair DNA damage from chemotherapy. All cells are able to fix DNA damage with special "repair enzymes," but cancer cells repair themselves quickly, says Dr. Del Priore. The drug *topotecan* (Hycamtin) is designed to interfere with a key repair enzyme in cancer cells called *topoisomerase 1*. Studies at NYU and elsewhere found the effects of topotecan to be equal to, or even greater than, Taxol. Topotecan was approved in 1996 for use in women who fail other chemotherapy agents.

CISPLATIN INTRAPERITONEAL THERAPY involves delivering cisplatin directly into the abdomen instead of injecting it into the bloodstream. "While ovarian cancer treatments are more successful in reducing the amount of disease, that doesn't equate with a cure. Delivering chemotherapy straight to where there's residual disease has the potential to save many more lives," says Franco M. Muggia, M.D., director of the Kaplan Cancer Center at NYU.

A 1996 randomized clinical trial of 654 patients with Stage III disease resulted in 24 percent fewer deaths and fewer side effects. Average survival was just over four years in those given intraperitoneal cisplatin plus intravenous cyclophosphamide, ten months longer than the women who got intravenous cisplatin-cyclophosphamide. Dr. Muggia believes adding an older drug, *5-fluorodeoxyuridine (FUDR)*, which interferes with the building blocks of DNA, "can add another 25 percent to the cure rate for ovarian cancer." Other intraperitoneal therapies under investigation include topotecan, and interleukin-2, an immune system stimulator.

FENRETINIDE (4-HPR), a synthetic vitamin A derivative, has been tested in Italy and found to prevent a recurrence of ovarian cancer. A trial of 4-HPR in centers around the United States will involve patients at high risk for recurrence.

No Easy Screen for Ovarian Cancer

The NIH Consensus Conference concluded that unlike the case of cervical or breast cancer, the value of routinely screening women for ovarian cancer has not been demonstrated. The panel of experts decided that the screening tests available—transvaginal ultrasound and CA-125—are often so inconclusive, and may lead to anxiety or unnecessary surgery. In fact, a woman may have a greater chance of complications from surgery than of finding a cancer, said Dr. Vicki Seltzer, who chaired the NIH panel. One recent study of 5,500 women screened with transvaginal ultrasonography detected ovarian cancer at an early stage in only five women. (However, some experts believe that women who've had breast cancer, who carry BRCA1 mutations, or who have a close family history of early onset breast or ovarian cancer, should be screened with pelvic exams, transvaginal ultrasound and CA-125.)

The NCI is sponsoring a large-scale study, the Prostate, Lung, Colorectal and Ovarian Cancer (PLCO) Screening Trial, to see if routine screening for ovarian and other cancers would have any benefit. Clinical trials are under way using more advanced ultrasound devices that could give three-dimensional pictures of the ovaries to help make diagnoses without surgery.

BRCA Genes and Ovarian Cancer

Two genes that may be responsible for more than one quarter of ovarian cancers are now under intensive study. Mutations in the gene BRCA1 play a role in both sporadic and inherited breast and ovarian cancers, especially in families where multiple members are affected. Initial studies of women in these families estimated that inheriting a flawed *BRCA1* gene could carry a lifetime risk of breast cancer as high as 85 percent. More recent data suggests that the lifetime risk of breast cancer among women in the general population with *BRCA1* mutations may be much lower, around 50 percent, with a 16 percent risk of ovarian cancer, and a slightly elevated risk of colon cancer. Preliminary studies suggest inherited mutations in BRCA1 may cause 20 percent of ovarian cancers. A second gene, BRCA2, is believed to be responsible for 5 percent of ovarian cancers.

The two BRCA genes appear to be tumor suppressor genes; when either gene is damaged, it does not produce (or produce properly) a protein that normally controls cell growth. There are two hundred or more mutations in the two BRCA genes, and different mutations may produce differing levels of risk. Three specific mutations in the BRCA genes are found in 2 percent of women of Eastern European Jewish descent, or Ashkenazic Jews, putting them at elevated risk of ovarian and breast cancers.

Unfortunately there are at present few options for otherwise healthy women identified as carriers other than preventive removal of the ovaries. However, new understanding of the genes and their function may lead to new therapies.

▪ Other Gynecological Cancers ▪

Cancer can also affect the vulva, vagina, peritoneum and fallopian tubes, but these malignancies are fairly uncommon. The rarest malignancy is cancer of the fallopian tube, accounting for only 0.2 to 1.6 percent of genital tract cancers; vulvar cancers account for 3 to 5 percent.

INTRAEPITHELIAL NEOPLASIA can occur on the vulva (*VIN*), progressing to squamous cell carcinoma in situ and invasive cancer. It can also be caused by human papilloma virus; VIN has the same sexual risk factors as cervical cancer. The vast majority of vulvar cancers are squamous cell, with the incidence ten times higher in women over seventy-five. Vulvar cancers cause about 500 deaths a year.

VAGINAL INTRAEPITHELIAL NEOPLASIA (VAIN) occurs most often in women over age sixty, most commonly in elderly women. Vaginal cancer accounts for 1 to 2 percent of genital tract malignancies. The squamous cells of the vagina are the same as those on the cervix and, as with cervical cancer, HPV infection is also a risk factor for vaginal dysplasia.

DES daughters are at high risk for *clear cell vaginal cancer*, a very rare cancer. The activist support group DES Action USA estimates that one out of every 1,000 DES daughters will develop clear cell vaginal (or cervical) cancer, frequently before age twenty. (For more on DES daughters, see page 313).

Vaginal and vulvar dysplasias are diagnosed and treated in a similar manner to cervical dysplasias. Application of 5-Fluorouracil cream is used for VAIN. Invasive cancers are treated with surgery, chemotherapy and/or radiation. For vaginal cancer, intracavitary therapy or radioactive implants can help avoid radical surgery of the vagina, says radiation oncologist Dr. Randy Stevens. "The trend is to use a combination of chemotherapy and radiation to shrink cancers so more limited surgery can be done and a woman can retain her vagina and other organs."

A Woman's Sexuality

Gynecological problems can cause a variety of sexual problems for women, and safeguarding your GYN health can help you hold on to a healthy sex life. Unfortunately sexual difficulties are all too common and suffered in silence.

A landmark sexual survey by researchers at the University of Chicago found that one in three women reported a lack of desire for sex for at least two months over a period of a year. The data, published in 1994, reported that one in five women had trouble reaching orgasm, while 13 percent had pain with sex for several months. Many of these women never discussed these problems with their partners, much less sought professional help.

One reason is that many women have never really been educated about sexuality. Religious, cultural and social beliefs about sex and sexual roles and the fact that a woman's genitalia are regarded as untouchable (and often unpleasant) all contribute to sexual ignorance and inhibition. Problems with sex are one of the areas women are least likely to discuss even with a physician. But before we talk about the things that can go wrong with sex, let's discuss what should go right.

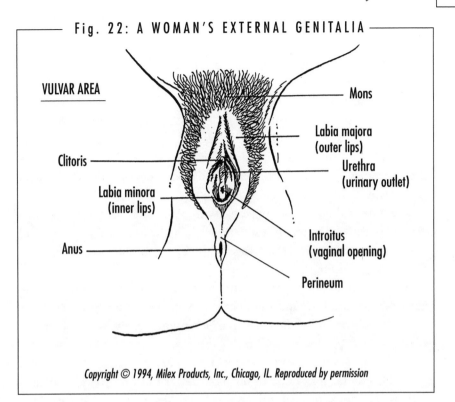

Fig. 22: A WOMAN'S EXTERNAL GENITALIA

VULVAR AREA

Mons

Labia majora
(outer lips)

Clitoris

Urethra
(urinary outlet)

Labia minora
(inner lips)

Anus

Introitus
(vaginal opening)

Perineum

Copyright © 1994, Milex Products, Inc., Chicago, IL. Reproduced by permission

A woman's physical sex organs are the vagina and clitoris. The clitoris is the only human organ that has no function other than bringing pleasure; there are more free nerve endings on the clitoris than any other part of the female body.

The entire genital area, including the vagina and clitoris, is eroticized by nerves that extend from the lower spine. These nerve endings also sensitize the upper thighs, buttocks and lower back. But the clitoris is the sexual nerve center. This small, sensitive shaft is protected by a mound of tissue called the *mons* and sheathed in a tiny hood just above where the inner lips of the vulva meet.

Tactile stimulation of the clitoris (by penile thrusting or manual or oral stimulation) results in an erection somewhat similar to that of the penis. Stimulation of nerve endings causes increased blood flow to the spongy erectile tissue in the clitoral shaft, and muscle contraction compresses a tiny vein, trapping blood in the erectile tissue, making the clitoris firm and exquisitely sensitive. Unlike an erect penis, which moves up and out, the clitoris moves up under its hood during arousal.

There are four phases to the sexual response cycle: desire, excitement (arousal), orgasm and resolution.

In sexual arousal, emotional and psychological responses in the brain send signals to the clitoris and vagina through the nerves in the spinal column. Those signals of desire cause a buildup of pressure in the blood vessels in the pelvis, clitoris and genital tissues. This *vasocongestion* causes the labia to swell and darken in color and triggers lubrication and dilation of the vaginal walls and engorgement and sensitization of the clitoral shaft. As the uterus becomes engorged with blood, it balloons upward and the cervical opening widens slightly.

The breasts also become congested with blood, and the nipples become erect and sensitive. During the excitement phase the heart beats faster, blood pressure increases and breathing speeds up. The skin may become flushed, and you may perspire.

As sexual excitement increases, the muscles around the entrance to the vagina become swollen, and the opening to the vagina narrows, the erect clitoris slides beneath its hood and muscle tension increases throughout the body.

If clitoral stimulation continues, orgasm occurs. During orgasm repeated pleasurable contractions pulse through the lower third of the vagina. Contractions also ripple through the uterus, beginning at the top and working their way down to the cervix. Some women may have more intense orgasms caused by pressure of the penis on the cervix and uterus or by the conscious contraction of their pelvic floor muscles. To some degree every muscle in the body contracts during climax. That's one reason you feel so relaxed after making love. It's a total body workout.

In the resolution phase the vasocongestion and muscle contractions dissipate, breathing and heart rates return to normal and you feel relaxed and peaceful.

For generations, traditional concepts of women's sexual responsiveness all but ignored the clitoris. Sigmund Freud taught that a woman became sexually mature only when she progressed from "infantile" focus on the clitoris (her inadequate substitute for a penis) to having vaginal orgasms. Unfortunately too many women went through life believing they were somehow inadequate (or abnormal) if they didn't have vaginal orgasms.

This notion was thankfully dispelled in 1953 by Alfred Kinsey in his landmark study on sex, based on interviews with nearly 6,000 women. *Sexual Behavior in the Human Female* revealed that the vast majority of women could not have orgasms without direct stimulation of their clitoris. More recent information from the Kinsey Institute shows that less than half of women are able to climax through penis-in-the-vagina intercourse alone.

One reason is that the timing of men's and women's sexual arousal and release is different, notes Virginia Sadock, M.D., who heads the Program in Human Sexuality and Sex Therapy at NYU Medical Center. A man can become aroused and climax in three or four minutes by physical stimulation alone. A woman's time from arousal to orgasm can be almost four times longer because her excitement phase is prolonged. Women generally need more stimulation than men to climax, including prolonged kissing, more caressing and oral sex.

Women do have the advantage over men in that once aroused, many can have multiple orgasms, while men have to wait to "recharge" after climaxing. Many women also have higher cycles of arousal linked to the hormonal changes of the menstrual cycle. Some women peak at mid-cycle or ovulation, others premenstrually.

It was the famous sexual research team of William Masters and Virginia Johnson that first studied the mechanics of orgasm and identified the arousal cycles of men and women in *Human Sexual Response*, published in 1966. During their studies involving more than 800 men and women in their laboratory, Masters and Johnson also uncovered some of the "hidden" aspects of a woman's sexual response, such as vaginal lubrication.

The works of Kinsey and Masters and Johnson proved that any woman can achieve orgasm through clitoral stimulation. One of the best ways is through masturbation; use of an electric vibrator can produce very intense orgasms. Unfortunately many women were taught in childhood that masturbation is wrong, shameful or mentally or physically harmful.

Once a woman learns to achieve orgasm, experts say it's rare to lose that capacity unless she experiences a trauma like rape or there's poor sexual communication or conflict in a relationship. Women can have just as intense orgasms with a female partner as they can with men, and orgasms vary in intensity. However, popular fiction and movies often depict women as having spectacular, multiple orgasms *every* time they make love. When reality doesn't measure up, some women may think they're abnormal, "frigid" or incapable of sexual response.

For a variety of reasons the earth doesn't always move every time, and it can be distressing if you get only a small tremor. Many women are reluctant to tell their partners they need more clitoral stimulation to climax. About 10 percent of women say they have never experienced an orgasm by any means. For some women, orgasm may not be the sole measure of sexual satisfaction or happiness in a relationship, notes Dr. Sadock.

Indeed what often fuels a woman's sexuality is a need for intimacy and emotional connection with a partner. For women, making love is about making connections on many levels, not just the physical. A 1995 study of 541 male and female college students found that more than 70 percent of the sexually active men, but only 36 percent of the women, said they'd had sex at least once with a person for whom they felt no emotional attachment. A majority of the women said having sex made them feel emotionally vulnerable and bond more closely with the person. In contrast, a high percentage of the men said they had no trouble having sex with women they were not emotionally attached to.

No surprise, then, that a recent survey of 400 heterosexual men and women aged eighteen to fifty-nine found that women were more likely to prefer activities associated with "romance," such as talking, holding hands, wearing sexy clothing, hugging, kissing and petting and affection after intercourse. On the other hand, the men were more focused on the physical, exploring new positions, performing and receiving oral sex, having both partners climax together and looking at erotic movies and books.

Cultural background, religious beliefs and upbringing may inhibit sexual functioning. In many cultures women are raised to be submissive to men, sexually pure, viewing sex for making babies, not pleasure. Women who are outwardly sexual or enjoy sex are seen as promiscuous. This madonna/whore conflict can result in an inability to reach orgasm and other sexual problems.

While just about every woman is physically capable of having orgasms (barring disease or anatomical problems), some women may not be psychologically capable of being aroused or coming to climax. Psychological factors, such as sexual or physical abuse, depression, stress and anxiety, can interfere with a woman's sexual desire and responsiveness, as can a lack of perceived intimacy.

"The entire life experience of a woman comes into play in her sexual response," comments Dr. Sadock. "Is she inhibited or is she open and responsive? Was she conditioned to be ashamed of her sexuality or her body? Does she perceive her partner as loving and concerned with her pleasure, or does she feel that he is insensitive to her needs? Does she feel emotionally connected to or distant from her partner?" If a man doesn't have an erection, he can't have sex. A woman can have intercourse with moderate vaginal lubrication and "fake it," without her partner ever knowing something is wrong, unless there's pain.

— ∞ *E l i s s a ' s   S t o r y ,   C o n t ' d* ∞ —

"My sex drive isn't what it was. I'm not sure if it's the fibroid surgery, my age, my workload or a combination of all three. I don't have the same erotic feelings. I don't have the same intense orgasms. That lusty feeling I had in my twenties, thirties and into my early forties just sort of died.

"I've been married to the same man for ten years. And it's not going to be the same as it was when we first met. You know, you get dressed up for him, your heart is pounding and you anticipate you're going to go to bed with him. You can't wait. Now it's like getting up and having breakfast.

"I don't have trouble getting mentally aroused. It's just that when I actually go to have sex, I don't have any feelings. And it's with the same man that I had tremendous feelings for just a few years ago. Maybe it's my age. I used to flirt like crazy. I was very aware of how attractive I was, but I don't feel desirable anymore. My husband says he still desires me, that I'm still attractive, but part of me wants to be that pretty young woman again with the firm breasts and tush.

"I guess you have to move on and find new ways of thinking about yourself, about expressing your sexuality. It's about growing older and closing doors. I know there are new doors to go through. But I feel sad that some of the old doors seem closed."

▪ When Gynecological Problems Interfere ▪

There are a number of gynecological problems that can interfere with a satisfying sex life. Among reproductive-age women, sex therapists often see vaginismus (muscle contractions which make vaginal penetration difficult or impossible) and lack of orgasm (*anorgasmia*). Women may have vulvodynia, chronic pain in the vulvar area, or vulvar vestibulitis, severe pain around the opening of the vagina. Some women with interstitial cystitis also experience pain with intercourse.

Chemotherapy can result in premature menopause and lowered sexual desire. Pelvic surgery can occasionally cause sexual problems. Some women who have had their ovaries removed find they lose interest in sex or have difficulty having orgasm (possibly because of loss of estrogen or androgens); other women who've had their uteri removed say they have less intense orgasms.

More commonly, problems with sex stem from low levels of estrogen that affect sexual functioning after menopause and sometimes in the years preceding it. As discussed in Chapter Twelve, as estrogen production slows, the vaginal tissue thins and becomes drier, and it may be slower to lubricate during sex. After menopause the vagina itself shrinks; this can make sex uncomfortable. Vaginal or clitoral irritation may also occur after orgasm. In addition, diabetes, hypertension and other medical conditions may affect lubrication and cause difficulty achieving orgasm.

During the years before and during menopause, testosterone production falls along with estrogen, dampening sexual desire and causing a decline in the orgasm intensity. Some women may need more clitoral stimulation. Estrogen cream can reverse dryness and vaginal atrophy, and systemic replacement hormones (along with a touch of testosterone) can restore lost libido in some women.

Interestingly, experts say sexual stimulation once or twice a week may help women avoid the age-related decrease in vaginal lubrication during arousal (lubrication occurs in response to sexual stimulation and does not appear to be dependent on high levels of estrogen). For women without partners, this may mean masturbation, an idea some older women may be uncomfortable with.

Since there's less fatty tissue in the pubic area after menopause, the urethra and bladder are less cushioned, and there can be irritation or frequency of urination after sexual contact.

Kegel exercises, which strengthen the muscles at the base of the pelvis, can help with urine leakage, and experts say the resulting improvement in muscle tone can tighten the "grip" of the vagina during intercourse. Some women report that awareness of the pelvic muscles and how to contract them enhances their ability to achieve orgasm and makes their climaxes more intense.

▪ Sexual Functioning Across the Life Span ▪

A woman's sexual functioning can be influenced by a host of factors over her life. Peer pressure often pushes teenage girls into sex before they're emotionally ready to handle their sexuality. A recent survey by the Alan Gutt-macher Institute found that around half of women (and three quarters of men) have had sexual intercourse before their eighteenth birthdays. It also found that a majority of teens who had intercourse before age fourteen said they had been forced to have sex. Experts say one of the biggest challenges for educating adolescent girls is to help them develop enough self-confidence to say no when they do not want to have sex.

Adolescence and early adulthood are also the times when we develop our sense of sexual adequacy and desirability or, unhappily, our sense of sexual inadequacy, says Dr. Sadock. "Our sexual self-esteem can be eroded by dislike or shame about our bodies, or bodily functions. We may love and desire someone who doesn't love us back, which makes us feel undesirable."

Healthy sexuality can also be damaged by sexual abuse that took place during childhood or adolescence, or by rape or domestic violence in adult-hood. Young adulthood is often the time some women come to terms with their homosexuality.

Some women may have satisfying sex lives up until they become preg-nant. While many women report an increase in desire and orgasmic potential during the early second trimester, most studies show a gradual decline in sexual interest as pregnancy progresses, with the biggest drop during the third trimester.

Some experts suggest hormonal shifts may be at fault, but cultural and psychological factors are more likely to blame. There are still physicians who believe that sexual intercourse during pregnancy, especially the first trimester, isn't a good idea, and there are still men who are afraid to touch their wives for fear of "hurting" the baby. While a few women who've had repeated preterm deliveries, preterm labor or miscarriages might be advised to refrain from sex because of the uterine contractions, for the majority of women, sex during pregnancy is safe and pleasurable, says Dr. Charles Lockwood.

For pregnant women, sensations during intercourse may be slightly dif-ferent. During the second trimester there may be an increase in sexual func-tioning and heightened arousal. And despite popular belief, there's no clinical evidence that sexual activity right up until the time of delivery is harmful or that it triggers labor in uncomplicated pregnancies.

Most women can physically resume making love three to six weeks after delivery, but some are simply not ready. Soreness from an episiotomy can linger, breast-feeding can temporarily cause a menopauselike low-estrogen state and many women are just too tired from the round-the-clock care of an infant. Experts stress that couples need to *make* time for sex after they become parents. If they neglect their sex lives or if sex becomes hurried and routine, it can lead to lack of interest.

∽ *S a r a ' s   S t o r y ,   C o n t ' d* ∽

"Your sex life gets shot to hell when you're trying hard to become pregnant. First of all, the drugs make you nuts. Then you have to keep track of your cycles. You know, this is 'D-day,' you're ovulating. And you have a three-year-old at home with a cold that day. If you miss, you have to take another round of drugs. The anxiety compounds the whole thing.

"It really messed up our marriage for a while. My husband felt like he was being asked to perform, and I felt guilty because the fault had to be with me, there was nothing wrong with his sperm. Being inseminated took some of the pressure off our sex life, even though I still had to be on Clomid.

"But my husband hated the whole thing of going into this little room and masturbating into a test tube. Every single man at the clinic felt the same way. It was humiliating for them. One couple finally took a room in a nearby motel and took the sample to the clinic in a urine container. We didn't live that far away, so one time we made love at home and I put the container under my coat to keep the sperm warm and drove to the clinic for the insemination. Maybe that's why it didn't take. But at least that time it seemed almost like normal."

As Sara found, the emotional process of coming to terms with infertility, or the strain and intrusiveness of using assisted reproductive technology, can take a toll on sexuality.

"There's a loss of privacy and control; people are looking at the most intimate part of your life. Sexual problems are very common. Sex ceases to be spontaneous and pleasurable," comments Gail Erlick Robinson, M.D., professor of psychiatry, obstetrics and gynecology at the University of Toronto and chair of the American Psychiatric Association's Committee on Women. "The husband may get a call at work that this is the day, come home right now. And nothing is more guaranteed to make a man impotent than to be told he *has* to perform."

Often the responsibilities of caring for children and aging parents, financial pressures, conflicts between jobs and home responsibilities, stress, fatigue and just the lack of time to relax together can lead to low sexual desire. Studies also show that almost half of all couples experience some waning of desire and sexual interest over the years, so often a special effort is needed to keep the sparks alive.

"We all have to adjust to the disappearance of the first euphoria of falling in love and the intense sexual desire of early intimacy," Dr. Sadock comments. But we don't have to lose emotional intimacy. "In order to maintain a healthy sex life, partners must maintain intimacy by talking and sharing. If we close down emotionally, we can't make love."

While many women find themselves sexually revitalized at midlife, men often find their sexual responsiveness slowed, and this can hamper a couple's sex life. Testosterone production declines in men by as much as 25 percent by age sixty. Because of changes in blood flow and muscle tone, a man's erections take longer to achieve and may not be as firm as he ages, and the refractory period between orgasms lengthens as well. Cardiovascular disease, smoking and diabetes also cause circulatory problems with erections. These factors can make men anxious about their virility and cause impotence. Added to the changes a woman experiences, it can strain or even break a relationship.

∾ Pat's Story, Cont'd ∾

"When my husband was alive, I would say we had a very satisfactory sex life. He was the only man I've ever been with, so I don't have anything to compare it to, but that part of our lives got better over the years.

"It's hard for me to imagine being with another man at this stage. My husband has been gone eight years, and I am now seventy-three, so I feel that part of my life is over. I have other friends who have lost their husbands, and they are much younger and I think maybe they might remarry. I don't think I would, but who knows?"

Older women may suffer from the lingering myths that they are no longer sexual beings. "In later life men often get trapped in performance anxiety. Women, on the other hand, are trapped in what might be called appearance anxiety," says Robert N. Butler, M.D., a noted expert on aging who heads the International Longevity Center at the Mt. Sinai Medical Center in New York. "Our culture promotes the image of a sexy woman as a young woman, so as women age, they may become trapped by the notion that older women are not sexual. But this is simply not true."

There is, however, a wide range of sexuality in people as they age, and personal health and the availability of a healthy partner are key factors. Around 80 percent of Americans aged sixty-five and older have at least one chronic disease that can potentially affect their sexual functioning. In addition, medications commonly taken for chronic diseases, such as antihypertensives, digitalis, diuretics and even antidepressants, can interfere with sexual functioning. An older woman's sex life can also be disrupted by the illness or death of a partner. One survey found that after age sixty-five, only about a third of unmarried women are in ongoing sexual relationships.

Divorced or widowed women (and men) may have to confront their children's reactions to their dating again. "Some of it relates to shock that there was such a thing as parent sexuality," notes Dr. Butler. "There's also loyalty to the deceased parent. There may be an unrealistic enshrinement of a former mate that interferes with sexual function."

But overall, older age does not have to shut the door on sexuality. Masters and Johnson found that 30 percent of seventy-year-olds continue to have sexual relations (not necessarily intercourse) once a week; 60 to 70 percent make love at least once a month. In a recent study of healthy upper-middle-class people aged eighty to one hundred and two living in a residential facility, the most common activities were touching and caressing without intercourse (a majority of the men and women still fantasized about sex).

There are special qualities of sex and intimacy that emotionally healthy people seem to discover in their later years, what Dr. Butler calls the second language of sex. "That is," he says, "a more respectful, mutual intimate concern with a partner and their needs, as opposed to only being concerned with our own selfish needs, as we sometimes were in our youth."

In fact, age-related changes can be a plus. Because older men need more time to achieve orgasm, the gender gap in the timing of arousal and climax becomes much narrower. Experts say slowing the pace of lovemaking, experimenting and restoring a sense of play can help women and their partners enjoy ever better sex lives in later life. "We know that in general, the principle holds: 'use it or lose it,' " concludes Dr. Butler.

⌘ *J u d y ' s   S t o r y* ⌘

"When I met girls in school for the first time, I knew that I was attracted to them. Nothing seemed wrong with it. I don't think I put it in a sexual context; who could at that age? I just knew that when I was around

girls, I couldn't talk. I would blush. All the awkward stuff that teenage boys go through when they fall for girls, I was feeling in first and second grade.

"I didn't realize what was 'wrong' until I was in high school and everybody started dating the opposite sex. I dated guys and enjoyed it, but when the pretty blond cheerleader types came near me, I would start to melt. With boys, even sexually, I always felt totally cool, in total control. I was very promiscuous for a while; I enjoyed the feeling of power I had over the guys. But I was never comfortable with girls, especially the ones I was attracted to.

"Sexually I felt like a normal teenager. That changed once I went out into the real world: going to college, meeting other gay women. I would have 'come out' if people had come out in those days. But this was the early 1960s. I didn't know there was a gay lifestyle.

"My parents found out when they read some love letters of mine. First there was screaming. They said things like 'Why did you do this to us?' After that they never wanted to talk about it again. That was sad. And it made me angry. Because once they denied what was one of the most important parts of my life, I felt that my parents lost their daughter.

"Sexually I think gay women are much more knowledgeable about their bodies and sexual responses because we're not out to please men; we're out to please ourselves. I don't know a gay woman who has ever faked an orgasm.

"I am very comfortable with being gay and saying that I am a lesbian, but it is really a very small part of who I am. I don't see my sexuality as a cause. I do get pissed off at some homophobic women who, as soon as they found out I was gay, were afraid to be my friend. I've wanted to say, 'Just because I'm gay doesn't mean I want you. Get over the ego trip.' I hate it when people automatically judge you, assume things and treat you differently. That's just fear and stupidity."

▪ Lesbian Sexuality ▪

It's estimated that between 4 and 10 percent of individuals in the United States are or will become predominantly or exclusively homosexual. One sexual survey of nearly 6,000 women found 2 to 3 percent identified themselves as exclusively lesbian, and 13 percent said they have had lesbian sexual experiences. Lesbian women come from all age-groups, cultural backgrounds, religions and nationalities and work in every occupation. But not every woman comes to terms with her sexual orientation as easily as Judy did.

"Behavior doesn't equal identity. Women who are in sexual relationships with women may or may not call themselves lesbian," emphasizes Marla Jean Gold, M.D., and assistant professor of medicine at the Medical College of Pennsylvania and a member of the advisory board of the Lesbian Health Fund. "Lesbian is more than just a sexual orientation; it has to do with psychological and emotional responses. While it's not a choice in *orientation*, it's an individualist choice in *identity*."

No one really understands how sexual orientation develops. Many women and men simply seem to be born with innate sexual preferences for members of their own sex. Researchers have been trying to find the genetic components of homosexuality for some time; some have been looking for physical differences in the brain. Whatever the source, homosexuality (or bisexuality) can emerge during adolescence or during later life. The University of Chicago sex survey found that a majority of lesbian women began same gender sexual activity after age eighteen.

Lesbian women experience the same physiological responses to sexual arousal and orgasm as do heterosexual women but concentrate more on caressing, specific erogenous zones and clitoral stimulation. Within monogamous relationships, their sex lives are not that different from those of heterosexuals.

It is important to understand that gay women want the same things in a relationship as do heterosexuals: love, commitment, mutual respect, caring and someone to share life with. Most gay women are in monogamous relationships and want society to acknowledge them in the same way as it does heterosexual couples.

Between one and five million lesbians have chosen to become parents, some by artificial insemination or, less frequently, by adoption. An estimated 6 to 14 million American children have one or more lesbian or gay parents. Recent studies find *no* differences in psychological development or the development of sexual or gender role identity in children raised by gay parents. Nor do these children grow up to be homosexual themselves.

Unfortunately some women who came to terms with their homosexuality later in life have had to fight legal battles over child custody. Many women continue to stay "in the closet" for fear of jeopardizing jobs, alienating families or losing their children in a divorce. The survey found almost 20 to 30 percent of lesbian women kept their sexual orientation a secret.

▪ Sexual Dysfunctions in Women ▪

Sexual dysfunction is usually a symptom of a medical or psychological problem. This can affect all phases of the sexual response cycle: desire for sex, sexual excitement, the physiological changes during arousal and the ability to have orgasm. Sexual dysfunction can be lifelong or acquired and can be due to specific situations or partners. It can be caused purely by psychological factors or by a combination of physical problems, affecting adults of any age and sexual orientation.

"Sexual difficulties can result from psychological conflict or interpersonal problems and may reflect relationship difficulties, stresses, chronic anxiety or depression as well as medical illness or medications," says Dr. Virginia Sadock.

Medications used to treat depression, high blood pressure, angina, cardiac arrhythmias, ulcers and irritable bowel syndrome may cause sexual dysfunction. Antihistamines which dry out the mucous membranes of the nose also dry the mucous membranes of the vagina and inhibit sexual function.

The same symptoms can be caused by physical and mental problems; there's no way to tell the difference between a woman who loses her desire because of hormone problems and one who loses her desire because of depression. So a woman experiencing sexual difficulties should have a complete medical evaluation.

For a *psychiatric* diagnosis of sexual dysfunction, the problem must be persistent and recurrent and cause mental distress and interpersonal problems. Types of sexual dysfunction include:

HYPOACTIVE SEXUAL DESIRE DISORDER is characterized by the absence (or deficiency) of sexual fantasies and desire for sex. It can affect all forms of sexual expression or may be limited to one sexual activity. A person with low sexual desire usually will not initiate lovemaking and may take part only reluctantly. It can occur after childbirth or the onset of menopause.

SEXUAL AVERSION DISORDER is an aversion to sex and an active avoidance of any sexual contact with a partner. Women with this disorder may feel disgust, anxiety or fear when faced with making love. People may go to great lengths to avoid sex, from a refusal to bathe to staying late at work.

FEMALE SEXUAL AROUSAL DISORDER is an inability to become excited sexually and maintain physical responses, such as vaginal lubrication. The problem should not be entirely due to menopause (vaginal dryness and atrophy), medical conditions or the effects of medications, and it excludes occasional arousal problems and inadequate sexual stimulation by a partner.

FEMALE ORGASMIC DISORDER means that a woman has a recurrent delay in achieving orgasm or does not achieve orgasm following a normal sexual excitement phase (in which all the physical signs of arousal are present). It's estimated that 10 to 15 percent of women may never have experienced an orgasm. Because a woman's orgasmic capacity may actually increase with age, most female orgasmic disorders are lifelong, rather than acquired (in fact, this problem may be more common in younger women).

VAGINISMUS is a recurrent, *involuntary* spasm of the muscles surrounding the vagina, which can be quite severe, resulting in constriction that prevents vaginal penetration. It can occur in response to pain, such as vulvodynia, or it can be psychological.

DYSPAREUNIA (SEXUAL PAIN DISORDER) results in genital pain associated with intercourse, usually during penile thrusting. Symptoms can range from mild discomfort to sharp pain. Thirty percent of women suffering from pain during intercourse have physical problems, including vaginal or urinary tract infections, vulvodynia, endometriosis and pelvic inflammatory disease.

▪ When You Need Help ▪

Many women are embarrassed to talk about sexual problems with their gynecologists. But some physical problems leading to sexual dysfunction are often treatable, for example, by using estrogen cream or vaginal lubricants or by clearing up a persistent urinary tract problem. If no medical problem is found, a referral may be given to a licensed sex therapist or other professional trained in treating sexual disorders.

However, sexual problems have to be handled as a couple. A recent study found that men with "nonorganic" impotence may often be reacting to a partner's sexual problem, such as pain during intercourse. The same may be true for women whose partners are having difficulties. Unlike women who see gynecologists on a regular basis, studies show that men avoid seeing physicians and are often reluctant to discuss impotence with their doctors. Men who do consult urologists about sexual problems too often come in alone, so information never gets to their partners, notes Andrew McCullough, M.D., an assistant professor of urology and director of the Male Sexual Health Program at NYU Medical Center. "Whenever possible, I like to see the couple as well as the individual. Whether the problem is physical or psychological, the couple invariably develop increasing fear and self-consciousness about their sexual performance. Sexual problems are frequently the pressure valve of other problem areas of the relationship."

For this reason, couples usually undergo sex therapy together. "The relationship as a whole is treated, but the emphasis is on sexual functioning as a part of that relationship," Dr. Sadock comments. Sex therapy does not involve engaging in any sexual activity in front of the therapist. Couples are usually seen once a week and are given special exercises to do at home, including masturbation. "The overall goal of sex therapy is to educate people about the physical and psychological aspects of sexual functioning, to diminish fears about performance and to establish or reestablish communication verbally as well as in sexual terms," Dr. Sadock adds.

The initial focus of therapy is not on intercourse but on getting partners to focus on each other sensually (*sensate focusing*), by touching and caressing, openly talking about desires and sexual fantasies. Through a gradual process of learning how to communicate and to understand each other's needs, partners progress through sensual exercises to the point where they can have intercourse. Older couples can also benefit.

Some therapists' strategies for maintaining a healthy sex life at any age:

- Talk to each other. Express your feelings and needs. While it's not always possible to put sensitive topics into words, try.

- Renew intimacy. Sex doesn't happen just in the bedroom. Intimacy is an ongoing process, involving sharing and expressing affection. Don't forget little gestures that say, "I love you."

- Learn to enjoy kissing and touching again. The less focused you are on intercourse, the more you can explore other needs in bed.

- If you'd like some changes in the way your partner makes love, start out by making positive statements like "I love it when you do this, but I'd also enjoy . . ."

- If your partner expresses a need that's different from your own, don't dismiss it as selfish or abnormal. If something makes you uncomfortable, speak up, but be open to new things.

- If your partner has lost interest in sex, don't blame yourself or get angry. Voice your love and concern in a tender way, and try to find out what may be wrong.

- If sex hurts for any reason, say so.

Each of us has uniquely individual emotional and sexual needs. In a fulfilling sexual relationship, both partners need to be aware of and accommodate those needs, stresses Dr. Sadock.

Remember, there is no "right way" to have an orgasm or "normal" way to make love. What feels right *is* right.

Getting the Best Gynecological Care

One of the most important steps a woman can take to safeguard her gynecological health is a regular GYN checkup.

There's no set age at which experts recommend a young girl see a gynecologist. An adolescent who is menstruating normally can be followed by a family physician or pediatrician. But a get-acquainted visit with a gynecologist may be a good idea sometime during the teenage years to discuss a girl's sexual maturation and gynecological health. A pelvic examination of a normal adolescent is rarely needed; progression through puberty can be assessed with standard measurements of breast and pubic hair development (Tanner staging).

"However, a pelvic examination is required every six to twelve months for all sexually active teenage girls," stresses Dr. Charles Lockwood, chairman of the Department of Obstetrics and Gynecology at NYU Medical Center. "A teenager who is sexually active should also see a gynecologist to obtain information on contraception and protecting herself from sexually transmitted diseases." One study found most teens are sexually active for six months to a year before they begin using contraceptives; often a teenager's first visit to a gynecologist is due to a suspected pregnancy.

In most states a parent must give consent for medical care of a minor until she is "emancipated" or is eighteen years of age (unless it's an emergency). However, 49 states permit minors to obtain confidential testing and treatment for STDs, and many others allow access to contraception, pregnancy-related care, mental health and substance abuse counseling without parental consent. But some conservative groups are pushing for federal and state laws limiting access to confidential health services for teens, saying it interferes with parents' rights to direct the upbringing of their children. At the same time medical organizations, led by the American Medical Association, are trying to improve teens' access to confidential care, citing high rates of serious health problems among young people, including STDs, alcohol and cigarette use and illicit drug abuse as well as depression, suicide and teenage pregnancy.

While every parent desires good communication with his or her children, experts say a young person may confide more readily in a health care professional. So while you need to accompany your daughter to the gynecologist, it's a good idea to allow her a private conversation to discuss her personal concerns.

"After age eighteen every woman should begin regular gynecological visits. *All* sexually active women should visit their gynecologists at least once a year for pelvic and breast exams," says Dr. Lockwood. STD testing should be performed if a woman has a new sexual partner, since some STDs are asymptomatic.

After menopause women may neglect gynecological checkups, wrongly believing that once their reproductive years are over they need not pay attention to their reproductive organs. But age is the single most important risk factor for gynecological cancers, which occur most often in women over sixty. Unfortunately up to 65 percent of older women do not have screening mammograms, and as many as 75 percent do not get regular Pap smears.

The American Cancer Society (ACS) and the American College of Obstetricians and Gynecologists (ACOG) recommend yearly Pap smears for all women eighteen and up who are (or have been) sexually active. The ACS also recommends that women have yearly clinical breast exams and begin screening mammography at forty.

Many women do not receive needed preventive and medical care because they lack health insurance or other coverage. But other factors can interfere with a woman's getting good gynecological care: cultural attitudes against doctors, disability and fear of disclosing homosexual status. This chapter will discuss such issues of special concern and offer advice on managing your health care in an era of managed care.

▪ What You Should Know About Your GYN Exam ▪

If you are menstruating, the best time to visit your gynecologist is in the middle of your cycle. There's no need to take any special cleansing measures other than a shower or a bath. Never douche before a GYN visit since it could affect the results of your Pap smear and other tests.

Before the actual exam your physician may request a urine specimen to check for the presence of bacteria, excess sugar, protein or red blood cells (a sign of a bladder infection or kidney disease). Even if you don't have to provide a urine sample, it's a good idea to urinate before your pelvic exam, as it will make the exam more comfortable, and if your bladder is not empty, its fullness could be mistaken for an abdominal mass, a pregnant uterus or an ovarian cyst during abdominal palpation, notes Louis A. Mucelli, M.D., a clinical instructor of obstetrics and gynecology at NYU Medical Center.

Before the physical, your physician should update your medical history or take a complete history if it is your first visit. Your weight and blood pressure will be checked, and your neck will be palpated for swollen glands (a sign of infection) and for any swelling or nodules in the thyroid (since thyroid disease may affect ovulation).

If you are using your gynecologist as a primary care physician, make sure you get a more complete physical, having your heart and lungs listened to and your eyes, ears, nose and throat examined. "By the same token, if you are past menopause and relying on an internist for your routine care, make sure you receive a pelvic exam and a Pap smear," stresses Dr. Mucelli. Blood tests, including a complete blood count (CBC) to check for anemia and other problems, may be ordered. If this visit is serving as a general physical, blood tests to check your cholesterol and other blood fats should be done on a regular basis to help assess your risk of heart disease.

The physical part of the exam should include an external and internal examination of the genitalia and a clinical breast exam. In a clinical breast exam a visual examination is done as you sit upright, with your arms raised above your head, then with your arms on your waist pushing down and in. Each breast (along with the underarm area and the area above the collarbone) is palpated as you sit up with your arm lifted. Then each breast is examined while you're lying down, first with your arms at your side, then with your arm behind your head. If you have large breasts, you may be asked to roll in the opposite direction of the breast being examined and put your arm in back of your head, so the breast is flattened against your ribs. If you have questions about doing breast self-exams, now's the time to ask.

The gynecological examination is performed while you are lying on the examining table in what's called the *lithotomy position*, with your buttocks extending over the end of the table, and your legs apart and elevated. The lithotomy position straightens the curvature of the lower spine and relaxes the abdominal muscles to aid the internal examination. Your legs will be raised either with foot or knee stirrups (preferably the latter, Dr. Mucelli advises, since this allows for maximum relaxation of the pelvic muscles and is more comfortable).

First, the doctor will palpate the abdomen and groin (where your thighs meet your pelvis), looking for lumps or tenderness; swelling or tenderness could indicate an infection. Then, donning latex surgical gloves, he or she will inspect the external genitalia, do an internal examination, perform a digital pelvic and rectal examination and take a Pap smear.

▪ What Your Doctor Can See ▪

During the external examination, the vulva and the perineum are inspected, and the labia majora and minora are spread apart to check the entrance to the vagina and the urethra for such conditions as inflammation, sores, warts or cysts.

"This part of the examination is important because a number of sexually transmitted diseases can manifest themselves on the external part of the vagina or the perirectal area without any symptoms. Lesions in the pubic area and on the vulva can alert us to a number of problems," says Dr. Mucelli. For example, carcinoma in situ of the vulva can show up as pink or whitish raised patches that may or may not be painful. Genital warts, which are painless, can show up anywhere in the genital area.

The gynecologist may also push up the urethral opening against the pubic bone with the tip of the forefinger, a procedure called *milking the urethra*. In acute urethritis or in gonorrhea, a few drops of pus can often be squeezed from the paraurethral or Skene's glands. The thumb and forefinger are used to palpate both sides of the labia majora to check the Bartholin's glands, which normally cannot be felt but when infected may be enlarged and tender.

In order to see the cervix and the vaginal mucosa, a stainless steel winged instrument called a speculum is used to separate and hold apart the walls of the vagina. Specula come in different sizes to match the size of the vaginal opening (introitus) and the depth of the vagina.

The type of speculum used depends on the individual patient. The *Graves speculum* widens at the tip; in a woman who has had children and where there's some relaxation of the area, it can open the vaginal walls a bit wider and help the physician see more, explains Dr. Mucelli. The *Pederson speculum,* which is narrow the entire length of the shaft, is used most often in very young or old women and women who have not had children, since it is easier to insert and opens the vaginal walls more gently.

The speculum is gently inserted up to its hilt in a closed position, then rotated and slowly opened, separating the walls of the vagina. For some women this may be slightly uncomfortable, but it is not painful, according to Dr Mucelli. If it hurts, say so.

Once the speculum is opened and its diameter fixed, the surface of much of the vagina and the entire circumference of the cervix can be seen. The color and texture of the cervix and the shape of the opening (os) can reveal a great deal.

The surface of the cervix is pale pink where it projects into the vagina, while the endocervical canal, which leads to the uterus, is darker in color (like the difference between the pink of your lips and the red inside your mouth). So redness from inflammation of the cervix (cervicitis) can be easily seen.

Other visible cervical conditions include: benign polyps (bulblike protrusions of cells from the cervical canal or uterine endometrium); *nabothian cysts* (blockage of glands that produce cervical mucus); cervical "erosions" (in which patches of the red inner lining appear on the exterior cervix) and warts. Cervical polyps may bleed, but erosions or warts may cause no symptoms and may be found incidentally during the exam.

Cervicitis due to an infection (most commonly STDs like chlamydia) can produce a thick, yellowish discharge. A sample will be taken, so appropriate treatment can be prescribed.

The next step is your Pap test, a simple procedure that involves taking cell samples from the external cervix (exocervix) with a tiny spatula and the endocervical canal with a tiny disposable cytobrush. The cytobrush may cause some momentary cramping or discomfort, but an accurate Pap smear must contain the columnar cells from the transformation zone where most cervical cancers begin, Dr. Mucelli points out. If your Pap test finds abnormal cells (or the doctor sees something suspicious), you will undergo colposcopy and biopsy.

As the speculum is slowly withdrawn, the vaginal walls are examined again to make sure that any irritation or other problem was not hidden by the blades and overlooked. If any vaginal irritation or inflammation is seen, your doctor may take a swab of vaginal cells or discharge to check for infections, or recommend estrogen cream after menopause.

■ What Your Doctor Can Feel ■

The next step is a bimanual examination of the vagina and cervix. The doctor will gently insert her or his middle and index fingers into the full length of the vagina, gently palpating the walls for any tenderness or masses. Then, using one hand to palpate the abdomen, the doctor gently pushes up on the cervix, so the entire mass of the uterus can be felt between the two hands, including the top, or fundus. The size and feel of the uterus can reveal if there are any fibroids, tenderness or other irregularities as well as reveal the progress of a pregnancy.

"About fifteen percent of women have a retroverted uterus, which is markedly tilted back, the so-called tipped uterus, as opposed to the normal uterus, which is slightly tilted forward, or anteverted. With a retroverted uterus, you slip your fingers behind the cervix, and the abdominal hand presses the uterus down. You can feel the bulk of the body of the uterus, but you cannot feel over the top," Dr. Mucelli explains. A tipped uterus has no medical significance, however.

Moving the fingers slightly to either side of the uterus, the physician palpates each ovary between the abdominal and vaginal hands, feeling for any irregularities or growths. "In a slender woman even slight enlargement of the ovary can often be felt. You can't determine whether a mass is fluid-filled or solid—for that you need ultrasound—but since ovarian cancer can be asymptomatic, a pelvic exam is one way we can detect it," says Dr. Mucelli. Palpating the ovaries can be very difficult in obese women because of abdominal wall and intra-abdominal fat. The fallopian tubes cannot be felt unless there's inflammation and enlargement.

During the internal exam you should be asked to hold your breath and "bear down" to increase intra-abdominal pressure and also to contract the muscles around the vagina. This can reveal any weakness in the pelvic floor, the muscular supports of the bladder, rectum or uterus and early signs of

Fig. 23: THE BIMANUAL EXAM

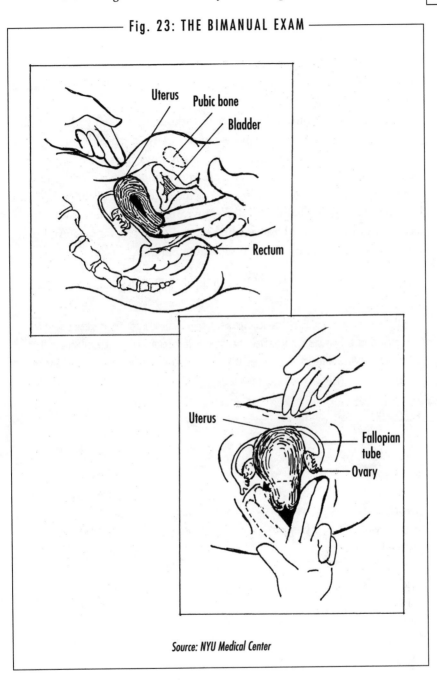

Source: NYU Medical Center

uterine prolapse. Many physicians are also using transvaginal ultrasound to assess pelvic organs. If a woman is over forty, a digital examination of the rectum is done to check for masses. Women over fifty may be given mail-in cards to take stool samples at home; microscopic blood in the stool can be an early sign of colorectal cancer.

No visit can be considered complete without a sit-down with your physician in his or her office after your exam to discuss any health concerns you have. With the advent of managed care, many physicians are being encouraged to cut this time short to increase the number of patients they see, according to Dr. Mucelli. So you need to make the most of the visit. Write down questions beforehand, and don't leave until you get the answers. If you need more time with a physician, make sure you get it, he says. And don't forget to get a referral for a screening mammogram.

WHAT TESTS YOU NEED AND WHEN

(This is a compilation of guidelines from various organizations, including: the American College of Obstetricians & Gynecologists; U.S. Preventive Services Task Force; American Cancer Society; The National Institutes of Health. These groups do not necessarily agree on the same guidelines. Discuss these tests and procedures with your physician.)

PROCEDURE	18–35	35–50	50+
Physical Exam			
Blood pressure	Every year	Every year	Every year
Thyroid exam	Every year	Every year	Every year
Clinical breast exam	Every year	Every year	Every year
Bimanual pelvic exam	Every year	Every year	Every year
Digital rectal exam		Every year	Every year
Laboratory Tests			
Pap smear*	Every year	Every year	Every year
Urinalysis	As needed		Yearly after 60
Fecal occult blood		Yearly after 40	Every year
Chlamydia/gonorrhea	Every year	With new sexual partner	
HIV	If high risk	If high risk	If high risk
Complete blood count	1–3 years	1–3 years	1–3 years
Glucose†	If symptomatic, at risk or a family history of diabetes		
Total Cholesterol/HDL**	Every 5 years	Every 5 years	Every 5 years

TSH	If symptomatic	If symptomatic	Periodically after 60
FSH		6 months–1 year after last period	
Rubella antibody titer	At preconception visit		

Other Procedures

Screening mammography	With family history	After 40	Every year
Bone densitometry			At menopause
Colposcopy	With abnormal Pap smear at any age		
Transvaginal ultrasound	As needed		Postmenopause

* According to the American Cancer Society (ACS), after three normal Pap smears a physician may elect to do the test every three years in selected low-risk women.

† According to new guidelines from the American Diabetes Association, all adults over the age of 45 should be given a fasting serum glucose test for non-insulin-dependent diabetes mellitus (NIDDM). The new threshold for NIDDM is a serum glucose level of 126 mg/dl.

** According to the National Cholesterol Education Program (NCEP), if total cholesterol is above 240, a total lipid breakdown should be done. Yearly total cholesterol/HDL testing may be done if a woman is not taking replacement hormones.

∞ Susan Wood's Story ∞

"My mother was very young when she had my oldest sister. But then she had six miscarriages and didn't have another successful pregnancy until eleven years later. She did two things to prevent further miscarriages: She went to bed for virtually her entire pregnancy each time, and she took DES.

"It was only in 1975, when the cancer stories were getting more attention, that mother remembered taking DES. Her OB/GYN checked her records and found out that she had taken DES while pregnant with my older sister, Betsy, with me and with my younger brother. First they had me go in and get checked, and I had vaginal adenosis (a benign condition). The next year Betsy was checked, and she also had vaginal adenosis. Then, in 1978, she was diagnosed with clear cell vaginal cancer; she was only twenty-one. She had surgery because it was caught very early. We really thought she was cured until about 1983, when she was rediagnosed. My sister died in 1991, two weeks shy of her thirty-fifth birthday.

"Meanwhile, my brother was diagnosed with testicular cancer when *he was around twenty-four. As a small child he had an undescended testicle, which we now know is common in DES sons. It's also correlated with cancer. The testicle was removed, and he was fine. But a few years later they found a recurrence. They blasted the hell out of him with chemotherapy for about six months. He still has some side effects left over from that, but we hope he's cured. . . .*

"In 1987 I had an ectopic pregnancy, and I had to have emergency surgery. I almost died. They found that I had a problem with my fallopian tubes related to the DES. They caught the ectopic pregnancy late, so one tube was totally destroyed. Then, a few years back, when I started actively trying to become pregnant, they found that I had a T-shaped uterus, which is a classic malformation associated with DES.

"Because I lacked one tube, it took me a couple of years of active trying finally to get pregnant—I did not want to use assisted reproduction—and because mine was a high-risk pregnancy, I went to my OB once every two weeks, instead of once a month, for internal exams, checking my cervix to make sure it was still closed. At twelve weeks they put a couple of stitches around the cervix to make sure it stayed closed for the pregnancy. Then, at about twenty-six weeks, they put me on twice daily home fetal monitoring to detect preterm labor. I was also at high risk for that because of DES.

"What upsets me the most is that long after they knew DES didn't work, they continued to give it to women. I don't blame my mother for taking it. She really thought she was doing the right thing. But this drug has ruined millions of lives.

"My next question is menopause. What happens then? What do you tell the DES daughters who are now getting close to menopause? All the baby boomers? There's no information. The first of the DES daughters are hitting fifty, when they're at higher risk of breast cancer and heart disease. I certainly wouldn't take hormones, not even estrogen cream. This generation of DES daughters will be the guinea pigs.

"It is hard not to be angry. Losing my sister was absolutely the worst thing in my entire life. I may never recover fully. I know DES has affected my biology, screwed up my reproductive system and destroyed my family. There's nothing I can do except hope for the best for my future. I will be happy just to have a healthy baby."

Susan F. Wood, Ph.D., is now acting deputy assistant U.S. secretary for Women's Health in the U.S. Department of Health and Human Services. In November 1995 Dr. Wood delivered a healthy baby girl by cesarean section because of cervical problems caused by DES and named her after her sister. The above remarks were taken from a personal interview and are printed with her permission.

▪ Special GYN Care for Women Exposed to DES ▪

Diethylstilbestrol (DES) is a nonsteroidal form of estrogen that was prescribed for women between 1938 and 1971 to prevent recurrent miscarriage, premature labor and other complications of pregnancy. In the early 1950s reports surfaced that DES was not effective in preventing miscarriage. But it was still given until 1971, when in utero exposure to DES was linked to a rare form of vaginal cancer, clear cell adenocarcinoma, in very young women.

Subsequent reports also linked the drug to an increase in breast cancer risk in DES mothers and serious malformations of the female reproductive tract in DES daughters, including an irregular T-shaped uterus, an incompetent cervix and misshapen or occluded fallopian tubes, which cause problems ranging from infertility to preterm delivery. (Sons exposed to DES before birth may have urogenital abnormalities, possible fertility problems and higher risk of testicular cancer.)

The use of DES during pregnancy was banned by the U.S Food and Drug Administration in 1973. But it's estimated that as many as ten million American women and their offspring were exposed.

According to DES Action USA, of the estimated 2.4 million DES daughters, about half have been born with some abnormality of the vagina, cervix, uterus or fallopian tubes. These reproductive abnormalities carry a fivefold higher risk of ectopic pregnancy, a twofold increase in the risk of miscarriage and three times higher risk of premature labor. It's estimated that 1 out of every 1,000 DES daughters will develop clear cell vaginal or cervical cancer, often around age nineteen, although there's no known upper age limit. Experts recommend that DES daughters see a gynecologist (one familiar with the effects of DES) at least *twice* a year.

In addition to a thorough external examination to look for such lesions, DES daughters should have twice yearly Pap smears and annual colposcopies to check for cellular changes in the vagina (more frequently if abnormalities are found). Abnormal cell growth can begin in the vagina in DES daughters right after puberty, eventually causing lesions that may be precursors to cancer. Because of malformations in the cervix, the vulnerable *squamocolumnar junction* may be larger and more exposed, promoting frequent vaginal infections and inflammation.

The healing process in women with prenatal exposure to DES may be altered, and even minor gynecological procedures or surgery in the vagina or cervix can cause problems. So if procedures such as cryoablation are needed, they should be performed by specialists familiar with treating DES daughters.

Studies show that DES not only harmed the reproductive system of those exposed in utero but may have also caused endocrine, immune and musculoskeletal problems. So DES daughters should also be screened for Hashimoto's thyroiditis (autoimmune hypothyroidism), pernicious anemia (caused by vitamin B_{12} malabsorption), *myasthenia gravis* (a degenerative muscle disorder) and possibly *multiple sclerosis*.

Like Susan Wood, DES daughters who become pregnant face a host of potential problems because of abnormalities in the uterus and cervix and need "high-risk" obstetric care, with more frequent office visits, according to NYU's Dr. Bruce Young. "We follow these women with serial sonograms so if there are any problems, we can take appropriate measures," he explains. "For example, in women with an incompetent cervix, we do a cerclage to maintain closure to prevent preterm birth." Serial sonographic measurements of the cervix and tests for fetal fibronectin as a sign of preterm labor may be particularly useful, adds Dr. Lockwood. Some women may be told to spend their pregnancies in bed; others may need at-home fetal monitoring.

Despite the best precautions, some DES daughters deliver prematurely and face an increased risk of having babies with serious problems, such as cerebral palsy. Fortunately 65 percent of DES daughters have successful pregnancies, according to Dr. Lockwood.

ஒ *J u d y ' s   S t o r y ,   C o n t ' d* ஒ

"There's this image that lesbian women don't visit doctors. I've been going to a gynecologist once a year since I was seventeen, and my friends all see gynecologists. We get Pap smears, we get mammograms and just because we're gay doesn't mean we don't see ourselves as women with the same health concerns as other women.

"The image that lesbian women don't take care of their health is there because basically we're not giving birth, we don't need birth control, so we don't have a reason to go to a gynecologist. Many doctors just assume a

woman is heterosexual, they never ask about sexuality and some are outright homophobic. I think that some lesbians just stay away from doctors in general. Maybe they don't want to be outed or have stupid, insensitive questions thrown at them.

"Some women do think that because they're not having sex with men, they don't get STDs or cancer, but I don't know a woman who isn't aware of breast cancer, and some of us are very much aware of STDs. I'm having an AIDS test because I do sleep with bisexual women, and I want to make sure I'm okay."

▪ Lesbian Health Concerns ▪

Most gynecologic health care is centered on reproductive concerns: whether or when to have children, contraception, prenatal care, diagnosing and treating infertility. Consequently, lesbian women may encounter problems when seeking GYN care.

For one thing, the health care system assumes every woman is heterosexual. Medical forms often use words like *husband* and *wife* instead of *partner*. So when a lesbian sits down to fill out the form, she immediately feels excluded, remarks Beverly Saunders Biddle, M.H.A., Executive Director of the National Lesbian and Gay Health Association based in Washington, D.C. "Two of the first questions often asked by a provider are: Are you sexually active? And if so, what type of birth control do you use? If the answer is none, a lecture usually follows about your irresponsibility and risk for unwanted pregnancy. For most lesbians, this entire situation is highly stressful," says Saunders Biddle. "She's faced with a choice: Does she take an unnecessary prescription for birth control pills or a diaphragm, or does she come out to a provider and put herself at risk for anything ranging from indifference to overt hostility?"

Indeed the homophobia of some physicians, and the fear of revealing their sexual identity to a provider, keep many lesbians away from the gynecologist's office. Surveys show that even if physicians are not homophobic, many are uncomfortable treating (or refuse to treat) gays and lesbians. Findings from 19 studies on lesbian health show that many women feared decreased quality of care if they revealed they were lesbian, and those who did disclose their identity often experienced negative reactions and even mistreatment from providers. As a consequence, many women delayed seeking care.

Many lesbian couples cannot share a partner's insurance coverage, so access to health care may be restricted. One survey showed that up to 40 percent of lesbians have no OB/GYN providers, and they may have gynecological exams as infrequently as every twenty-one months, compared with every eight months for heterosexual women. Other surveys show that up to 50 percent of lesbians have not had Pap smears in the past year, were less likely to have mammograms or breast exams and were not receiving any care for existing gynecological problems. (However, some lesbians may get Pap smears and pelvic exams from internists or family practioners.)

Gay women should be aware of their special risks. Although lesbians have children, they have fewer pregnancies and take oral contraceptives less often than straight women, so they experience long years of uninterrupted ovulation, known to be risk factors for breast, ovarian and endometrial cancer. A 1993 report suggested that lesbians may have a two to three times greater risk of developing breast cancer than women in the general population. But many lesbians erroneously believe that these cancers are linked to heterosexual sex. Experts say lesbians should follow the same mammography screening and breast self-exam guidelines as do heterosexual women.

But there are no recommendations for cervical cancer screening among women who are sexually active with women or who are celibate. Although cervical cancer appears to be less common among lesbians, new data shows that women who had been sexually active *only* with women can get human papilloma virus (HPV) from their sexual partner and develop cervical cancer.

"A woman's sexual history is more important than her sexual identity in determining her risk for HPV and the frequency of Pap smears," stresses Jocelyn C. White, M.D., an internist at the Oregon Health Sciences Center and a researcher on lesbian health. "Risk factors include early sexual activity, having numerous partners, smoking, a history of genital warts or known history of HPV and abnormal Pap smears." Women who have had significant heterosexual or bisexual contact (or past histories of such contact) should also have yearly Pap tests. Low-risk lesbians can have Pap smears every three years if they've had three normal tests in a row (as current guidelines permit for low-risk women).

While there is a lower incidence of STDs among lesbians, studies show transmission of chlamydia and genital herpes, as well as HPV, does occur between women. Lesbians are at risk for STDs and HIV, especially those who have sexual contact with men. "You can't just assume that because your partner identifies as lesbian she is 'safe.' She may have had sexual contact with IV drug users or gay men, who are at HIV risk," Dr. White warned the Third Annual Congress on Women's Health. So lesbians do need STD testing.

Infections like *Trichomonas,* bacterial vaginosis (BV) and *Candida* are as common among lesbians as heterosexual women (a recent study showed that BV can be transmitted during female-to-female sexual contact). Symptoms of vaginitis and abnormal discharge should be seen and treated by a gynecologist; a woman's partner may need to be treated as well.

There are no GYN problems unique to lesbians, so information about gynecological health should be applicable to *all* women.

▪ Race, Culture, Ethnicity and Health Care ▪

Our cultural and ethnic backgrounds can be a powerful force in our feelings about sex, childbirth, menstruation and menopause, influencing our health behaviors. Beliefs may be so deeply ingrained that we may not even be aware of them.

Because of historical factors, blacks and Latinos often have a mistrust of doctors, which may delay women from seeking care. A study by the Chicago gynecologist Dr. Donald Chatman found that 40 percent of black women who complain of pelvic pain are misdiagnosed as having pelvic inflammatory disease instead of endometriosis because of misperceptions resulting from skewed heath statistics showing that black women are more at risk for STDs.

Surveys show that Native Americans, older African Americans and Asian Americans tend to believe that cancer is a death sentence (Asian culture attaches a stigma to it). The journal *Cancer Practice* notes that Latinos are also more likely than whites to believe that cancer is always fatal and that little can be done to prevent it.

These are major factors (along with cost) in low rates of mammography screening among these groups, causing delays in care that contribute to higher death rates from breast cancer. Hispanic and Native-American women are twice as likely as white women to develop cervical cancer, yet screening rates among these women remain fairly low.

Modesty may be a major issue among many Asian, Latina, Islamic and some Orthodox Jewish women, who may feel inhibited from seeking care and screening, especially from male providers.

A report by the National Asian Women's Health Organization (NAWHO) says gynecological health may be viewed by some women as important only when it concerns childbearing. "The perception that gynecological care is only acceptable after marriage . . . prevents many girls and women . . . from accessing the services they need for routine procedures such as Pap smears and pelvic exams," reported NAWHO. Indeed rates of cervical cancer screening are low among Asian-American women. (But the report notes that most younger women actively seek care.)

Latinos, Native Americans and Asian Americans frequently see their own practitioners and "healers" for herbal medicines and treatments for everyday complaints or to supplement mainstream medical treatments. But they might never discuss alternative treatments with a physician.

Cultural beliefs might even contribute to a woman's choice of contraception. Dr. Chatman says many of his African-American patients prefer not to take birth control pills, citing a folk belief that monthly menstrual flow "cleans a woman out" and that the pill produces scantier periods. On the other hand, NAWHO notes that the pill is the most common form of contraception among Asian-American women because sex is never discussed and they do not feel comfortable asking their partners to use condoms.

Cultural beliefs can also determine whether a woman uses assisted reproduction and which technique is employed. For example, Islamic and Orthodox Jewish beliefs permit IVF, but view insemination with donated sperm as tantamount to adultery.

There is a high awareness of sexually transmitted diseases in some minority communities, but surveys show that many Latina and Asian-American women believe they are not at risk, assuming their partners to be monogamous. So they may take fewer precautions and be tested less frequently.

While many health care professionals have become more aware of these issues, you need to help your provider understand your particular feelings, beliefs and needs and discuss alternative therapies you may be using. This can be difficult, but it's necessary for you to be an active partner in your health care.

▪ Disabled Women and GYN Care ▪

More than 27 million women in the U.S. have some sort of disability and often have trouble obtaining basic gynecological care. Reasons include limited mobility, fewer pregnancies and a care system more geared to men with traumatic injuries, as well as psychosocial and economic barriers, notes Dr. Ilona Brandeis, who heads a new center for disabled women's reproductive health care at the NYU-affiliated Hospital for Joint Diseases.

A 1997 study of disabled women aged eighteen to seventy-nine conducted by the YWCA of New York City found that while over half visited a gynecologist at least yearly, 22 percent had never seen an OB/GYN, with the number rising to 37 percent among women thirty-five or younger. Half the women rated their doctors' knowledge of their disabilities as poor, and many did not know how that disability affected reproduction. Many providers wrongly assume that disabled women cannot have children, and a woman's other problems may overshadow her need for GYN care and cancer screening, says Dr. Brandeis.

A small study of 319 women who underwent basic gynecological screening, presented to the Fourth Annual Congress on Women's Health, found the most common diagnoses included dysfunctional uterine bleeding, secondary amenorrhea (lack of periods), postmenopausal bleeding, benign breast masses and osteoporosis. Other studies show that disabled women often have more urinary tract problems but may not have symptoms because of nerve damage.

She advises women to look for gynecologists with handicapped access and new, specially designed examining tables which have handrails and special footrests which can be adjusted to the needs of disabled patients. Disabled women also need physicians who can refer them to assisted reproductive services, if desired.

▪ Managing Your Own Health Care ▪

According to a 1993 Commonwealth Fund Survey on Women's Health, 13 percent of women report they do not get needed medical care in a given year; 36 percent of uninsured women do not get needed care in a given year. More than a third report not having had physician exams within the last year. Some can't *afford* to take good care of themselves.

While many poor women are covered by Medicaid, some women may not qualify because their incomes exceed the limit; perhaps a third of poor women lack coverage. Around 19 percent of all American women lack health insurance altogether.

Insurance doesn't always cover the preventive and reproductive services most frequently needed by women. Women often have to pay out of pocket for routine GYN exams as well as for contraception, mammograms, Pap smears and infertility services, so many forgo these services because of cost. Managed care plans and health maintenance organizations (HMOs) can be beneficial because they typically cover well care, routine GYN visits, cancer screening (but at less frequent intervals) and birth control, have low out-of-pocket costs and allow women to self-refer to a gynecologist.

However, a 1995 conference on managed care and women's health convened by the Jacobs Institute for Women's Health noted that managed care does not guarantee access to needed care or to quality care. A physician may act as a "gatekeeper" for referrals to specialists in areas like infertility. While shorter hospital stays are becoming the norm, in 1996 a federal law was passed mandating a two-day hospital stay after a routine vaginal delivery and four days after a C-section.

One fourth of privately insured women and women receiving Medicaid are enrolled in HMOs. Efforts are under way to set federal guidelines to establish minimum standards for managed care organizations, monitor access and quality of care and abolish gag rules that prevent doctors from disclosing financial incentives to limit tests and procedures. In the interim, women will have to be aggressive in making sure they receive the care they need. "You need to be a savvy consumer, especially in this era of managed care, when so many physicians are being encouraged or often given a financial incentive to do less for their patients," says Dr. Sandra Kammerman. "On the other hand, too many women focus on getting a Pap smear and don't access all the other things a doctor can do for them during that GYN visit, especially if he or she is their primary care provider."

∞ *Tina's Story, Cont'd* ∞

"I think it's extremely important to find a doctor who will listen to you. I never would have gotten treated for my PMS with my first gynecologist. I never had the impression that he really listened when I talked, and he didn't encourage me to discuss my concerns with him. He just gave me my pelvic exam, did the Pap, and that was that.

"When I was in my twenties, I was convinced I did not want kids. Absolutely, positively not. I told my gynecologist I wanted to get my tubes tied. He flat out refused. He said I was much too young, and I might change my mind. That was the reason I found a new gynecologist. But he was right. I did change my mind. So I'm grateful that he said no, but he was not the right doctor for me."

▪ Finding a Good Gynecologist ▪

As Tina notes, it's important to feel comfortable with your physician, not only during a physical gynecological exam but also while talking about the intimate details of your life.

Finding a good gynecologist may be as simple as getting a recommendation from a friend. Managed care plans provide lists of participating doctors. Before you go for an actual exam, schedule a brief visit to meet the physician, so you can see if there's a good "fit." Some women feel more comfortable with female OB/GYNs or physicians of their own racial or ethnic groups.

Does having a woman gynecologist ensure you'll get better care? Some studies suggest that it can. A 1993 study in the *New England Journal of Medicine* examined patient records of almost 98,000 women in Minnesota and found that those who had women doctors were twice as likely to have Pap smears and 40 percent more likely to get mammograms. Studies also suggest that women doctors listen to patients more and interrupt less and that younger physicians tend to practice more preventive medicine.

Some women may also need a broader range of services than routine GYN exams. They may be struggling with infertility or need surgery for fibroids. So they may need to see a gynecologist who is board-certified not only in obstetrics and gynecology but also in reproductive endocrinology and infertility or gynecologic surgery, says Dr. Charles Lockwood.

Becoming board certified by the American Board of Obstetricians and Gynecologists takes several years after completing medical school, Dr. Lockwood points out. First, there is a residency in OB/GYN, followed by written and oral examinations. After passing *both* examinations, a physician is board-certified as an obstetrician-gynecologist. An OB/GYN can also elect to do an approved three-year fellowship in reproductive endocrinology and fertility, gynecological oncology or maternal and fetal medicine, also followed by written and oral examinations; once he or she passes, he or she is doubly board-certified. *Board-eligible* means only that the physician is eligible to take the exams. If you need a specialist, you can contact the professional organizations listed in Appendix I to find a qualified physician in your area.

Many medical schools have also established special training programs so that physicians are better educated in the issues affecting women's health, whether they end up in gynecology or not. At the same time increasing numbers of physicians may be practicing at facilities specializing in women's health.

▪ What About Women's Health Centers? ▪

There's nothing new about the idea of a medical facility solely for women. In the nineteenth century there were scores of hospitals that admitted only women, although the concept of a "woman's doctor" or gynecologist was unknown. As the health care climate changed and the number of specialty hospitals declined, only a dozen or so women's hospitals remain in the U.S.

In recent years, however, many hospitals have established separate facilities specializing in women's health care. It's estimated there are now around 4,000 such centers; 80 percent of the newer facilities are affiliated with hospitals. The American Hospital Association reports that almost one third of its members now have some sort of women's health center.

Will a woman receive *better* care from such a facility? That depends. These centers vary widely in the types of services they offer, cautions Carol S. Weisman, Ph.D., professor of health management and policy at the University of Michigan School of Public Health. Some facilities calling themselves women's health centers do provide "one-stop shopping" for comprehensive primary and preventive care, while others offer only specialized services, such as breast imaging and bone density scans.

"A woman looking in the phone book or seeing an advertisement for a hospital-sponsored women's health center may think it will provide all her health needs. But that's not always the case. Women need to beware and find out what services are provided *before* they go," says Dr. Weisman, who surveyed almost 500 women's health centers around the country. She found that reproductive health centers were more likely to provide contraceptive counseling and abortion services than were primary care centers, but both were equally likely to offer general GYN care. Since there is no accrediting body for women's health centers, if a center is hospital-based, the hospital must be accredited. "You also need to know if the center has any other accreditations for services provided," advises Dr. Weisman. Other tips:

- ◆ Ask whether all its physicians are board-certified in their respective specialties; if providers are internists, ask if they have training in gynecology and if the gynecologists have training in primary care.

- ◆ Ask whether a facility will accept your health insurance or Medicare. If not, find out whether your insurer will reimburse *you* for care at a women's health center.

- If there is a mammography facility, make sure it is certified by the FDA. Under federal regulations, facilities must have doctors, certified radiologists and radiology technologists and other staff members who are specially trained to do breast X rays. Each center also must have high-quality equipment designed specifically for mammography, calibrated on a regular basis and submit to annual auditing visits and quality testing.

- Find out where the center sends Pap smears. Under federal law, the more than 12,000 cytopathology labs which analyze Pap smears (and receive Medicare and Medicaid reimbursements) must be certified every two years by the Health Care Financing Administration of the U.S. Department of Health and Human Services.

- If the center provides infertility services, find out if it belongs to the Society for Assisted Reproductive Technology (SART), which requires its members to meet strict standards and submit yearly reports on pregnancy rates (see Appendix I).

- If the center provides gynecological and obstetrical ultrasound, determine if it has the rigorous quality control checks required for certification by the American Institute for Ultrasound in Medicine (AIUM).

"It's wonderful to have the option of getting all your care in one place. But the important thing is making sure you *go*," says Dr. Kammerman. "Women are often so busy caring for others they forget to care for *themselves*. Don't neglect this important part of your health."

Where to Go for Help—Information and Support Groups

▪ AIDS and HIV ▪

National AIDS Hot Line (CDC)

800-342-2437 (English, 7 days a week, 24 hours a day)

800-344-7432 (Spanish, 7 days a week, 8 A.M.–2 A.M., eastern time)

800-243-7889 (TTY Service for the Deaf, M–F 10 A.M.–10 P.M., eastern time)

National Indian AIDS Hot Line

800-283-2437 (7 days a week, 8:30 A.M.–12 P.M., 1 P.M.–5 P.M., Pacific time)

American Foundation for AIDS Research (AmFAR)

733 3d Avenue, 12th Floor

New York, NY 10017

212-682-7440

http://www.amfar.org

Centers for Disease Control and Prevention National AIDS
  Clearinghouse
800-458-5231
http://www.cdcnac.org/

AIDS Treatment Data Network
http://www.aidsnyc.org/network/

Newsletters for HIV-Positive Women

Women Being Alive [monthly]
3626 Sunset Boulevard
Los Angeles, CA 90026
213-667-3262

Women's Information Services and Exchange [monthly]
125 5th Street, NE
Atlanta, GA 30308
404-817-3441

Women's AIDS Network [WAN, monthly]
San Francisco AIDS Foundation
584 Castro, Suite 321
San Francisco, CA 94114
415-621-4160

Mothers' Voices [quarterly]
165 W. 46th Street, Suite 1310
New York, NY 10036
212-730-2777
http://www.mvoices.org

▪ Cancer ▪

AMERICAN CANCER SOCIETY
National Office
1599 Clifton Road, NE
Atlanta, GA 30329
404-320-3333
http://www.cancer.org/

ACS TOLL-FREE HOT LINE
1-800-ACS-2345

NATIONAL CANCER INSTITUTE INFORMATION SERVICE
National Institutes of Health
Bethesda, MD 20205
1-800-4-CANCER
Alaska: 1-800-638-6070
Hawaii: 1-800-524-1234

NATIONAL OVARIAN CANCER COALITION
1-888-OVARIAN
www.ovarian.org
   Ovarian cancer survivors' organization formed in 1997.

GILDA RADNER FAMILIAL OVARIAN CANCER REGISTRY
Roswell Park Cancer Institute
Elm and Carrolton Streets
Buffalo, NY 14263
1-800-OVARIAN
www.rpci.med.buffalo.edu/clinic/gynonc/grwp.html

NATIONAL COALITION FOR CANCER SURVIVORSHIP
1010 Wayne Avenue, 5th Floor
Silver Spring, MD 20910
301-650-8868

CANCER CARE, INC.
National Office
1180 Avenue of the Americas
New York, NY 10036
212-221-3300
http://cancercareinc.org

Counseling Line
800-813-HOPE (4673)

SHARE
1501 Broadway, Suite 1720
New York, NY 10036
212-719-0364
http://www.noah.cuny.edu/providers/share.html

OncoLink
http://www.oncolink.upenn.edu/

This is a University of Pennsylvania Web site providing information on diagnosis and treatment of most types of cancer. Has links to other cancer-related Web sites.

▪ Childbirth and Postpartum ▪

ASPO/LAMAZE
American Society for Psychoprophylaxis in Obstetrics, Inc.
1200 19th Street, NW, Suite 300
Washington, DC 20036
800-368-4404
http://www.lamaze-childbirth.com

Depression After Delivery
P.O. Box 1282
Morrisville, PA 19067
800-944-4PPD

Post-Partum Support International
927 N. Kellogg Avenue
Santa Barbara, CA 93111
805-967-7636

Prenatal Care Hot Line
1-800-331-BABY

■ DES National Consumer Organizations ■

DES Action USA
National Office
1615 Broadway, Suite 510
Oakland, CA 94612
Nora Cody, Executive Director
800-DES-9288
http://www.desaction.org

DES Cancer Network
P.O. Box 10185
Rochester, NY 14610
800-DES-NET-4

DES Third Generation Network
Box 328
Mahwah, NJ 07430

Local DES Hot Lines

DES hot lines operate in the following areas and can be accessed by calling: 800-DES-NEWS (800-337-6397).

CALIFORNIA (San Francisco Bay Area only)
California Public Health Foundation

ILLINOIS, IOWA, MINNESOTA, NEBRASKA and WISCONSIN
University of Wisconsin

MASSACHUSETTS
Education Development Center, Inc.

NEW YORK CITY, NASSAU and SUFFOLK COUNTIES
Long Island Jewish Medical Center
New England Research Institutes

TEXAS and LOUISIANA
The Southwest DES Center
Baylor College of Medicine

▪ Endometriosis ▪

National Endometriosis Association
8585 N. 76th Place
Milwaukee, WI 53223
800-992-3636
http://www.endometriosisassn.org

▪ Hysterectomy ▪

Hysterectomy Educational Resources and Services Foundation (HERS)
422 Bryn Mawr Avenue
Bala Cynwyd, PA 19004
610-667-7757
http://www.dca.net~hers/

▪ Incontinence ▪

The Simon Foundation for Continence
P.O. Box 815
Wilmette, IL 60091
800-237-4666

National Association for Continence (NAFC)
P.O. Box 8310
Spartanburg, SC 29305
800-BLADDER (252-3337)
http://www.nafc.org/

American Foundation for Urologic Disease
300 W. Pratt Street, Suite 401
Baltimore, MD 21201
800-242-2383
410-727-2908

American Urogynecologic Society
401 N. Michigan Avenue
Chicago, IL 60611-4267
312-644-6610

International Foundation for Bowel Dysfunction (IFBD)
P.O. Box 17864
Milwaukee, WI 53217
414-964-1799

National Kidney and Urologic Diseases Information Clearinghouse
3 Information Way
Bethesda, MD 20892
301-654-4415
http://www.niddk.nih.gov/

For an educational pamphlet, *Let's Talk About Bladder Control for Women*, call: 800-891-5388.

• Infertility •

American Society for Reproductive Medicine
1209 Montgomery Highway
Birmingham, AL 35216
205-578-5000
http://www.asrm.com

RESOLVE
1310 Broadway
Somerville, MA 02144-1731
617-623-1156
617-623-0744 (help line)
http://www.resolve.org

CDC Assisted Reproductive Technology Success Rates:
http://www.cdc.gov/nccdphp/drh/arts/index.htm

• Interstitial Cystitis •

Interstitial Cystitis Association
P.O. Box 1553
Madison Square Station
New York, NY 10159
212-979-6057
http://ichelp.com

National Kidney and Urological Diseases Information Clearinghouse
3 Information Way
Bethesda, MD 20892
301-654-4415

▪ Lesbian Health ▪

National Lesbian and Gay Health Association
Lesbian Health Advocacy Network
1407 S Street, NW
Washington, DC 20009
202-939-7880
www.serve.com/nlgha/index.html

Lesbian Health Project
8235 Santa Monica Boulevard, Suite 308
Los Angeles, CA 90099-5575
213-650-1508

National Latino Lesbian & Gay Organization
Leticia Gomez, Director
703 G Street, SE
Washington, DC 20003
202-554-0092

Gay and Lesbian Medical Association
211 Church Street
San Francisco, CA 94114
415-255-4547
http://glma.org

Lesbian Health Issues Newsletter
National Center for Lesbian Rights
870 Market Street, Suite 570
San Francisco, CA 94102
415-392-6257

▪ Menopause and Beyond ▪

North American Menopause Society
c/o University Hospitals of Cleveland
Department of OB/GYN
11100 Euclid Avenue
Cleveland, OH 44106
216-844-8748 (provides names of local specialists)
http://www.menopause.com

Older Women's League (OWL)
666 11th Street, NW, Suite 700
Washington, DC 20001
202-783-6686

American Association of Retired Persons (AARP)
1909 K Street, NW
Washington, DC 20024
202-872-4700
http://www.aarp.org/

American Society on Aging
833 Market Street, Suite 511
San Francisco, CA 94103
800-537-9728

▪ Miscarriage ▪

Pregnancy and Infant Loss Center
1421 E. Wayzata Boulevard
Wayzata, MN 55391
612-473-9372

▪ Reproductive Choices ▪

Planned Parenthood Federation of America
810 7th Avenue
New York, NY 10019
212-261-4701
http://www.ppfa.org/ppfa

Alan Guttmacher Institute
120 Wall Street
New York, NY 10005
212-248-1111
www.agi-usa.org

National Family Planning and Reproductive Health Organization
122 C Street, NW, Suite 380
Washington, DC 20001
202-628-3535

Emergency Contraception Hot Line & Website
1-888-NOT-2-LATE (1-888-668-2528)
http://opr.princeton.edu/ec/

Norplant Hot Line
800-934-5556

▪ Sexual Abuse and Domestic Violence ▪

National Domestic Violence Hot Line
800-799-SAFE (7233)
800-787-3224 (TDD)

The National Victim Resource Center
2111 Wilson Boulevard, Suite 300
Arlington, VA 22201
703-276-2880

National Organization for Victim Assistance (NOVA)
1757 Park Road, NW
Washington, DC 20010
800-TRY-NOVA (800-879-6682)
http://www.access.nova.digex.net

National Clearinghouse on Marital and Date Rape
2325 Oak Street
Berkeley, CA 94708
510-524-1582

▪ Sexuality ▪

American Association of Sex Educators, Counselors and Therapists
435 N. Michigan Avenue, Suite 1717
Chicago, IL 60611-4067

Sex Information and Education Council of the U.S.
130 W. 42d Street, Suite 350
New York, NY 10036
212-817-9770
http://www.siecus.org/

▪ Sexually Transmitted Diseases ▪

American Social Health Association (ASHA)
P.O. Box 13827
Research Triangle Park, NC 27709
919-361-8400
www.sunsite.unc.edu./ASHA/

ASHA/CDC National STD Hot Line
Palo Alto, CA
800-227-8922 (M–F, 8 A.M.–11 P.M., eastern time)
800-243-7012 (TTY/TDD)

ASHA Herpes Resource Center
800-230-6039

National Herpes Hot Line
919-361-8488 (M–F, 9 A.M.–7 P.M., eastern time)

National Hepatitis B Hot Line
800-437-2872

Office of Minority Health Resource Center
800-444-6472 (M–F 9 A.M.–5 P.M., eastern time)

▪ Vaginitis and Vaginal Infections ▪

National Vaginitis Association
220 S. Cook Street, Suite 201
Barrington, IL 60010
708-847-6066

▪ Vulvodynia ▪

Vulvar Pain Foundation
Post Office Drawer 177
Graham, NC 27253
910-226-0704 (Tu & Th 8:30 A.M.–4:30 P.M.)

International Society for the Study of Vulvar Disease
930 N. Meacham Road
Schaumburg, IL 60173

National Vulvodynia Association
P.O. Box 19288
Sarasota, FL 34276
301-299-0775

▪ Women's Health (General Information) ▪

American College of Obstetricians and Gynecologists (ACOG)
Office of Public Information
409 12th Street, SW
Washington, DC 20024–2188
202-484-3321
www.acog.org

National Maternal and Child Health Clearinghouse
Health Resources and Services Administration
8201 Greensboro Drive, Suite 600
McLean, VA 22102
703-821-8955, ext. 254

Society for the Advancement of Women's Health Research
1920 L Street, NW, Suite 510
Washington, DC 20036
202-223-8224
http://www.womens-health.org

National Women's Health Network
514 10th Street, NW, No. 400
Washington, DC 20004
202-347-1140

▪ Women of Color ▪

National Black Women's Health Project
1237 Ralph David Abernathy Boulevard, SW
Atlanta, GA 30310
404-758-9590

National Latina Health Organization
P.O. Box 7567
Oakland, CA 94601
510-534-1362

National Asian Women's Health Organization
250 Montgomery Street, Suite 410
San Francisco, CA 94104
415-989-9747

Office of Minority Health Resource Center
800-444-6472 (M–F 9 A.M.–5 P.M., eastern time)

▪ A Sampling of Women's Health Sites on the Web ▪

Ask a Woman Doctor
www.healthwire.com/woman/ask.htm

Guide to Women's Health Issues
www.asa.ugl.lib.umich.edu/chdocs/womenhealth/womens___
health.html

Women's Medical Health Page
www.best.com/~sirlou/wmhp.html

Endometriosis Information and Links
www.ivf.com/witsend.html

Obstetrics and Gynecology Links
www.bris.ac.uk/Depts/ObsGyn/og__links.html

Atlanta Reproductive Health Centre WWW
www.ivf.com//index.html

Pap Test
www.erinet.com/fnadoc/pap.html

Pregnancy and Childbirth Info
www.efn.org/~djz/birth/birthindex.html

American Autoimmune and Related Diseases Association, Inc.
www.aarda.org

Women's Health Weekly
http://www.newsfile.com/1w.htm

Additional Reading
on Women's Health

Woman to Woman: A Leading Gynecologist Tells You All You Need to Know About Your Body and Your Health, by Yvonne S. Thornton, M.D., M.P.H., with Jo Coudert, Dutton, 1997.

Listening to Your Hormones: From PMS to Menopause, Everywoman's Complete Guide, by Gillian Ford, Prima Publishing, 1996.

The Good News About Women's Hormones: Complete Information and Proven Solutions for the Most Common Hormonal Problems, by Geoffrey Redmond, M.D., Warner Books, 1995.

Perimenopause: Preparing for the Change, by Nancy Lee Teaff, M.D., and Kim Wright Wiley, Prima Publishing, 1996.

Menopause Naturally: Preparing for the Second Half of Life, by Sadja Greenwood, M.D., Volcano Press, 1996.

Menopause Without Medicine, Linda Ojeda, Ph.D., Hunter House, 1995.

Estrogen: The Facts Can Change Your Life, by Lila E. Nachtigall and Joan Ratner Heilman, HarperPerennial, 1995.

What Every Woman Needs to Know About Menopause: The Years Before, During and After, by Mary Jane Minkin, M.D., and Carol V. Wright, Ph.D., Yale University Press, 1996.

The Complete Book of Menopause: Every Woman's Guide to Good Health, by Carol Landau, Ph.D., Michele G. Cyr, M.D., and Anne W. Moulton, M.D., Putnam Grosset, 1994.

Managing Your Menopause, by Wulf Utian, M.D., and Ruth Jacobowitz, Simon & Schuster, 1990.

The Birth Control Book: A Complete Guide to Your Contraceptive Options, by Samuel A. Pasquale, M.D., and Jennifer Cadoff, Ballantine, 1996.

The Endometriosis Sourcebook, by Mary Lou Ballweg and the Endometriosis Association, Contemporary Books, 1995.

Coping with Miscarriage: A Simple, Reassuring Guide to Emotional and Physical Recovery, by Mimi Lieberman, Prima Publishing, 1996.

The Planned Parenthood Women's Health Encyclopedia, Crown, 1996.

Women with Disabilities: Achieving and Maintaining Health and Well-Being, by Danuta M. Krotoski, Ph.D., Margaret A. Nosek, Ph.D., and Margaret A. Turk, M.D., Paul Brookes, 1995.

Women's Sexual Health: An Up-to-Date, Comprehensive Guide to Female Sexuality and Sexual Health, by Ruth Steinberg, M.D., and Linda Robinson, R.N., C.N.M., Primus/Donald L. Fine, 1995.

The Biology of Women, by Ethel Sloane, 3d ed., Delmar Publishing, 1993.

The Woman's Guide to Hysterectomy: Expectations and Options, by Adelaide Haas, Ph.D., and Susan Puretz, Ed.D., Celestial Arts, 1995.

The No-Hysterectomy Option: Your Body Your Choice, by Herbert A. Goldfarb, M.D., and Judith Greif, M.S., R.N.C., John Wiley & Sons, 1997.

Overcoming Infertility: 12 Couples Share Their Success Stories, by Herbert A. Goldfarb, M.D., with Zoe Graves, Ph.D., and Judith Greif, M.S., R.N.C., John Wiley & Sons, 1995.

The Couple's Guide to Fertility: How Medical Advances Can Help You Have a Baby, by Gary S. Berger, M.D., Marc Goldstein, M.D., and Mark Fuerst, Doubleday, 1995.

From Infertility to In Vitro Fertilization: A Personal and Practical Guide to Making the Decision That Could Change Your Life, by Geoffrey Sher, M.D., and Virginia A. Marriage, R.N., M.N., with Jean Stoess, M.A., McGraw-Hill, 1995.

To Be Alive: A Woman's Guide to a Full Life After Cancer, by Carolyn D. Runowicz, M.D., and Donna Haupt, Henry Holt, 1995.

Women's Cancers: How to Prevent Them, How to Treat Them, How to Beat Them, by Kerry A. McGinn, R.N., and Pamela J. Haylock, R.N., Hunter House, 1993.

Managing Herpes: How to Live and Love with a Chronic STD, by Charles Ebel, American Social Health Organization, 1993.

Love and Sex After 60, by Robert N. Butler, M.D., and Myrna I. Lewis, M.S.W., rev. ed., Ballantine Books, 1994.

Managing Incontinence: A Guide to Living with Loss of Bladder Control, edited by Cheryle B. Gartley, Jameson Books, 1985.

Overcoming Bladder Disorders, by Kristene E. Whitmore, M.D., Harper-Collins, 1990.

Staying Dry: A Practical Guide to Bladder Control, by Kathryn Burgio, Ph.D., K. Lynette Pearce, R.N., and Angelo Lucco, M.D., Johns Hopkins University Press, 1989.

Fibroid Tumors and Endometriosis, by Susan Lark, M.D., Simon & Schuster, 1995.

Complete Candida Yeast Guidebook: Everything You Need to Know About Prevention, Treatment and Diagnosis, by Jeanne Marie Marti with Zotan Rona, M.D., Prima Publishing, 1996.

The Woman's HIV Sourcebook, by Patricia Kloser, M.D., and Jane MacLean Craig, University of Massachusetts Press, 1994.

The Invisible Epidemic: The Story of Women and AIDS, by Gena Corea, HarperCollins, 1992.

The Good Housekeeping Guide to Pregnancy and Childbirth, William Morrow, 1994.

The Gynecological Sourcebook, by M. Sara Rosenthal, Contemporary Books–Lowell House, 1995.

A Gynecologist's Second Opinion: The Questions and Answers You Need to Know to Take Charge of Your Health, by William H. Parker, M.D., and Rachel L. Parker, Plume, 1996.

Index